Diagnosis and Management of Femoroacetabular Impingement

Olufemi R. Ayeni • Jón Karlsson
Marc J. Philippon • Marc R. Safran
Editors

Diagnosis and Management of Femoroacetabular Impingement

An Evidence-Based Approach

Springer

Editors
Olufemi R. Ayeni
Division of Orthopaedic Surgery
McMaster University
Hamilton, Ontario
Canada

Jón Karlsson
Departement of Orthopaedics
Sahlgrenska University Hospital
Sahlgrenska Academy
Gothenburg University
Gothenburg
Sweden

Marc J. Philippon
Orthopaedic Surgeon
Steadman Clinic and Steadman
Philippon Research Institute
Vail, Colorado
USA

Marc R. Safran
Dept. of Orthopaedic Surgery
Stanford University
Redwood City, California
USA

ISBN 978-3-319-31998-8 ISBN 978-3-319-32000-7 (eBook)
DOI 10.1007/978-3-319-32000-7

Library of Congress Control Number: 2016947959

Printed on acid-free paper

This Springer imprint is published by Springer Nature
The registered company is Springer International Publishing AG Switzerland

Preface

Using Evidence to Power Surgical Decision-Making: It Is the Right Time!

Evidence-based orthopedics (EBO) is part of a broader movement known as evidence-based medicine, a term first coined at McMaster University in 1990 for applicants to the internal medicine residency training program. Clinicians at McMaster described EBM as "an attitude of enlightened skepticism" toward the application of diagnostic, therapeutic, and prognostic technologies. While orthopedic surgeons were generally slow to adopt this new approach, the last 5 years have experienced an increasing popularity of the language and practice of EBO.

Evidence-based orthopedics does not accept the traditional "eminence-based" paradigm as being sufficiently adequate to address clinical problems, especially when considering the large quantity of valuable information available to surgeons to help them in their problem-solving process. Today, lesser emphasis is placed on the surgeon's own professional authority. The new EBO approach posits that surgeons' experiences, beliefs, and observations alone are not enough to make satisfactory decisions with respect to patient care. Evidence-based orthopedics promotes the need to evaluate the evidence available in the surgical literature from published research and integrate it into clinical practice. Practicing EBO requires, in turn, a clear delineation of relevant surgical questions, a thorough search of the literature relating to the questions, a critical appraisal of available evidence, its applicability to the surgical situation, and a balanced application of the conclusions to the problem at hand. The balanced application of the evidence (i.e., the surgical decision-making) is the central point of practicing evidence-based orthopedics and involves, according to EBO principles, integration of our surgical expertise and judgment with patients' values (or preferences) with the best available research evidence.

The paradigm of EBO is particularly important in the uptake of surgical procedures in the cycle of innovation. Orthopedics is a breeding ground for innovation often led by surgical pioneers and early adopters. The challenge, however, to broad adoption of novel techniques in surgery is sufficient evidence of patient safety and compelling data for treatment efficacy. A recent systematic review evaluating sources and quality of literature available for hip arthroscopy indicated that although there has been a fivefold increase in publications related to hip arthroscopic procedures from 2005 to 2010, lower-quality research studies (Level IV and Level V studies) accounted for more than half of the available literature with no randomized control studies identified [1].

How do surgeons evaluate novel techniques purported to improve outcomes in femoroacetabular impingement in a time when good evidence always trumps surgeon "eminence"? Practicing EBO is not easy. Surgeons must know how to frame a clinical question to facilitate use of the literature in its resolution. Typically, a question should include the population, the intervention, and relevant outcome measures. Evidence-based practitioners must know how to search the literature efficiently to obtain the best available evidence bearing on their question, evaluate the strength of the methods of the studies they find, extract the clinical message, apply it back to the patient, and store it for retrieval when faced with similar patients in the future. Because becoming a regular EBM practitioner comes at the cost of time, effort, and other priorities, surgeons can also seek information from sources that explicitly use EBM approaches to select and present evidence. Given the paucity of clinical trials, surgeons aiming to understand the evidence must resort to time-consuming searches of the medical literature to collate current best observational studies.

Ayeni, Karlsson, Philippon, and Safran in this evidence-based approach to femoroacetabular impingement provide a highly efficient solution to the surgical community. Using the tenets of EBO, they bring together a wonderfully talented group of authors and researchers to collate the world's knowledge on this rapidly changing specialty area in orthopedic surgery. To the busy surgeon, this text is one critical must-have resource. While modern approaches to EBO are sometimes perceived as a blinkered adherence to only randomized trials, it more accurately involves informed and effective use of all types of evidence to inform patient care. The approaches and evidence in this text, despite a lack of randomized trial evidence, still represent the state of the art in the field. What we learn most from this important work is an ever-present need for a shift from traditional opinion-based textbooks to ones which involve question formulation, validity assessment of available studies, and appropriate application of research evidence to individual patients.

Mohit Bhandari, MD, PhD, FRCSC
Evidence-Based Orthopaedics
McMaster University
Hamilton, ON, Canada

Reference

1. Ayeni OR, Chan K, Al-Asiri J, et al. Sources and quality of literature addressing femoroacetabular impingement. Knee Surg Sports Traumatol Arthrosc. 2013;21(2):415–9.

Contents

1 Historical Background of the Treatment of Femoroacetabular Impingement

Edwin R. Cadet

Contents

E.R. Cadet, MD
Raleigh Orthopaedic Clinic, 3001 Edwards Mill Road, Raleigh, NC 27608, USA
e-mail: ecadet@raleieghortho.com

1.1 Historical Background

Early degenerative hip disease has often been noted in patients with abnormal acetabular morphology usually secondary to developmental dysplasia of the hip (DDH), and it has been hypothesized to be the consequence of abnormal edge loading on the anterosuperior acetabular cartilage from an eccentrically centered femoral head. However, the role femur morphology played in the development of degenerative hip disease was not as defined. In 1936, Smith-Petersen classically described a concept of impingement in which hip pain was theorized to be caused the femoral neck impinged against anterior acetabular margin [1]. Surgical correction, by way of impingement correction, was successful in his small case series. Decades later, Murray et al. described a tilt deformity of the proximal femur and its association with the development of osteoarthritis of the hip [2]. In 1986, Harris described his theory on how derangements in femoral anatomy development caused primary or "idiopathic osteoarthrosis of the hip" in the non-dysplastic hip [3]. Harris wrote that based on his numerous radiographic observations, the convex, "pistol grip" femoral deformity at the femoral head-neck junction following the sequelae of a recognized or undetected slipped capital femoral epiphysis (SCFE), Legg-Calve-Perthes disease, or the congenital epiphyseal dysplasia was a common pathway for

O.R. Ayeni et al. (eds.), *Diagnosis and Management of Femoroacetabular Impingement*,
DOI 10.1007/978-3-319-32000-7_1

development of the so-called "idiopathic" degenerative hip disease. Although Harris reported of the association of abnormal femoral head-neck deformity and osteoarthritis, he did not elaborate on the underlying mechanisms that such deformity can result in the development of primary degenerative hip disease.

In this early report, Harris also implied that the acetabular labrum may play an important role in the development of primary osteoarthritis. Harris described what he termed the "intra-acetabular" labrum. He viewed the labrum as an extra-articular structure, and any presence of labrum within the intra-articular space should be considered abnormal and represented an "internal derangement" of the hip, analogous to a torn glenoid labrum in the shoulder or meniscus in the knee [3, 4]. Such observations were early suggestions that acetabular labral pathology could play a part in the development of primary degenerative hip disease.

Subsequently to the assertions made by Harris, McCarthy et al. reported that chondral injury was noted in 73 % of 436 consecutive hip arthroscopies where labral fraying or tears were present, thus suggesting the role of labral pathology in the development of degenerative hip disease in a patient population. These findings were further supported in the authors' cadaveric examination of 52 acetabula in the same report [5, 6]. Subsequently, basic science studies further demonstrated that the labrum was found to be a critical structure in hip joint preservation by maintaining a "fluid seal" that prevents the efflux of synovial fluid from the central compartment, thus maintaining hydrostatic pressure to lower contact stresses between the femoral and acetabular cartilage surfaces [7–9].

The interplay between the femoroacetabular anatomy, labral and chondral injury, and the development of degenerative hip disease in the non-dysplastic hip was best narrated in the work done by Ganz et al. and Lavigne et al. [11, 12]. In 2003, Ganz and colleagues outlined the biomechanical rationale on how the disease they coined "femoroacetabular impingement" can cause labral and articular cartilage degradation in the non-dysplastic hip [11]. The authors suggested that the mechanism of articular cartilage and labral damage and degradation in these hips was that of aberrant hip motion rather than isolated, abnormal eccentric axial loading of the anterosuperior acetabulum that was hypothesized to occur in hip dysplasia. The authors arrived at their hypothesis based on the observations seen of labral injury and cartilage wear patterns in over 600 surgical dislocations performed for patients with hip pain without dysplasia. The authors proposed three mechanisms of femoroacetabular impingement: (1) CAM impingement, (2) pincer impingement, or (3) a combination of both. CAM impingement resulted from decreased clearance of the acetabulum from a convex, femoral head-neck junction, particularly during flexion. The "abutment," as the authors described it, between the diminished femoral head-neck offset and acetabulum is thought to cause shear injury to the adjacent cartilage and labro-chondral junction, thus leaving the bulk of the labrum undisturbed. Pincer impingement was described to originate from the acetabular side, where general (coxa profunda) or regional acetabular retroversion may cause direct, crushing injury to the labrum with a normal femoral head-neck surface. The continuous labral injury could cause intra-labral substance degeneration or labral ossification. Moreover, the premature impact on the femoral head-neck junction could cause chondral injury to the posteroinferior acetabulum secondary to abnormal shear stresses from the excessive premature levering, which the authors termed the "contrecoup" lesion. Finally, there can be a combination of both, which we now know occurs most commonly in clinical practice. The authors found that pincer impingement was more commonly seen in middle-aged women, and CAM impingement was more often observed in young, athletic male populations.

Moreover, the authors outlined the principles for successful surgical management of femoroacetabular impingement: (1) establishing a safe and reproducible approach to the hip joint that would respect and protect the femoral head vascularity and viability, (2) improving femoral head clearance by reestablishing normal femoral neck and acetabular anatomy via femoral and/or acetabular osteoplasty, and (3) addressing labral and chondral injury with repair or debridement. To accomplish these principles, Ganz et al. in a previous report described an anterior surgical hip dislocation technique via a posterior approach by using a "trochanteric flip" osteotomy that would preserve the medial femoral circumflex arteries [13].

Over the last decade, the surgical management of femoroacetabular impingement has evolved from open surgical dislocations to more minimally invasive techniques such as mini-open exposures and arthroscopic techniques. The importance of labral preservation and restoration has also been stressed as critical factor for successful management of femoroacetabular impingement [10, 14–18]. Although open surgical dislocation has yielded good to excellent results [19], the advent of advanced arthroscopic instruments designed to accommodate the complex anatomy of the hip has contributed to equal, and in some cases surpassed, clinical outcomes historically reported with open techniques [20–22] with less morbidity, thus increasingly becoming the "gold standard" for the management of femoroacetabular impingement. With this historical description laying the foundation of diagnosis and treatment, the next chapters will introduce contemporary approaches to addressing FAI. Evidence-based approaches for the comprehensive management for FAI and associated disorders will be focused upon highlighting the best strategies, opportunities, and challenges of current practice.

Key Evidence Related Sources

1. Smith-Petersen MN. Treatment of malum coxaesenilis, old slipped upper capital femoral epiphysis, intrapelvic protrusion of the acetabulum, and coxae plana by means of acetabuloplasty. J Bone Joint Surg Am. 1936;18:869–80.
2. Murray RO. The aetiology of primary osteoarthritis of the hip. Br J Radiol. 1965;38(455):810–2.
3. Harris WH. Etiology of osteoarthritis of the hip. Clin Orthop Relat Res. 1986; 213:20–33.
4. Ferguson SJ, et al. The acetabular labrum seal: a poroelastic finite element model. Clin Biomech (Bristol, Avon). 2000;15(6):463–8.
5. Ganz R, et al. Femoroacetabular impingement: a cause for osteoarthritis of the hip. Clin Orthop Relat Res. 2003; 417:112–20.

References

1. Smith-Petersen MN. Treatment of malum coxaesenilis, old slipped upper capital femoral epiphysis, intrapelvic protrusion of the acetabulum, and coxae plana by means of acetabuloplasty. J Bone Joint Surg Am. 1936;18:869–80.
2. Murray RO. The aetiology of primary osteoarthritis of the hip. Br J Radiol. 1965;38(455):810–2.
3. Harris WH. Etiology of osteoarthritis of the hip. Clin Orthop Relat Res. 1986;213:20–33.
4. Harris WH, Bourne RB, Oh I. Intra-articular acetabular labrum: a possible etiological factor in certain cases of osteoarthritis of the hip. J Bone Joint Surg Am. 1979;61(4):510–4.
5. McCarthy JC, Noble PC, Schuck MR, Wright J, Lee J. The Otto E. Aufranc Award: the role of labral lesions to development of early degenerative hip disease. Clin Orthop Relat Res. 2001;393:25–37.
6. McCarthy JC, Noble PC, Schuck MR, Wright J, Lee J. The watershed labral lesion: its relationship to early arthritis of the hip. J Arthroplasty. 2001;16(8 Suppl 1):81–7.
7. Ferguson SJ, Bryant JT, Ganz R, Ito K. The influence of the acetabular labrum on hip joint cartilage consolidation: a poroelastic finite element model. J Biomech. 2000;33(8):953–60.
8. Ferguson SJ, Bryant JT, Ganz R, Ito K. The acetabular labrum seal: a poroelastic finite element model. Clin Biomech (Bristol, Avon). 2000;15(6):463–8.
9. Ferguson SJ, Bryant JT, Ganz R, Ito K. An in vitro investigation of the acetabular labral seal in hip joint mechanics. J Biomech. 2003;36(2):171–8.
10. Cadet ER, Chan AK, Vorys GC, Gardner T, Yin B. Investigation of the preservation of the fluid seal effect in the repaired, partially resected, and reconstructed acetabular labrum in a cadaveric hip model. Am J Sports Med. 2012;40(10):2218–23.
11. Ganz R, Parvizi J, Beck M, Leunig M, Nötzli H, Siebenrock KA. Femoroacetabular impingement: a

cause for osteoarthritis of the hip. Clin Orthop Relat Res. 2003;417:112–20.
12. Lavigne M, Parvizi J, Beck M, Siebenrock KA, Ganz R, Leunig M. Anterior femoroacetabular impingement: part I. Techniques of joint preserving surgery. Clin Orthop Relat Res. 2004;418:61–6.
13. Ganz R, Gill TJ, Gautier E, Ganz K, Krügel N, Berlemann U. Surgical dislocation of the adult hip a technique with full access to the femoral head and acetabulum without the risk of avascular necrosis. J Bone Joint Surg Br. 2001;83(8):1119–24.
14. Larson CM, Giveans MR. Arthroscopic debridement versus refixation of the acetabular labrum associated with femoroacetabular impingement. Arthroscopy. 2009;25(4):369–76.
15. Philippon MJ, Briggs KK, Hay CJ, Kuppersmith DA, Dewing CB, Huang MJ. Arthroscopic labral reconstruction in the hip using iliotibial band autograft: technique and early outcomes. Arthroscopy. 2010; 26(6):750–6.
16. Murphy KP, Ross AE, Javernick MA, Lehman RA Jr. Repair of the adult acetabular labrum. Arthroscopy. 2006;22(5):567.e1–3.
17. Philippon MJ, Weiss DR, Kuppersmith DA, Briggs KK, Hay CJ. Arthroscopic labral repair and treatment of femoroacetabular impingement in professional hockey players. Am J Sports Med. 2010;38(1): 99–104.
18. Sierra RJ, Trousdale RT. Labral reconstruction using the ligamentum teres capitis: report of a new technique. Clin Orthop Relat Res. 2009;467(3):753–9.
19. Beck M, Leunig M, Parvizi J, Boutier V, Wyss D, Ganz R. Anterior femoroacetabular impingement: part II. Midterm results of surgical treatment. Clin Orthop Relat Res. 2004;418:67–73.
20. Bedi A, Chen N, Robertson W, Kelly BT. The management of labral tears and femoroacetabular impingement of the hip in the young, active patient. Arthroscopy. 2008;24(10):1135–45.
21. Philippon MJ, Briggs KK, Yen YM, Kuppersmith DA. Outcomes following hip arthroscopy for femoroacetabular impingement with associated chondrolabral dysfunction: minimum two-year follow-up. J Bone Joint Surg Br. 2009;91(1):16–23.
22. Philippon MJ, Stubbs AJ, Schenker ML, Maxwell RB, Ganz R, Leunig M. Arthroscopic management of femoroacetabular impingement: osteoplasty technique and literature review. Am J Sports Med. 2007; 35(9):1571–80.

Differential Diagnosis of Hip Pain

2

Filippo Randelli, Fabrizio Pace, Daniela Maglione, Paolo Capitani, Marco Sampietro, and Sara Favilla

Contents

A description of other conditions that may present like or with FAI

F. Randelli (✉) • F. Pace • D. Maglione • P. Capitani
M. Sampietro • S. Favilla
Hip Department and Trauma, I.R.C.C.S. Policlinico San Donato, Piazza Malan 1, San Donato Milanese, Milan 20097, Italy
e-mail: filippo.randelli@fastwebnet.it

2.1 Introduction

Since the introduction of femoroacetabular impingement (FAI) [1–3] and new diagnostic tools, such as intra-articular injections and more advanced magnetic resonance imaging (MRI) [4–6], a number of previously unexplained causes of hip pain have been revealed.

Nevertheless a comprehensive diagnosis of hip pain is not always easy to obtain for a variety of reasons. First, radiographic signs of FAI are found in a high percentage of the asymptomatic population [7, 8]. Consequently, radiographic signs of FAI alone should not be considered as the only cause of pain around the hip. Second, a variety of possible associated pathologies may be found in patients with hip pain. Sometimes these associated pathologies represent the real cause of hip pain, and FAI is secondary or not related to the hip pain. That is why a careful history, a thorough clinical evaluation, and knowledge of the other possible clinical entities should be considered. This chapter will provide an overview of the more frequent and/or insidious causes of hip pain (Table 2.1) that may be confused or associated with FAI.

Pathologies have been divided in the classical three major groups: intra-articular pathologies, extra-articular pathologies and hip mimickers.

O.R. Ayeni et al. (eds.), *Diagnosis and Management of Femoroacetabular Impingement*,
DOI 10.1007/978-3-319-32000-7_2

Table 2.1 Differential diagnosis of hip pain

Intra-articular	Extra-articular	Hip mimickers
Femoroacetabular impingement	Greater trochanteric pain syndrome	Adductor-rectus abdominis tears
Isolated labral tears	External snapping hip	Osteitis pubis
Loose bodies	Internal snapping hip	Sports hernia
Chondral damage	Bursitis	Obturator neuropathy
Ligamentum teres tears	Osteoid osteoma	Piriformis syndrome
Capsular laxity	Bone marrow edema syndrome	Meralgia paresthetica (Roth)
Developmental dysplasia of the hip	Avascular necrosis of the femoral head	Spine-derived cruralgia
Slipped capital femoral epiphysis	Stress fractures	SI joint disease
Post Perthes disease	Bone and soft-tissue neoplasms	Buttock claudication
Septic arthritis	Ischiofemoral impingement	
Inflammatory arthritis and synovitis		

2.2 Intra-articular Pathologies

Different intra-articular pathologies may be associated or mistaken for FAI. The most important are ligamentum teres tears and inflammatory synovitis as synovial chondromatosis and pigmented villonodular synovitis (PVNS).

2.2.1 Ligamentum Teres Tears

2.2.1.1 Introduction

Lesions of the ligamentum teres have been increasingly recognized as a source of pain. Byrd reported them as the third most common diagnosis in athletes undergoing hip arthroscopy [9]. A complete lesion is usually associated with traumatic dislocation but may be also seen in high-impact athletes [10, 11].

2.2.1.2 Diagnosis

Clinical diagnosis can be difficult. Symptoms are nonspecific during clinical evaluation, characterized by a reduced or painful range of motion, a painful straight leg raise test, and locking of the joint [12]. O'Donnell et al. [13] have proposed a diagnostic test for ligamentum teres tears with a sensitivity and specificity of 90% and 85%, respectively. The clinician passively flexes the hip fully and then extends 30°, leaving the hip at about 70° flexion (knee is flexed 90°); the hip is then abducted fully and then adducted 30°, typically leaving it at about 30° abduction; the leg is then passively internally and externally rotated to available end range of motion; the test is positive when there is reproduction of pain either upon internal or external rotation [14].

Imaging rarely identifies ligamentum teres injuries and a preoperative diagnosis varies from 1 to 5% [15]. MRI and MRA (magnetic resonance arthrography) appear to be accurate diagnostic tools [16, 17], while arthroscopy remains the gold standard in identifying these lesions.

2.2.1.3 Treatment

In case of failure of conservative treatment such as physiotherapy, arthroscopic debridement [18] is indicated in patients with pain caused by partial-thickness lesions, while reconstruction with autografts [19], allografts, or synthetic grafts may be indicated in patients with full-thickness lesions that cause instability or in which debridement was not effective in reducing symptoms [11].

2.2.2 Pigmented Villonodular Synovitis

2.2.2.1 Introduction

Pigmented villonodular synovitis (PVNS) is a rare proliferative disorder of the synovium. Eventhough PVNS is a benign disease, it may be aggressive in certain cases. PVNS may also occur in a localized or more diffused form.

2.2.2.2 Diagnosis

Patients typically present with mild to severe pain and impaired joint function. Recurrent hemarthrosis is typical. The concurrent presence of FAI can mistakenly lead to a diagnosis of a secondary synovial reaction instead of PVNS. Diagnosis is suspected through MRI and confirmed by histology.

2.2.2.3 Treatment

Treatment is often surgical, either via open or arthroscopic synovectomy, or, in more severe cases, a total hip arthroplasty (THA) is indicated once significant degenerative changes are present. Treatment with radiation and intra-articular injections of radioisotope are indicated in incomplete synovectomy or recurrences. Treatment of hip PVNS presents a high rate of failure. Hip arthroscopy has been shown to be effective but with a recurrence rate of 12 % and a conversion rate to THA ranging from 8 to 46 %. A high rate (31 %) of aseptic loosening in THA after PVNS has been also reported. An open transtrochanteric approach has been recently suggested with some success [20–24].

2.3 Extra-articular Pathologies

These disorders affect structures surrounding the joint or the bone itself. It is not rare to find them in association with FAI.

2.3.1 Bone Marrow Edema Syndromes

2.3.1.1 Introduction

The term bone marrow edema syndrome (BMES) refers to several different clinical conditions. They are usually self-limiting (may take up to 24 months) and they are best seen on MRI [25].

Different clinical entities have been reported, such as transient osteoporosis of the hip (TOH), transient marrow edema, regional migratory osteoporosis (RMO), and reflex sympathetic dystrophy (RSD) also known as complex regional pain syndrome (CRPS) [25, 26].

The main differential diagnosis is avascular necrosis of the femoral head (AVN), and it is still controversial, whether BMES represents a distinct self-limiting disease or merely reflects a subtype of AVN [25].

Etiology remains unclear in most patients, but appears to be multifactorial and related to increased intraosseous pressure with increased bone turnover, a diminished perfusion, and subsequent hypoxia producing pain [27].

2.3.1.2 Diagnosis

TOH mainly affects male patients who are 30–50 years old and women in the third trimester of pregnancy, without history of trauma. The main symptoms are severe hip pain with weight bearing and functional disability. Radiographs may show diffuse osteoporosis in the hip after several weeks from the onset of hip pain. In addition, MRI shows bone marrow edema in the femoral head, sometimes involving the femoral neck. MRI is also useful in differentiating between BME, FAI, and greater trochanteric pain syndrome (GTPS) that may present as localized bone marrow edema but with different edema patterns [28].

A bone scan may differentiate BME from AVN at its initial stage where a "cold in hot" image is seen. A "cold" zone of decreased tracer uptake (the necrotic zone) is surrounded by a half-moon-shaped area of increased uptake (crescent) [29].

Regional migratory osteoporosis presents a similar clinical course but is characterized by a polyarticular involvement.

RSD, also called algodystrophy, complex regional pain syndrome (CRPS), or Sudeck's dystrophy, is characterized by a history of trauma and presents three phases: acute, dystrophy, and atrophy. Symptoms are dull and burning pain with a rapid onset and subsequently skin atrophy, sensorimotor alteration, and joint contractures. Osteoporosis is early visible radiographically [29].

2.3.1.3 Treatment

The recommended treatment is often nonsurgical, with protected weight bearing and analgesics. Once diagnosed, to shorten the duration of symptoms, hyperbaric oxygen therapy, bisphosphonates, and, more recently, prostaglandin inhibitors have been used with encouraging results. In a controlled randomized study, hyperbaric oxygen therapy showed a significant resolution of bone marrow edema in 55.0 % of the patients compared to 28 % in the control group [30, 31]. In a series of 186 patients treated with prostaglandin inhibitors, there was a significant decrease in bone marrow edema on MRI and an increase in the mean Harris Hip Score from 52 points to 79 at latest follow-up [32].

2.3.2 Osteonecrosis

2.3.2.1 Introduction

Avascular necrosis or osteonecrosis (AVN or ON) of the femoral head is caused by inadequate blood supply [33, 34] and can be idiopathic or secondary to different predisposing factors such as trauma, alcoholism, use of steroids, barotraumas, and hematological or coagulation diseases [35, 36]. Different classification systems have been developed with the aim to provide guidelines for treatment. Ficat and Arlet published the first classification system based on radiographic changes [37]. Subsequently the ARCO classification system was introduced [38]. Steinberg et al. introduced an MRI classification subdivided in six stages [39].

2.3.2.2 Diagnosis

The suspicion of osteonecrosis should be always high in case of a deep groin pain with a history of trauma (femoral neck fracture or fracture dislocation) or other predisposing factors. Standardized radiography is the first step to evaluate the presence of the pathognomonic "crescent sign" (sign of early femoral head collapse due to necrotic subchondral bone). It is not rare to find FAI signs that may divert attention from the real cause of the pain. MRI is the gold standard to confirm the diagnosis with a high sensitivity and specificity [40]. The use of bone scan is debated and mainly used to aid with determining the definitive diagnosis [41].

2.3.2.3 Treatment

The treatment of AVN is still controversial and depends on the stage and the location of the pathology following the different classification systems.

Nonsurgical treatment alternatives such as shock wave therapy (still debated [42]), intravenous iloprost, bisphosphonates, pulsed electromagnetic fields, hyperbaric oxygen [41, 43, 44], enoxaparin [45], and, more recently, injection of stem cells and platelet-rich plasma have been reported in the literature [46].

Intravenous use of iloprost, a prostacyclin derivate with vasoactive action, appears to give good results in some studies, both if used alone and in combination with core decompression [43, 44].

Surgical salvage procedures, in the early stages of AVN, include core decompression, rotational osteotomies, and vascularized bone grafting [47, 48]. Stem cell therapy in adjunction of core decompression is growing; in a review by Houdek et al., MRI showed a decrease in the zone of marrow edema from 32 % to more than 75 % in patients treated with core decompression and stem cells [49].

In more advanced stages, total hip replacement is the only alternative treatment to achieve pain relief and improved function [50].

2.3.3 Greater Trochanteric Pain Syndrome/Trochanteric Bursitis

2.3.3.1 Introduction

Greater trochanteric pain syndrome (GTPS) is a term used to describe chronic pain localized at the lateral aspect of the hip [51]. This pain syndrome, once described as "trochanteric bursitis" (TB), is also known as the "great mimicker" because its clinical features overlap with several other conditions including myofascial pain, degenerative joint disease, and some spinal pathologies [52]. Typical presentation is pain and tenderness over the greater trochanter region. GTPS is very common, reported to affect between 10 and 25 % of the general population. The most affected population is middle aged (ages 40–60 years) with a high female predominance (4:1) [53].

2.3.3.2 Pathogenesis

The pathogenesis is still unclear. It could be related anatomical factors such as a wide pelvis, stresses on the iliotibial band, hormonal effects on bursal irritation, or alteration in physical activities [54, 55]. Gluteus minimus and medius tendinopathy is also one of the primary causes of greater trochanteric pain [56, 57].

2.3.3.3 Clinical Presentation

A history of lateral hip pain and pain on palpation of the lateral hip are the most common clinical findings of GTPS. Other symptoms are pain during weight bearing and lying on the affected side during nighttime [58]. On examination, patients complain of pain during direct compression of the peritrochanteric area, often reproducible with a FABER test (flexion, abduction, and external rotation). The Ober test is useful to assess iliotibial band (ITB) tightness [58–61]. Kaltenborn et al. [62] have described the hip lag sign as useful to identify gluteal musculo-tendinous lesions.

2.3.3.4 Diagnosis

Plain radiographs are useful to exclude other concurrent pathologies (osteoarthritis, FAI, coxa profunda, avulsion fractures). Calcification adjacent to the greater trochanter may be seen in up to 40 % of patients presenting with GTPS. Insertional tendinopathic calcification rather than bursal calcification is usually present [54]. Several studies have demonstrated the association between a low femoral neck-shaft angle or an increased acetabular anteversion and GTPS [63, 64]. Small-field MRI is very useful to assess tendon insertions and surroundings [54].

2.3.3.5 Treatment

Greater trochanteric bursitis should initially be managed nonoperatively with rest, stretching, physical therapy, and weight loss (when indicated). Other treatment options are extracorporeal shock wave therapy and steroid injections [54, 60, 65–68].

About one-third of the patients suffer chronic pain. In these patients there may be an indication for surgical intervention [69–72]. Currently, there are different endoscopic techniques for local decompression (ITB release), bursectomy, and suture of torn gluteal tendons. Unfortunately there are only few studies and no long-term follow-up for these treatments. Good results have been shown in endoscopic gluteus medius repair at minimum 2-year follow-up in more than 90 % of 15 patients. Interestingly, 100 % of those patients had concomitant intra-articular pathologies (labral tears and cartilage damages). A recent study [72] on endoscopic treatment of GTPS in 23 patients demonstrated significant improvement in pain and functional score at 12-month follow-up [43, 59, 61, 73–76].

2.3.4 Snapping Hip Syndrome

2.3.4.1 Introduction

Snapping hip, or coxa saltans, is a condition that involves an audible or palpable snap during movement of the hip, with or without pain. It was first described at the beginning of the last century [77, 78]. The iliotibial band was usually considered the only cause until Nunziata and Blumenfeld suggested the psoas tendon, slipping over the iliopectineal eminence, as another source [79].

An important contribution was by Allen and Cope [80] who described three different etiologies of the snapping hip: intra-articular, internal, or external. They also introduced the use of coxa saltans as a general term [79, 80].

In the general population, the incidence of asymptomatic snapping hip is 5–10 % with a female predominance. In most cases the condition is associated with sporting activities, such as soccer/football, weight lifting and dance (up to 90 and 80 % of these bilaterally), and running [77, 78].

2.3.4.2 Diagnosis

Radiographs are usually negative and useful only to rule out other diseases or to identify predisposing factors such as coxa vara, prominence of the greater trochanter, and reduced bi-iliac width for the external or hip dysplasia for the internal. MRI usually may reveal a cause of an intra-articular snap. Dynamic ultrasound can identify the snapping tendon and may give additional information, such as the presence of inflammation, tendinopathy, or bursitis [77, 79].

2.3.4.3 Treatment

Initial treatment includes rest, ice, anti-inflammatory medications, and activity modification avoiding triggering the snap. Physical therapy, stretching of the involved structures, and a reduced training usually lead to good results. Many symptomatic snapping hips, between 36 and 67 %, resolve without surgery [77, 79, 81].

2.3.4.4 External Snapping Hip

External snapping hip is caused by the thickening of the posterior aspect of the iliotibial band (ITB) or anterior aspect of the gluteus maximus close to its insertion. The greater trochanter bursa may become inflamed because of the recurrent snapping and causes pain [77].

Patients with external snapping hip often report a sensation of subluxation or dislocation of the hip (pseudosubluxation).

The goal of surgery, when needed, is the releasing or lengthening of the ITB [77]. A Z-plasty of the ITB transects, transposes and reattaches the ITB with resolution of symptoms in most patients. A reported complication is a Trendelenburg gait that in an athlete or dancer takes on added importance [82]. Usually an endoscopic ITB diamond-shaped release at the level of the greater trochanter is successful [83]. A new interesting technique, the endoscopic gluteus maximus tendon release, has recently been introduced [84].

2.3.4.5 Internal Snapping Hip

In the internal snapping hip, the iliopsoas tendon snaps over a bony prominence, usually the iliopectineal eminence or the anterior femoral head. The snap usually occurs when extending the flexed hip or with moving the hip from external to internal rotation or moving the hip from abduction to adduction. Running and standing up from a seated position are difficult for patients with this condition [77, 79].

The aim of surgery is to release the iliopsoas tendon. Today the preferred approaches to perform a tenotomy are endoscopic, at the lesser trochanter, or arthroscopic, at the joint level. A high rate of associated labral tears have been reported [81, 85–89]. Particular attention should be paid to bifid or trifid psoas tendons that may result in an unsuccessful procedure [90, 91]. It was reported that arthroscopic surgery had better results than open techniques with fewer complications and less pain. Open fractional lengthening could lead to an increased postoperative pain than open transection at the lesser trochanter, but it is more efficacious. These results must be read considering the deficiency of high-quality literature evidence or direct comparison [81].

2.3.4.6 Intra-articular Snapping Hip

Intra-articular snapping hip has a variety of causes, including synovial chondromatosis, loose bodies, labral tears, (osteochondral) fracture fragments, and recurrent subluxation [77, 79, 80]. Intra-articular lesions may create a snap, click or pop, but, usually, it is the sensation of catching, locking, or sharp stabbing pain that is first reported by the patient [77, 79, 92]. The injection of anesthetic into the iliopsoas bursa (internal snapping hip) or the hip joint (intra-articular pathology) helps in diagnosis and in identifying the involved structure [77, 79].

2.3.5 Ischiofemoral Impingement

2.3.5.1 Introduction

Ischiofemoral impingement (IFI) is an uncommon cause of hip pain caused by an abnormal contact between the ischium and the lesser trochanter with compression of the quadratus femoris muscle [93]. It was first described in 1977 by Johnson [94] in patients previously treated with hip replacement or osteotomy of the femur. Only recently it has been diagnosed and described as a stand-alone pathology [95–97]. This disease is more common in women, is bilateral in about a third of cases, and usually occurs later in life compared with femoroacetabular impingement (mean age at presentation 51–53 years) [95, 98].

2.3.5.2 Clinical Presentation

The typical symptoms are pain localized to the hip, groin or buttock level and sometimes irradiation to the lower extremities, probably caused by irritation of the adjacent sciatic nerve [95, 98]. There is pain upon direct palpation of the ischiofemoral space and when the hip is in extension and adduction. Clinical tests are the long-stride walking test, in which the patient feels pain during extension of the hip (the pain is relieved by walking in short strides or by abduction of the hip during walking), and the ischiofemoral impingement test, which is performed with the patient in contralateral decubitus, extending the affected hip passively in adduction or neutral position [99].

2.3.5.3 Diagnosis

Imaging studies include a standing anteroposterior view of the pelvis and a frog-leg projection [96, 99] where a reduction of the ischiofemoral distance can be seen (normal 23 ± 8 mm, pathological 13 ± 5 mm) [95]. Moreover, there are a variety of possible associated malformations, such as coxa breva, coxa valga, or others that lead to medialization of the femoral head in the acetabulum [99]. MRI can be valuable to detect diffuse edema of the quadratus femoris muscle [95, 98].

2.3.5.4 Treatment

Treatment includes guided steroid infiltrations. In some patients surgical decompression of the quadratus femoris with resection, either by endoscopy or by open surgery, of the lesser trochanter may be indicated, but there is still low-quality evidence about the success of this procedure [93, 99, 100].

2.4 Hip Mimickers

These diseases affect structures away from the joint (either anatomically or functionally), with pain in the hip region.

2.4.1 Osteitis Pubis

2.4.1.1 Introduction

Osteitis pubis is a painful, noninfectious, inflammatory process involving the pubic bone, the symphysis, and the surrounding structures, such as cartilage, muscles, tendons, and ligaments [101, 102].

The true incidence and prevalence of osteitis pubis are unknown. The condition was first described as a complication of suprapubic surgery in 1924 [103] and then in a fencer athlete in 1932 [104]. Usually, osteitis pubis is a self-limiting inflammatory condition secondary to trauma, pelvic surgery, childbirth, pelvic functional instability, or overuse (particularly in athletes). It also has the potential to turn into a chronic pain problem in the pelvic region [105–107].

2.4.1.2 Pathogenesis

FAI appears to represent a major predisposing factor for this condition. Reduced hip rotation associated with FAI may result in increased stress to the rest of the pelvis generating an osteitis pubis as loads are applied to adjacent joints [108]. In a study on 125 American collegiate football players (239 hips), there was a high prevalence of osteitis pubis in FAI symptomatic hips [109]. The only independent factor, for hip or groin pain in these athletes, was an increased alpha angle [108].

2.4.1.3 Clinical Presentation

A gradual onset of pain in the pubic region is the main symptom. The pubic symphysis or the superior pubic ramus may be painful upon palpation. The pain typically radiates to the inner thigh (adductor musculature), to the groin, or upward to the abdomen. The perineal region and scrotum may also be involved. Running, hip flexion or adduction against resistance and abdominal eccentric exercises usually aggravate the pain. Later in the disease a reduction in the internal and external rotation of the hip joint, muscular weakness, and sacroiliac joint dysfunction are reported. In severe cases, pain limits walking capability promoting an antalgic or waddling gait. Pain can be also be evoked when getting up from a sitting position [110–112].

2.4.1.4 Diagnosis

Standard anteroposterior radiographs usually show widening of the symphysis and sclerosis, rarefaction, cystic changes, or marginal erosions in the subchondral bone of the symphysis. In acute cases, or in mild form, radiographs may also be normal in some cases. Instability can be evaluated with "flamingo view" radiographs. However, the correlation with symptoms is always necessary, because similar radiographic findings may be seen also in asymptomatic persons [111].

Bone scan may show an increased uptake at the symphysis, but this is a late sign, and may take months to appear.

CT scan may show marginal stamp erosions of the parasymphyseal pubis bone, insertional bony spur or periarticular microcalcifications.

MRI has a superior role in visualization of soft-tissue abnormalities (e.g., microtears of the adductor tendons) and changes within the bone marrow (e.g., bone edema) and is useful for differential diagnosis of osteitis pubis, bursitis and stress fractures [111, 112].

2.4.1.5 Treatment

Because osteitis pubis is normally self-limiting, initial treatment is nonoperative. In highly competitive athletes, activity modification is recommended. Many different therapeutic modalities and rehabilitation protocols have been successfully used [113]. Corticosteroid injections may be beneficial.

Surgical treatment includes open curettage of the symphysis pubis with or without subsequent fusion of the joint, wedge resection, posterior wall mesh repair and a variety of procedures to reinforce or repair the abdominal and pelvic floor musculature, with or without adductor tendon release with an average return to sports of 6 months [111, 112].

Recently an arthroscopic technique has been described to debride the symphysis and, eventually, to divide and reattach the degenerated origin of adductor tendon. With this technique the stability of the symphysis pubis is maintained and time to return to sports is supposed to be shorter. More recent reports document that five competitive nonprofessional soccer players were able to return to full-activity sports in an average period of 14.4 weeks after the arthroscopic surgery with satisfactory results [114–116].

2.4.2 Sports Hernia

2.4.2.1 Introduction

Sports hernia (also called "athletic pubalgia") is a condition characterized by a strain or a tear of any soft tissue (such as muscle, tendon and ligament) in the lower abdomen or groin area. Unlike a traditional hernia, the sports hernia doesn't create a defect in the abdominal wall. As a result, there is no visible bulge under the skin and a definitive diagnosis is often difficult. It often occurs where the abdominal muscles/tendons and adductors attach at the pubic bone at the same location.

Groin pain caused by sports hernia can be disabling, and it most often occurs during sports that require sudden changes of direction, intense twisting movements, cutting and/or kicking [117, 118].

Sports hernias typically affect young males who actively participate in sports. Females are affected, but much less commonly than males, comprising just 3–15 % of cases [119]. Sports hernia is a frequent cause of acute and chronic groin pain in athletes [120] and there is a high incidence of symptoms of sports hernia in professional athletes with FAI [121].

2.4.2.2 Pathogenesis

The exact cause of sports hernia is not completely known and remains heavily debated. The soft tissues most frequently affected are the oblique muscles in the lower abdomen (especially vulnerable are the tendons of the internal and external oblique muscles). When both oblique and adductor muscles contract at the same time, there is a disequilibrium between the upward and oblique pull of the abdominal muscles on the pubis against the downward and lateral pull of the adductors on the inferior pubis. This imbalance of forces can lead to injuries of the lower central abdominal muscles and the upper common insertion of the adductor muscles [122].

Muschaweck and Berger described sports hernias as a weakness of the transversalis fascia portion of the posterior wall of the inguinal canal [123]. This weakness of the pelvic floor can lead to localized bulging and compression of the genital branch of the genitofemoral nerve. Compression of this nerve appears to be the major reason of pain in these patients [124].

2.4.2.3 Clinical Examination

Although the physical examination reveals no detectable inguinal hernia, a tender, dilated superficial inguinal ring and tenderness of the posterior wall of the inguinal canal are often found. The patient typically presents with an insidious onset of activity-related, unilateral, deep groin pain that abates with rest, but returns upon sports activity, especially with twisting movements [125]. The pain may be more severe with resisted hip adduction, but the most specific finding is pain in the inguinal floor with a resisted sit-up. Pain can also be elicited in the "frog position" [126]. Gentle percussion over the pubic symphysis is performed to assess concurrent presence of osteitis pubis. Next, the patient is asked to adduct the thighs against resistance. Alternatively, the athlete can suspend the ipsilateral straight leg in external rotation, against resistance, and then perform the abdominal crunch and test the medial inguinal floor for tenderness.

2.4.2.4 Diagnosis

Experienced clinicians will identify this condition only from history and physical examination [127]. Even if the role of imaging studies is unclear [125], plain radiographs, bone scans, ultrasound, computed tomography scans and, especially, magnetic resonance imaging (MRI) may be necessary to rule out related or associated pathology [127]. Shortt et al. have imaged over 350 patients. In their experience, patients with a clinical sports hernia almost always exhibit abnormalities on MRI. The two dominant patterns of injury include the lateral rectus abdominis/adductor aponeurotic injury just adjacent to the external inguinal ring and the midline rectus abdominis/adductor aponeurotic plate injury [127, 128].

2.4.2.5 Treatment

The available literature favors early surgical management [129, 130] for those athletes who are unable to return to sports at their desired level after a trial of nonsurgical treatment for 6–8 weeks [118, 131–136].

Nonsurgical treatment consists primarily of rest and cryotherapy. Two weeks after the injury, the physical therapy exercises can improve strength and flexibility in the abdominal and inner thigh muscles. The nonsteroidal anti-inflammatory therapy can be useful to reduce swelling and pain [118].

Surgery is indicated as either a traditional open procedure or as an endoscopic procedure. Some surgeons perform also an inguinal neurectomy to relieve pain or an adductor tenotomy to release tension and increase range of motion [124, 135].

Continued groin pain after surgery may be caused by an underlying concurrent FAI; Economopoulos et al. have demonstrated a high prevalence of radiographic FAI signs in patients with athletic pubalgia that should be always closely evaluated [137].

Most studies have reported that 90–100 % of patients returned to full activity in 6 months [122].

2.4.3 Piriformis Muscle Syndrome

2.4.3.1 Introduction

Piriformis muscle syndrome (PMS) is an entrapment neuropathy caused by sciatic nerve compression in the infrapiriformis canal [138, 139]. Some researchers account PMS for up to 5 % of all cases of low back, buttock and leg pain [140]. Other anatomical anomalies have been reported to explain its etiology [141]. Similar sciatic compression-type pathology has also been referred to the obturator internus, evocating the obturator internus syndrome (OIS) [142].

Yeoman in 1928 first reported that sciatica may be caused by sacroiliac periarthritis and piriformis muscle entrapment [143]. Freiberg and Vinke in 1934 stated that sacroiliac joint inflammation may primarily cause reaction of the piriformis muscle and its fascia that may secondarily irritate the overlying lumbosacral plexus [144].

Based on cadaveric dissections, Beaton and Anson 1938 hypothesized that a piriformis muscle spasm could be responsible for the irritation of the sciatic nerve [145]. Robinson in 1947 has introduced the term "piriformis syndrome" [146].

2.4.3.2 Clinical Presentation

The classic features of piriformis syndrome include "sciatica-like pain," aggravated by sitting, buttock pain, external tenderness over the greater sciatic notch and augmentation of the pain with maneuvers that increase piriformis tension [147]. Other clinical features may be pain with straight leg raise test, a positive Pace test (pain with resisted hip abduction in a seated position) [148], and a positive Freiberg test (pain upon forceful internal rotation of the extended hip) [144].

2.4.3.3 Diagnosis

The piriformis entrapment is often diagnosed via exclusion. The diagnosis is often difficult to establish. There are no laboratory or radiographic methods for diagnosing the syndrome. An MRI may in some cases show variations in anatomy, muscle hypertrophy, as well as abnormal signal of the sciatic nerve [149].

EMG may provide findings for sciatic nerve compression at the level of the piriformis muscle [142]. A "piriformis syndrome" may be confirmed through a positive response to the injection of a local anesthesia [150].

2.4.3.4 Treatment

Traditional treatment is nonsurgical with physical therapy, stretching, extracorporeal shock wave therapy (ESWT) and steroid or analgesic injections [151, 152]. Open tenotomy has been reported [153]. Recently, botulinum toxin [154, 155] and arthroscopic release have been used with promising results in selected cases [156, 157].

2.4.4 Meralgia Paresthetica

2.4.4.1 Etiology and Epidemiology

Meralgia paresthetica is a clinical condition characterized by paresthesia and burning pain over the anterolateral thigh, due to entrapment of the lateral femoral cutaneous nerve (LFCN) [158].

It was first described by Martin Bernhardt in 1878, but the term meralgia paresthetica (MP) was coined by Vladimir Roth, a Russian neurologist, in 1895 who noticed this condition in a horseman who wore tight belts [159].

It most commonly occurs in 30–40-year-old men with an incidence of 1–4.3 per 10,000 patients in the general population [160, 161].

Other than idiopathic, causes of meralgia paresthetica are mechanical factors as obesity, pregnancy, and other factors that increase abdominal pressure, such as strenuous exercise, sports and tight belts. Lower limb-length discrepancy has also been associated with this neuropathy and also different metabolic factors, as diabetes mellitus, alcoholism, lead poisoning and hypothyroidism [160, 162]. Iatrogenic causes are due to surgical procedures, such as ilioinguinal approach for acetabular fracture fixation, iliac crest bone graft, anterior approach for total hip replacements, laparoscopy for cholecystectomy or inguinal hernia, coronary artery bypass grafting, aortic valve surgery and gastric reduction [160].

2.4.4.2 Pathophysiology

The lateral femoral cutaneous nerve originates from different combinations of lumbar nerves (L1–L3); its course is extremely variable. Passing from the pelvis to the thigh, the nerve crosses a tunnel between the ileopubic tract and the inguinal ligament, where it enlarges its diameter developing, in some cases, the meralgia paresthetica [160, 163, 164].

2.4.4.3 Clinical Presentation

Patients usually present with paresthesia, dysesthesia, numbness, pain, burning, buzzing, muscle aches and coldness on the lateral or anterolateral thigh. Prolonged standing or long walking exacerbates symptoms. Pain relief is usually obtained with sitting [160].

Clinical tests are represented by the pelvic compression (described by Nouraei et al. [165]) executed with the patient lying on the contralateral side; a manual compression is applied downward to the pelvis for 45 seconds to achieve inguinal ligament relaxation. The maneuver is positive if there is a relief of the symptoms. Another test described by Butler is the neurodynamic testing executed with the patient lying on the contralateral side with the knee flexed; with one hand the pelvis is stabilized and with other hand the affected leg is sustained, and then the knee is flexed and adduction is performed obtaining the tension of the inguinal ligament. The test is positive if the neurological symptoms are evoked [158].

2.4.4.4 Diagnosis

Differential diagnosis includes lumbar stenosis, disc herniation, nerve root radiculopathy, iliac crest metastasis and anterior superior iliac spine avulsion fracture. Ahmed has speculated about a possible association between meralgia paresthetica and FAI: the anatomical variability of LFCN could be compressed by abnormal hip structures typical of FAI [160, 166].

Neurophysiological studies can help to confirm the diagnosis, especially somatosensory evoked potential and sensory nerve conduction, even if they have some limitations and a sensitivity and specificity of 81.3 % and 65.2 %, respectively. In recent times, magnetic resonance neurography (MRN) has been introduced and appears to produce better results with an accuracy >90 % [158, 167]. Nerve block with local anesthetics is a good diagnostic test [162].

2.4.4.5 Treatment

Nonsurgical treatment includes nonsteroidal anti-inflammatory drugs and to avoid compression to the area and physical therapy as the first step.

In case of continuous pain, ultrasound-guided nerve block with a combination of corticosteroids and lidocaine appears to give good results in some patients [168, 169]. Usually the course of this condition is benign and in most cases the resolution is within 4–6 months of nonsurgical treatment.

Pulse radiofrequency ablation of the nerve is infrequently used [158].

Surgical treatment is indicated only in refractory cases. The most common procedures are neurolysis and resection of the lateral cutaneous femoral nerve. Best results are obtained with nerve resection, but patients must accept a permanent change of thigh skin sensation. Some cases of recurrence have been described with neurolysis [158, 160, 165].

2.4.5 Obturator Neuropathy

2.4.5.1 Introduction

Obturator neuropathy is an uncommon mononeuropathy that usually occurs acutely after a well-defined event (surgery or trauma). The pain related to obturator neuropathy can be difficult to distinguish from the pain due to the recent surgical procedure or trauma [170, 171].

2.4.5.2 Pathogenesis

Injury to the obturator nerve is rare because the nerve is located deep and protected in the pelvis and medial thigh [172]. The injury can result from entrapping, sectioning, stretching, or crushing the nerve. Other common injury mechanisms are electrocoagulation, ligation, or neuroma formation [172]. Reports have described obturator nerve injury during total hip replacement (poor acetabular screw placement or cement extrusion) and after abdominal procedures or major pelvic surgery [171, 173–181].

2.4.5.3 Clinical Presentation

The most prominent symptom of obturator neuropathy is pain radiating from the groin into the medial upper aspect of the thigh. Dysesthesia (less frequent) and weakness of the muscles supplied by the obturator nerve can occur in some cases [170, 171, 173].

2.4.5.4 Diagnosis

Ultrasonography, MRI, and plain radiographs can be useful for a complete diagnosis and a proper differential diagnosis. The most accurate diagnostic investigation to confirm obturator neuropathy is needle electromyography (EMG) [170, 171].

2.4.5.5 Treatment

Acute obturator neuropathy tends to have good prognosis after nonsurgical treatment [171] that should be initiated as soon as possible to prevent motor deficits or permanent hypotrophy of the muscle group innervated by the nerve [174]. Rest, NSAIDs, and modification of the activities may offer relief too [170, 171]. Surgery, which includes nerve decompression or repair with grafting or end-to-end anastomosis, should be considered in those patients with pain and weakness resistant to nonsurgical treatment and documented EMG changes or response to nerve block [170, 172, 182].

2.4.6 Osteoid Osteoma

2.4.6.1 Introduction

Osteoid osteoma was described in the literature for the first time in 1935 by Jaffe [183] as a benign bone tumor and it is a small nonprogressive osteoblastic lesion characterized by pain. It is the third most common benign bone tumor (11–14%) [184, 185]. This tumor can affect either sex at any age and it is estimated that about 50% of the patients are aged between 10 and 20 years [5, 186]. The most characteristic presentation is at the level of the femoral neck or the intertrochanteric region, and, when intra-articular, the hip is one of the most affected regions [186, 187]. There is an interesting concurrent diagnosis of FAI and hip osteoid osteoma in a series of patients treated either with a CT-guided thermoablation or hip arthroscopy [188].

2.4.6.2 Clinical Presentation

Patients with osteoid osteoma may complain of articular pain at rest and during physical activity [189]. The most common clinical feature is a dull pain that becomes worse over time, frequently with nocturnal exacerbations and resolution after taking acetylsalicylic acid or NSAIDs. These features are more pronounced in intra-articular localizations producing symptoms that may mimic an inflammatory monoarthritis [187, 190].

2.4.6.3 Diagnosis

The diagnosis is usually delayed. Plain radiograph is the first diagnostic approach even if it is difficult to diagnose intra-articular osteomas due to the absence of periosteal reaction [191, 192]. Bone scan typically shows intense uptake in the arterial phase, because of the vascularization of the nidus, and in the delayed phase, because of the reactive bone: this pattern is pathognomonic for osteoid osteoma (double density sign) [193]. SPECT (single-photon emission computed tomography) can be used when bone scan does not provide a diagnosis [194]. After bone scan, CT is the diagnostic method of choice because it will give precise localization of the nidus and its surrounding sclerotic margin [187]. Usually in MRI the nidus has a low T1 and high T2 signal in the early stages [195–197]. In intra-articular localization, however, the nidus may not be easily detectable on MRI, because it is often hidden by perilesional edema or due to an atypical presentation [192].

2.4.6.4 Treatment

Today CT-guided percutaneous procedure, such as radiofrequency, cryoablation or thermocoagulation, appears to be the method of choice for extra-articular osteomas [198]. In case of intra-articular and subchondral localization, percutaneous procedure could damage the healthy cartilage surrounding the lesion. In such intra-articular lesions, surgery, either arthroscopic [188, 199, 200] or open excision [201, 202], is recommended. Shoji et al. [203] proposed T2-mapping MRI as a method to evaluate and treat arthroscopically an osteoid osteoma of the acetabular wall.

2.4.7 Cruralgia/Leg Pain

2.4.7.1 Introduction

Leg pain (cruralgia) is defined as referred pain in the area of the femoral nerve innervation that includes the anteromedial part of the thigh and leg. The most frequent cause of leg pain/cruralgia is lumbar disc herniation (L2–L3, L3–L4 or L4–L5). Because of the similar distribution, it can be difficult to distinguish cruralgia from pain originating in the hip [204, 205]. Low back and associated radiation pain is a common problem: it is estimated that 15–20 % of adults have back pain every year and 50–80 % experience at least one episode of back pain during a lifetime. Low back pain afflicts all ages, and it is a major cause of disability in the adult working population [206].

2.4.7.2 Clinical

Wasserman [207, 208], in 1918, described the main clinical signs to assess leg pain/cruralgia also known as femoral nerve stretch test (FNST): the examiner passively flexes the knee of the patient in the prone position approaching the heel to the buttock. The test is positive if the usual groin and anterior thigh pain, reported by the patient, is reproduced. The sensitivity of this test can be increased by ipsilateral hip extension [208]. Other clinical tests are the CFNST (crossed femoral nerve stretch test); the "hip flexion test," where the patient is asked to flex the hip against resistance (the test is positive when the patient is unable to overcome the resistance); and the "sit-to-stand" test, in which the patient is unable to get up from sitting using the single stance on the affected side. Additional clinical manifestations of leg pain (cruralgia) can be dysesthesia or hypoesthesia in the region innervated by the femoral nerve and decreased patellar reflex [209–211]. The persistence of pain even at rest, the absence of pain in hip rotational movement, the presence of sensory and motor disturbances, and positivity of provocative tests may lead to the diagnosis.

2.4.7.3 Diagnosis

The first radiological examination is plain radiographs of the lumbosacral spine in standard projections, which may be followed by a dynamic study (flexion-extension in lateral views) to rule out instability and other major pathologies. The most important test is the MRI. CT scan has also high sensitivity and specificity in the diagnosis of herniated lumbar discs and spinal stenosis.

2.4.7.4 Treatment

The treatment varies according to the presence of peripheral deficits and symptoms. In acute manifestations, the first approach is a conservative treatment with rest, NSAIDs, neuromodulators and neurotrophic vitamin supplements. In the subacute phase manual or physical therapies of support are recommended [212]. Surgical treatment should be performed in acute cases where there are major neurological deficits or in chronic cases with poor outcome from conservative treatment or a poor control of the pain [213].

2.4.8 Buttock Claudication

2.4.8.1 Introduction

Buttock claudication is defined as an intermittent and invalidating buttock or thigh pain, usually related to walking, and is due to a stenosis, of at least 50 % of the area, of the internal iliac artery (IIA) on the affected side [214].

Buttock claudication is usually underdiagnosed because buttock or thigh pain is usually investigated as an orthopedic or neurological disease rather than a vascular disease. Only a few case reports [215–218] and small case series have been reported [214, 219].

2.4.8.2 Diagnosis

Physical examination may rule out most hip pathologies, but less spine involvement. The most characteristic symptoms are buttock or thigh pain and claudication after less than 200 meters of walking. Pain disappears at rest. Fatigue of the lower limb is often present and impotence [215, 219] is another possible symptom. Distal pulses are normal in case of isolated stenosis of the internal iliac artery and this is a possible cause of missed diagnosis.

The diagnosis is confirmed with iliac axis angiography and ultrasound investigation of gluteal arteries (branches of IIA).

2.4.8.3 Treatment

Treatment is surgical with percutaneous transluminal angioplasty. Good results, with relief from pain and claudication, are reported in the majority of patients [214, 219].

Take-Home Points

1. Many different pathologies may present with pain around the hip joint.
2. FAI radiographic signs are very frequent and might hide the real cause of pain and disability.
3. Different conditions may be present at the same time and present concurrently.
4. Some of these pathologies are outside the usual orthopedic knowledge and require multiple specialties collaborating.
5. A careful history, a thorough clinical evaluation, and knowledge of other possible clinical entities are critical to make an accurate diagnosis.

Key Evidence Related Sources

1. Hack K, Di Primio G, Rakhra K, Beaulé PE. Prevalence of cam-type femoroacetabular impingement morphology in asymptomatic volunteers. J Bone Joint Surg Am. 2010;92:2436–44.
2. de Sa D, Phillips M, Philippon MJ, Letkemann S, Simunovic N, Ayeni OR. Ligamentum teres injuries of the hip: a systematic review examining surgical indications, treatment options, and outcomes. Arthroscopy. 2014;30(12):1634–41.
3. Byrd JW, Jones KS, Maiers 2nd GP. Two to 10 Years' follow-up of arthroscopic management of pigmented villonodular synovitis in the hip: a case series. Arthroscopy. 2013; 29(11):1783–7.
4. Hofmann S, Engel A, Neuhold A, Leder K, Kramer J, Plenk Jr H. Bone-marrow oedema syndrome and transient osteoporosis of the hip. An MRI-controlled study of treatment by core decompression. J Bone Joint Surg Br. 1993;75:210–6.
5. Ficat RP. Idiopathic bone necrosis of the femoral head. Early diagnosis and treatment. J Bone Joint Surg Br. 1985;67:3–9.
6. Strauss EJ, Nho SJ, Kelly BT. Greater trochanteric pain syndrome. Sports Med Arthrosc. 2010;18(2):113–9.
7. Khan M, Adamich J, Simunovic N, Philippon MJ, Bhandari M, Ayeni OR. Surgical management of internal snapping hip syndrome: a systematic review evaluating open and arthroscopic approaches. Arthroscopy. 2013;29(5):942–8.
8. De Sa D, Alradwan H, Cargnelli S, Thawer Z, Simunovic N, Cadet E, Bonin N, Larson C, Ayeni OR. Extra-articular hip impingement: a systematic review examining operative treatment of psoas, subspine, ischiofemoral, and greater trochanteric/pelvic impingement. Arthroscopy. 2014;30(8):1026–41. doi:10.1016/j.arthro.2014.02.042.
9. Hölmich P. Long-standing groin pain in sportspeople falls into three primary patterns, a "clinical entity" approach: a prospective study of 207 patients. Br J Sports Med. 2007;41(4):247–52.
10. Hammoud S, Bedi A, Magennis E, Meyers WC, Kelly BT. High incidence of athletic pubalgia symptoms in professional athletes with symptomatic femoroacetabular impingement. Arthroscopy. 2012;28(10):1388–95 [Epub 2012 May 19].
11. Michel F, Decavel P, Toussirot E, Tatu L, Aleton E, Monnier G, Garbuio P, Parratte B, Piriformis muscle syndrome: diagnostic criteria and treatment of a monocentric series of 250 patients. J Rehab. 2013.
12. Cheatham SW, Kolber MJ, Salamh PA. Meralgia paraesthetica: a review of the literature. Int J Sports Phys Ther. 2013;8(6):883–93.

13. Sorenson EJ, Chen JJ, Daube JR. Obturator neuropathy: causes and outcome. Wiley Periodicals, Inc. Muscle Nerve. 2002;25:605–7.
14. Cassar-Pullicino VN, McCall IW, Wan S. Intra-articular osteoid osteoma. Clin Radiol. 1992;45:153–60.
15. Suri P, Hunter DJ, Katz JN, Li L, Rainville J. Bias in the physical examination of patients with lumbar radiculopathy. BMC Musculoskelet Disord. 2010;11:275.
16. Smith G, Train J, Mitty H, Jacobson J. Hip pain caused by buttock claudication. Relief of symptoms by transluminal angioplasty. Clin Orthop Relat Res. 1992;284:176–80. PubMed: 1395290.

References

Introduction

1. Reynolds D, Lucas J, Klaue K. Retroversion of the acetabulum. A cause of hip pain. J Bone Joint Surg Br. 1999;81(2):281–8.
2. Myers SR, Eijer H, Ganz R. Anterior femoroacetabular impingement after periacetabular osteotomy. Clin Orthop Relat Res. 1999;363:93–9.
3. Ito K, Minka 2nd MA, Leunig M, Werlen S, Ganz R. Femoroacetabular impingement and the cam-effect. A MRI-based quantitative anatomical study of the femoral head-neck offset. J Bone Joint Surg Br. 2001;83(2):171–6.
4. Byrd JW, Jones KS. Diagnostic accuracy of clinical assessment, magnetic resonance imaging, magnetic resonance arthrography, and intra-articular injection in hip arthroscopy patients. Am J Sports Med. 2004;32(7):1668–74.
5. Schmaranzer F, Klauser A, Kogler M, Henninger B, Forstner T, Reichkendler M, Schmaranzer E. Diagnostic performance of direct traction MR arthrography of the hip: detection of chondral and labral lesions with arthroscopic comparison. Eur Radiol. 2014; [Epub ahead of print].
6. Reurink G, Jansen SP, Bisselink JM, Vincken PW, Weir A, Moen MH. Reliability and validity of diagnosing acetabular labral lesions with magnetic resonance arthrography. J Bone Joint Surg Am. 2012; 94(18):1643–8.
7. Laborie LB, Lehmann TG, Engesæter IØ, Eastwood DM, Engesæter LB, Rosendahl K. Prevalence of radiographic findings thought to be associated with femoroacetabular impingement in a population-based cohort of 2081 healthy young adults. Radiology. 2011;260:494–502.
8. Hack K, Di Primio G, Rakhra K, Beaulé PE. Prevalence of cam-type femoroacetabular impingement morphology in asymptomatic volunteers. J Bone Joint Surg Am. 2010;92:2436–44.

Ligamentum Teres

9. Byrd JW, Jones KS. Hip arthroscopy in athletes. Clin Sports Med. 2001;20(4):749–61.
10. Philippon MJ, Kuppersmith DA, Wolff AB, Briggs KK. Arthroscopic findings following traumatic hip dislocation in 14 professional athletes. Arthroscopy. 2009;25(2):169–74.
11. de Sa D, Phillips M, Philippon MJ, Letkemann S, Simunovic N, Ayeni OR. Ligamentum teres injuries of the hip: a systematic review examining surgical indications, treatment options, and outcomes. Arthroscopy. 2014;30(12):1634–41.
12. Cerezal L, Kassarjian A, Canga A, Dobado MC, Montero JA, Llopis E, Rolón A, Pérez-Carro L. Anatomy, biomechanics, imaging, and management of ligamentum teres injuries. Radiographics. 2010;30(6):1637–51.
13. O'Donnell J, Economopoulos K, Singh P, Bates D, Pritchard M. The ligamentum teres test: a novel and effective test in diagnosing tears of the ligamentum teres. Am J Sports Med. 2014;42(1):138–43.
14. Reiman MP, Thorborg K. Clinical examination and physical assessment of hip joint-related pain in athletes. Int J Sports Phys Ther. 2014;9(6): 737–55.
15. Byrd JW, Jones KS. Traumatic rupture of the ligamentum teres as a source of hip pain. Arthroscopy. 2004;20(4):385–91.
16. Chang CY, Gill CM, Huang AJ, Simeone FJ, Torriani M, McCarthy JC, Bredella MA. Use of MR arthrography in detecting tears of the ligamentum teres with arthroscopic correlation. Skeletal Radiol. 2014. [Epub ahead of print].
17. Datir A, Xing M, Kang J, Harkey P, Kakarala A, Carpenter WA, Terk MR. Diagnostic utility of MRI and MR arthrography for detection of ligamentum teres tears: a retrospective analysis of 187 patients with hip pain. AJR Am J Roentgenol. 2014; 203(2):418–23.
18. Haviv B, O'Donnell J. Knee arthroscopic debridement of the isolated ligamentum teres rupture. Surg Sports Traumatol Arthrosc. 2011;19(9): 1510–3. doi:10.1007/s00167-010-1318-7. Epub 2010 Nov 13.

19. Amenabar T, O'Donnell J. Arthroscopic ligamentum teres reconstruction using semitendinosus tendon: surgical technique and an unusual outcome. Arthrosc Tech. 2012;1(2):e169–74.

Pigmented Villonodular Synovitis

20. Byrd JW, Jones KS, Maiers 2nd GP. Two to 10 Years' follow-up of arthroscopic management of pigmented villonodular synovitis in the hip: a case series. Arthroscopy. 2013;29(11):1783–7.
21. Mankin H, Trahan C, Hornicek F. Pigmented villonodular synovitis of joints. J Surg Oncol. 2011;103(5):386–9.
22. Jaffe HL, Lichtenstein L, Sutro CJ. Pigmented villonodular synovitis, bursitis and tenosynovitis. Arch Pathol. 1941;31:731–65.
23. Ma X, Shi G, Xia C, Liu H, He J, Jin W. Pigmented villonodular synovitis: a retrospective study of seventy five cases (eighty one joints). Int Orthop. 2013;37(6):1165–70.
24. Shoji T, Yasunaga Y, Yamasaki T, Nakamae A, Mori R, Hamanishi M, Ochi M. Transtrochanteric rotational osteotomy combined with intra-articular procedures for pigmented villonodular synovitis of the hip. J Orthop Sci. 2014.

Bone Marrow Edema Syndromes

25. Hofmann S. The painful bone marrow edema syndrome of the hip joint. Wien Klin Wochenschr. 2005;117(4):111–20.
26. Hofmann S, Engel A, Neuhold A, Leder K, Kramer J, Plenk Jr H. Bone-marrow oedema syndrome and transient osteoporosis of the hip. An MRI-controlled study of treatment by core decompression. J Bone Joint Surg Br. 1993;75:210–6.
27. Plenk Jr H, Hofmann S, Eschberger J, Gstettner M, Kramer J, Schneider W, et al. Histo- morphology and bone morphometry of the bone marrow edema syndrome of the hip. Clin Orthop Relat Res. 1997;334:73–84.
28. Karantanas AH. Acute bone marrow edema of the hip, role of MR imaging. Eur Radiol. 2007;17(9): 2225–36.
29. Korompilias AV, Karantanas AH, Lykissas MG, Beris AE. Bone marrow edema syndrome. Skeletal Radiol. 2009;38:425–36.
30. Patel S. Primary bone marrow oedema syndromes. Rheumatology. 2014;53:785–92.
31. Capone A, Podda D, Ennas F, Iesu C, Casciu L, Civinini R. Hyperbaric oxygen therapy for transient bone marrow oedema syndrome of the hip. Hip Int. 2011;21(2):211–6.
32. Jager M, Zilkens C, Bittersohl B, Matheney T, Kozina C, Blondin D, Krauspe R. Efficiency of iloprost treatment for osseus malperfusion. Int Orthop. 2011;35:761–5.

Osteonecrosis

33. Yamamoto T, Bullough PG. Spontaneous osteonecrosis of the knee: the result of subchondral insufficiency fracture. J Bone Joint Surg A. 2000;82:858–66.
34. Gil HC, Levine SM, Zoga AC. MRI findings in the subchondral bone marrow: a discussion of conditions including transient osteoporosis, transient bone marrow edema syndrome, SONK, and shifting bone marrow edema of the knee. Semin Musculoskelet Radiol. 2006;10:177–86.
35. Fernández-Cantón G. From bone marrow edema to osteonecrosis. New concepts. Reumatol Clin. 2009;5(5):223–7.
36. Jones Jr JP. Risk factors potentially activating intravascular coagulation and causing nontraumatic osteonecrosis. In: Urbaniak JR, Jones Jr JP, editors. Osteonecrosis, etiology, diagnosis and treatment. Rosemont: American Academy of Orthopaedic Surgeons; 1997. p. 89–96.
37. Ficat RP. Idiopathic bone necrosis of the femoral head. Early diagnosis and treatment. J Bone Joint Surg Br. 1985;67:3–9.
38. ARCO (Association Research Circulation Osseous). Committee on terminology and classification. ARCO News. 1992;4:41–6.
39. Steinberg ME, Hayken GD, Steinberg DR. A quantitative system for staging avascular necrosis. J Bone Joint Surg Br. 1995;77:34–41.
40. Liebermann J, Berry D, Mont M, Aaron R, Callaghan J, Rayadhyaksha A, Urbaniak J. Osteonecrosis of the hip: management in the twenty-first century. J Bone Joint Surg. 2002;84-A:833–53.
41. Malizos K, Karantanas A, Varitimidis S, Dailiana Z, Bargiotas K, Maris T. Osteonecrosis of the femoral head: etiology, imaging and treatment. Eur J Radiol. 2007;63:16–28.
42. Alves EM, Angrisani AT, Santiago MB. The use of extracorporeal shock waves in the treatment of osteonecrosis of the femoral head: a systematic review. Clin Rheumatol. 2009;28:1247–51.
43. Beckmann J, Schmidt T, Shaumburger J, Rath B, Luring C, Tingart M, Grifka J. Infusion, core decompression, or infusion following core decompression in the treatment of bone edema syndrome and early avascular osteonecrosis of the femoral head. Rheumatol Int. 2013;33:1561–5.
44. Disch AC, Matziolis G, Perka C. The management of necrosis- associated and idiopathic bone-marrow oedema of the proximal femur by intravenous iloprost. J Bone Joint Surg Br. 2005;87:560–4.

45. Glueck CJ, Freiberg RA, Sieve L, Wang P. Enoxaparin prevents progression of stages I and II osteonecrosis of the hip. Clin Orthop Relat Res. 2005;435:164–70.
46. Rackwitz L, Eden L, Reppenhagen S, Reichert JC, Jakob F, Walles H, Pullig O, Tuan RS, Rudert M, Nöth U. Stem cell and growth factor-based regenerative therapies for avascular necrosis of the femoral head. Stem Cell Res Ther. 2012;3(1):7.
47. Sugioka Y, Yamamoto T. Transtrochanteric posterior rotational osteotomy for osteonecrosis. Clin Orthop. 2008;466:1104–9.
48. Castro FP, Barrack RL. Core decompression and conservative treatment for avascular necrosis of the femoral head: a meta-analysis. Am J Orthop. 2000;29:187–94.
49. Houdek MT, Wyles CC, Martin JR, Sierra RJ. Stem cell treatment for avascular necrosis of the femoral head: current perspectives. Stem Cells Cloning. 2014;7:65–70.
50. Solarino G, Piazzolla A, Notarnicola A, Moretti L, Tafuri S, De Giorgi S, Moretti B. Long-term results of 32-mm alumina-on-alumina THA for avascular necrosis of the femoral head. J Orthop Traumatol. 2012;13(1):21–7.

Greater Trochanteric Pain Syndrome

51. Karpinski MR, Piggott H. Greater trochanteric pain syndrome. A report of 15 cases. J Bone Joint Surg Br. 1985;67(5):762–3.
52. Tortolani PJ, Carbone JJ, Quartararo LG. Greater trochanteric pain syndrome in patients referred to orthopedic spine specialists. Spine J. 2002; 2(4):251–4.
53. Strauss EJ, Nho SJ, Kelly BT. Greater trochanteric pain syndrome. Sports Med Arthrosc. 2010;18(2): 113–9.
54. Chowdhury R, et al. Imaging and management of greater trochanteric pain syndrome. Postgrad Med J. 2014;90:576–81.
55. Segal NA, Felson DT, Torner JC, Zhu Y, Curtis JR, Niu J, Nevitt MC, Multicenter Osteoarthritis Study Group. Greater trochanteric pain syndrome: epidemiology and associated factors. Arch Phys Med Rehabil. 2007;88(8):988–92.
56. Klauser AS, Martinoli C, Tagliafico A, Bellmann-Weiler R, Feuchtner GM, Wick M, Jaschke WR. Greater trochanteric pain syndrome. Semin Musculoskelet Radiol. 2013;17(1):43–8.
57. Tibor LM, Sekiya JK. Differential diagnosis of pain around the hip joint. Arthroscopy. 2008;24(12): 1407–21.
58. Fearon AM, et al. Greater trochanteric pain syndrome: defining the clinical syndrome. Br J Sports Med. 2013;47:649–53.
59. Baker CL, Massie V, Hurt WG, Savory CG. Arthroscopic bursectomy for recalcitrant trochanteric bursitis. Arthroscopy. 2007;23:827–32.
60. Walker P, Kannangara S, Bruce WJM, Michael D, Van der Wall H. Lateral hip pain: does imaging predict response to local injection? Clin Orthop Relat Res. 2006;457:144–9.
61. Farr D, Selesnick H, Janecki C, Cordas D. Arthroscopic bursectomy with concomitant iliotibial band release for the treatment of recalcitrant trochanteric bursitis. Arthroscopy. 2007;23:905.e1–5.
62. Kaltenborn A, Bourg CM, Gutzeit A, Kalberer F. The hip lag sign – prospective blinded trial of a new clinical sign to predict hip abductor damage. PLoS One. 2014;9(3), e91560.
63. Fearon A, Stephens S, Cook J, Smith P, Neeman T, Cormick W, Scarvell J. The relationship of femoral neck shaft angle and adiposity to greater trochanteric pain syndrome in women. A case control morphology and anthropometric study. Br J Sports Med. 2012;46(12):888–92.
64. Moulton KM, Aly AR, Rajasekaran S, Shepel M, Obaid H. Acetabular anteversion is associated with gluteal tendinopathy at MRI. Skeletal Radiol. 2015;44(1):47–54. doi:10.1007/s00256-014-1991-6. Epub 2014 Aug 27.
65. Ho GW, Howard TM. Greater trochanteric pain syndrome: more than bursitis and iliotibial tract friction. Curr Sports Med Rep. 2012;11(5):232–8.
66. McEvoy JR, Lee KS, Blankenbaker DG, del Rio AM, Keene JS. Ultrasound-guided corticosteroid injections for treatment of greater trochanteric pain syndrome: greater trochanter bursa versus subgluteus medius bursa. AJR Am J Roentgenol. 2013;201(2):W313–7.
67. Mani-Babu S, Morrissey D, Waugh C, Screen H, Barton C. The effectiveness of extracorporeal shock wave therapy in lower limb tendinopathy: a systematic review. Am J Sports Med. 2014. [Epub ahead of print].
68. Rompe JD, Segal NA, Cacchio A, Furia JP, Morral A, Maffulli N. Home training, local corticosteroid injection, or radial shock wave therapy for greater trochanter pain syndrome. Am J Sports Med. 2009;37(10):1981–90. doi:10.1177/0363546509334374. Epub 2009 May 13.
69. Reich MS, Shannon C, Tsai E, Salata MJ. Hip arthroscopy for extra-articular hip disease. Curr Rev Musculoskelet Med. 2013;6(3):250–7.
70. Barnthouse NC, et al. Greater trochanteric pain syndrome: endoscopic treatment options. Oper TechSports Med. 2012;20(4):320–4.
71. Ebert JR, Bucher TA, Ball SV, Janes GC. A review of surgical repair methods and patient outcomes for gluteal tendon tears. Hip Int. 2014.
72. Domínguez A, Seijas R, Ares O, Sallent A, Cuscó X, Cugat R. Clinical outcomes of trochanteric syndrome endoscopically treated. Arch Orthop Trauma Surg. 2015;135(1):89–94.

73. Govaert LH, van Dijk CN, Zeegers AV, Albers GH. Endoscopic bursectomy and iliotibial tract release as a treatment for refractory greater trochanteric pain syndrome: a new endoscopic approach with early results. Arthrosc Tech. 2012;1(2):e161–4.
74. Voos JE, Rudzki JR, Shindle MK, Martin H, Kelly BT. Arthroscopic anatomy and surgical techniques for peritrochanteric space disorders in the hip. Arthroscopy. 2007;23(11):1246.
75. Ilizaliturri Jr VM, Martinez-Escalante FA, Chaidez PA, Camacho-Galindo J. Endoscopic iliotibial band release for external snapping hip syndrome. Arthroscopy. 2006;22(5):505–10.
76. Domb BG, Botser I, Giordano BD. Outcomes of endoscopic gluteus medius repair with minimum 2-year follow-up. Am J Sports Med. 2013;41(5):988–97.

Snapping Hip

77. Lewis CL. Extra-articular snapping hip: a literature review. Sports Health. 2010;2(3):186–90.
78. Winston P, Awan R, Cassidy JD, Bleakney RK. Clinical examination and ultrasound of self-reported snapping hip syndrome in elite ballet dancers. Am J Sports Med. 2007;35(1):118–26.
79. Byrd JW. Snapping hip. Oper Tech Sports Med. 2005;13:46–54.
80. Allen WC, Cope R. Coxa saltans: the snapping hip revisited. J Am Acad Orthop Surg. 1995;3:303–8.
81. Khan M, Adamich J, Simunovic N, Philippon MJ, Bhandari M, Ayeni OR. Surgical management of internal snapping hip syndrome: a systematic review evaluating open and arthroscopic approaches. Arthroscopy. 2013;29(5):942–8.
82. Provencher MT, Hofmeister EP, Muldoon MP. The surgical treatment of external coxa saltans (the snapping hip) by Z-plasty of the iliotibial band. Am J Sports Med. 2004;32(2):470–6.
83. Ilizaliturri Jr VM, Martinez-Escalante FA, Chaidez PA, Camacho-Galindo J. Endoscopic iliotibial band release for external snapping hip syndrome. Arthroscopy. 2006;22(5):505–10.
84. Polesello GC, Queiroz MC, Domb BG, Ono NK, Honda EK. Surgical technique: endoscopic gluteus maximus tendon release for external snapping hip syndrome. Clin Orthop Relat Res. 2013;471(8):2471–6.
85. Anderson SA, Keene JS. Results of arthroscopic iliopsoas tendon release in competitive and recreational athletes. Am J Sports Med. 2008;36(12):2363–71.
86. Flanum ME, Keene JS, Blankenbaker DG, Desmet AA. Arthroscopic treatment of the painful "internal" snapping hip: results of a new endoscopic technique and imaging protocol. Am J Sports Med. 2007;35(5):770–9.
87. Ilizaliturri Jr VM, Buganza-Tepole M, Olivos-Meza A, Acuna M, Acosta-Rodriguez E. Central compartment release versus lesser trochanter release of the iliopsoas tendon for the treatment of internal snapping hip: a comparative study. Arthroscopy. 2014;30(7):790–5.
88. Nelson IR, Keene JS. Results of labral-level arthroscopic iliopsoas tenotomies for the treatment of labral impingement. Arthroscopy. 2014;30(6):688–94.
89. El Bitar YF, Stake CE, Dunne KF, Botser IB, Domb BG. Arthroscopic iliopsoas fractional lengthening for internal snapping of the hip: clinical outcomes with a minimum 2-year follow-up. Am J Sports Med. 2014;42(7):1696–703.
90. Shu B, Safran MR. Case report: Bifid iliopsoas tendon causing refractory internal snapping hip. Clin Orthop Relat Res. 2011;469(1):289–93.
91. Philippon MJ, Devitt BM, Campbell KJ, Michalski MP, Espinoza C, Wijdicks CA, Laprade RF. Anatomic variance of the iliopsoas tendon. Am J Sports Med. 2014;42(4):807–11.
92. Byrd JW. Hip arthroscopy: patient assessment and indications. Instr Course Lect. 2003;52:711–9.

Ischiofemoral Impingement

93. Safran M, Ryu J. Ischiofemoral impingement of the hip: a novel approach to treatment. Knee Surg Sports Traumatol Arthrosc. 2014;22(4):781–5. doi:10.1007/s00167-013-2801-8. Epub 2013 Dec 18.
94. Johnson KA. Impingement of the lesser trochanter on the ischial ramus after total hip arthroplasty: report of three cases. J Bone Joint Surg Am. 1977;59:268–9.
95. Torriani M, Souto SC, Thomas BJ, Ouellette H, Bredella MA. Ischiofemoral impingement syndrome: an entity with hip pain and abnormalities of the quadratus femoris muscle. AJR Am J Roentgenol. 2009;193:186–90.
96. Patti JW, Ouellette H, Bredella MA, Torriani M. Impingement of lesser trochanter on ischium as a potential cause for hip pain. Skeletal Radiol. 2008;37:939–41.
97. Stafford GH, Villar RN. Ischiofemoral impingement. J Bone Joint Surg Br. 2011;93-B:1300–2.
98. Tosun O, Algin O, Yalcin N, Cay N, Ocakoglu G, Karaoglanoglu M. Ischiofemoral impingement: evaluation with new MRI parameters and assessment of their reliability. Skeletal Radiol. 2012;41:575–87.
99. De Sa D, Alradwan H, Cargnelli S, Thawer Z, Simunovic N, Cadet E, Bonin N, Larson C, Ayeni OR. Extra-articular hip impingement: a systematic review examining operative treatment of psoas, subspine, ischiofemoral, and greater trochanteric/pelvic impingement. Arthroscopy. 2014;30(8):1026–41. doi:10.1016/j.arthro.2014.02.042.
100. Hatem MA, Palmer IJ, Martin HD. Diagnosis and 2-year outcomes of endoscopic treatment for ischiofemoral impingement. Arthroscopy. 2014. pii: S0749-8063(14)00704-X. doi:10.1016/j.arthro.2014.07.031. [Epub ahead of print].

Osteitis Pubis

101. Choi H, McCartney M, Best TM. Treatment of osteitis pubis and osteomyelitis of the pubic symphysis in athletes: a systematic review. Br J Sports Med. 2011;45:57–64.
102. Lentz SS. Osteitis pubis: a review. Obstet Gynecol Surv. 1995;50(4):310–5.
103. Beer E. Periostitis of symphysis and descending rami of pubes following suprapubic operations. Int J Med Surg. 1928;37:224–5.
104. Spinelli A. Nuova malattia sportive: la pubalgia degli schernitori. Ortop Traumatol Appar Mot. 1932;4:111–27.
105. Andrews SK, Carek PJ. Osteitis pubis: a diagnosis for the family physician. J Am Board Fam Pract. 1998;11(4):291–5.
106. Radic R, Annear P. Use of pubic symphysis curettage for treatment-resistant osteitis pubis in athletes. Am J Sports Med. 2008;36(1):122–8.
107. Hölmich P. Long-standing groin pain in sportspeople falls into three primary patterns, a "clinical entity" approach: a prospective study of 207 patients. Br J Sports Med. 2007;41(4):247–52.
108. Hammoud S, Bedi A, Voos JE, Mauro CS, Kelly BT. The recognition and evaluation of patterns of compensatory injury in patients with mechanical hip pain. Sports Health. 2014;6(2):108–18.
109. Larson CM, Sikka RS, Sardelli MC, Byrd JW, Kelly BT, Jain RK, Giveans MR. Increasing alpha angle is predictive of athletic-related "hip" and "groin" pain in collegiate National Football League prospects. Arthroscopy. 2013;29(3):405–10.
110. Holt MA, Keene JS, Graf BK, Helwig DC. Treatment of osteitis pubis in athletes. Results of corticosteroid injections. Am J Sports Med. 1995;23(5):601–6.
111. Hiti CJ, Stevens KJ, Jamati MK, Garza D, Matheson GO. Athletic osteitis pubis. Sports Med. 2011;41(5):361–76.
112. Tibor LM, Sekiya JK. Differential diagnosis of pain around the hip joint. Arthroscopy. 2008;24(12):1407–21.
113. Rodriguez C, Miguel A, Lima H, Heinrichs K. Osteitis pubis syndrome in the professional soccer athlete: a case report. J Athl Train. 2001;36:437–40.
114. Hopp S, Tumin M, Wilhelm P, Pohlemann T, Kelm J. Arthroscopic pubic symphysis debridement and adductor enthesis repair in athletes with athletic pubalgia: technical note and video illustration. Arch Orthop Trauma Surg. 2014;134(11):1595–9.
115. Hopp S, Culemann U, Ojodu I, Pohlemann T, Kelm J. Arthroscopic debridement of the pubic symphysis: an experimental study. Knee Surg Sports Traumatol Arthrosc. 2015;23:2568–75.
116. Hopp SJ, Culemann U, Kelm J, Pohlemann T, Pizanis A. Osteitis pubis and adductor tendinopathy in athletes: a novel arthroscopic pubic symphysis curettage and adductor reattachment. Arch Orthop Trauma Surg. 2013;133(7):1003–9.

Sports Hernia

117. Meyers WC, McKechnie A, Philippon MJ, Horner MA, Zoga AC, Devon ON. Experience with "sports hernia" spanning two decades. Ann Surg. 2008;248(4):656–65 [PubMed].
118. Kachingwe A, Grech S. Proposed algorithm for the management of athletes with athletic pubalgia: a case series. J Orthop Sport Phys Ther. 2008; 38(12):768–81 [PubMed].
119. Brown A, Abrahams S, Remedios D, Chadwick SJ. Sports hernia, a clinical update. Br J Gen Pract. 2013;63(608):e235–7.
120. Anderson K, Strickland S, Warren R. Hip and groin injuries in athletes. Am J Sports Med. 2001;29(4):521–33 [PubMed].
121. Hammoud S, Bedi A, Magennis E, Meyers WC, Kelly BT. High incidence of athletic pubalgia symptoms in professional athletes with symptomatic femoroacetabular impingement. Arthroscopy. 2012; 28(10):1388–95 [Epub 2012 May 19].
122. Holmich P, Uhrskou P, Ulnits L, et al. Effectiveness of active physical training as treatment for longstanding adductor related groin pain in athletes: a randomised trial. Lancet. 1999;353:439–43 [PubMed].
123. Muschaweck U, Berger L. Minimal repair technique of sportsmen's groin: an innovative open-suture repair to treat chronic inguinal pain. Hernia. 2010;14:27–33 [PubMed].
124. Minnich JM, Hanks JB, Muschaweck U, Brunt LM, Diduch DR. Sports hernia: diagnosis and treatment highlighting a minimal repair surgical technique. Am J Sports Med. 2011;39:1341–9 [PubMed].
125. Farber AJ, Wilckens JH. Sports hernia: diagnosis and therapeutic approach. J Am Acad Orthop Surg. 2007;15:507–14 [PubMed].
126. Le Blanc E, LeBlanc KA. Groin pain in athletes. Hernia. 2003;7(2):68–71.
127. Preskitt JT. Sports hernia: the experience of Baylor University Medical Center at Dallas. Proc (Bayl Univ Med Cent). 2011;24(2):89–91.
128. Shortt CP, Zoga AC, Kavanagh EC, Meyers WC. Anatomy, pathology, and MRI findings in the sports hernia. Semin Musculoskelet Radiol. 2008;12(1):54–61 [PubMed].
129. Woodward JS, Parker A, MacDonald RM. Non-surgical treatment of a professional hockey player with the signs and symptoms of sports hernia: a case report. Int J Sports Phys Ther. 2012;7(1):85–100 [PubMed].
130. Ekstrand J, Ringborg S. Surgery versus conservative treatment in soccer players with chronic groin pain: a prospective randomised study in soccer players. Euro J Sport Trauma Relat Res. 2001;23(4):141–5.
131. Susmallian S, Ezri T, Ellis M, et al. Laparoscopic repair of "sportsman's hernia" in soccer players as treatment of chronic inguinal pain. Med Sci Monit. 2004;10:CR52–4 [PubMed].
132. Swan Jr K, Wolcott M. The athletic hernia: a systematic review. Clin Ortho Relat Res. 2007;455:78–87 [PubMed].

133. Lynch S, Renström P. Groin injuries in sport. Sports Med. 1999;28(2):137–44 [PubMed].
134. Diaco JF, Diaco DS, Lockhart L. Sports hernia. J Oper Tech Sports Med. 2005;13(1):68–70.
135. Joesting DR. Diagnosis and treatment of sportsman's hernia. Curr Sports Med Rep. 2002;1(2):121–4.
136. Meyers W, Foley D, Garrett W, et al. Management of severe lower abdominal or inguinal pain in high performance athletes. Am J Sports Med. 2000;28(1):2–8 [PubMed].
137. Economopoulos KJ, Milewski MD, Hanks JB, Hart JM, Diduch DR. Radiographic evidence of femoroacetabular impingement in athletes with athletic pubalgia. Sports Health. 2014;6(2):171–7 [PubMed].

Piriformis Muscle Syndrome

138. Michel F, Decavel P, Toussirot E, Tatu L, Aleton E, Monnier G, Garbuio P, Parratte B, Piriformis muscle syndrome: diagnostic criteria and treatment of a monocentric series of 250 patients. J Rehab. 2013.
139. Michel F, Decavel P, Toussirot E, Tatu L, Aleton E, Monnier G, Garbuio P, Parratte B. The piriformis muscle syndrome: an exploration of anatomical context, pathophysiological hypotheses and diagnostic criteria. Ann Phys Rehabil Med. 2013;56(4):300–11.
140. Papadopoulos EC, Khan SN. Piriformis syndrome and low back pain: a new classification and review of the literature. Orthop Clin North Am. 2004;35(1):65–71 [PubMed].
141. Jawish RM, Assoum HA, Khamis CF. Anatomical clinical and electrical observations in piriformis syndrome. J Orthop Surg Res. 2010;5:3.
142. Meknas K, Johansen O. Jüri Kartus Retro-trochanteric sciatica-like pain: current concept. Knee Surg Sports Traumatol Arthrosc. 2011;19(11):1971–85.
143. Yeoman W. The relation of arthritis of the sacro-iliac joint to sciatica, with an analysis of 100 cases. Lancet. 1928;2:1119–22.
144. Freiburg AH, Vinke TA. Sciatica and the sacroiliac joint. J Bone Joint Surg. 1934;16:126–36.
145. Beaton LE, Anson BJ. The sciatic nerve and the piriformis muscle. Their interrelation and possible cause of coccygodynia. J Bone Joint Surg Am. 1938;20:686–8.
146. Robinson D. Piriformis syndrome in relation to sciatic pain. Am J Surg. 1947;73:356–8.
147. Hopayian K, Song F, Riera R, Sambandan S. The clinical features of the piriformis syndrome: a systematic review. Eur Spine J. 2010;19(12):2095–109.
148. Pace JB, Nagle D. Piriform syndrome. West J Med. 1976;124(6):435–9 [PubMed].
149. Pecina HI, Boric I, Smoljanovic T, Duvancic D, Pecina M. Surgical evaluation of magnetic resonance imaging findings in piriformis muscle syndrome. Skeletal Radiol. 2008;37(11):1019–23.
150. Niu CC, Lai PL, Fu TS, Chen LH, Chen WJ. Ruling out piriformis syndrome before diagnosing lumbar radiculopathy. Chang Gung Med J. 2009;32(2):182–7.
151. Naja Z, Al-Tannir M, El-Rajab M, et al. The effectiveness of clonidine-bupivacaine repeated nerve stimulator-guided injection in piriformis syndrome. Clin J Pain. 2009;25(3):199–205 [PubMed].
152. Ozisik PA, Toru M, Denk CC, Taskiran OO, Gundogmus B. CT-guided piriformis muscle injection for the treatment of piriformis syndrome. Turk Neurosurg. 2014;24(4):471–7.
153. Indrekvam K, Sudmann E. Piriformis muscle syndrome in 19 patients treated by tenotomy – a 1 to 16 year follow-up study. Int Orthop. 2002;26(2):101–3.
154. Jeynes LC, Gauci CA. Evidence for the use of botulinum toxin in the chronic pain setting: a review of the literature. Pain Pract. 2008;8(4):269–76 [PubMed].
155. Kirschner JS, Foye PM, Cole JL. Piriformis syndrome, diagnosis and treatment. Muscle Nerve. 2009;40(1):10–8 [PubMed].
156. Dezawa A, Kusano S, Miki H. Arthroscopic release of the piriformis muscle under local anesthesia for piriformis syndrome. Arthroscopy. 2003;19:554–7.
157. Martin HD, Shears SA, Johnson JC, Smathers AM, Palmer IJ. The endoscopic treatment of sciatic nerve entrapment/deep gluteal syndrome. Arthroscopy. 2011;27:172–81.

Meralgia Paraestetica

158. Cheatham SW, Kolber MJ, Salamh PA. Meralgia paraesthetica: a review of the literature. Int J Sports Phys Ther. 2013;8(6):883–93.
159. Pearce JM. Meralgia paraesthetica (Bernhardt-Roth syndrome). J Neurol Neurosurg Psych. 2006;77(1):84.
160. Harney D, Patijn J. Meralgia paresthetica: diagnosis and management strategies. Pain Med. 2007;8(8):669–77.
161. van Slobbe AM, Bohnen AM, Bernsen RM, et al. Incidence rates and determinants in meralgia paresthetica in general practice. J Neurol. 2004;251(3):294–7.
162. Grossman MG, Ducey SA, Nadler SS, et al. Meralgia paresthetica: diagnosis and treatment. J Am Acad Orthop Surg. 2001;9(5):336–44.
163. Aszmann OC, Dellon ES, Dellon AL. Anatomical course of the lateral femoral cutaneous nerve and its susceptibility to compression and injury. Plast Reconstr Surg. 1997;100(3):600–4.
164. De Ridder VA, de Lange S, Popta JV. Anatomical variations of the lateral femoral cutaneous nerve and

the consequences for surgery. J Orthop Trauma. 1999;13:207–11.
165. Nouraei SA, Anand B, Spink G, et al. A novel approach to the diagnosis and management of meralgia paresthetica. Neurosurgery. 2007;60(4):696–700.
166. Ahmed A. Meralgia paresthetica and femoral acetabular impingement: a possible association. J Clin Med Res. 2010;2(6):274–6.
167. Chhabra A, Del Grande F, Soldatos T, et al. Meralgia paresthetica: 3-Tesla magnetic resonance neurography. Skeletal Radiol. 2013;42(6):803–8.
168. Tagliafico A, Serafini G, Lacelli F, et al. Ultrasound-guided treatment of meralgia paresthetica (lateral femoral cutaneous neuropathy): technical description and results of treatment in 20 consecutive patients. J Ultrasound Med. 2011;30(10):1341–6.
169. Hurdle MF, Weingarten TN, Crisostomo RA, et al. Ultrasound-guided blockade of the lateral femoral cutaneous nerve: technical description and review of 10 cases. Arch Phys Med Rehabil. 2007;88(10):1362–4.

Obturator Neuropathy

170. Tipton JS. Obturator neuropathy. Curr Rev Musculoskelet Med. 2008;1:234–7.
171. Sorenson EJ, Chen JJ, Daube JR. Obturator neuropathy: causes and outcome. Wiley Periodicals, Inc. Muscle Nerve. 2002;25:605–7.
172. Kitagawa R, Kim D, Reid N, Kline D. Surgical management of obturator nerve lesions. Neurosurgery. 2009;65:A24–8.
173. Yukata K, Arai K, Yoshizumi Y, Tamano K, Imada K, Nakaima N. Obturator neuropathy caused by an acetabular labral cyst: MRI findings. AJR Am J Roentgenol. 2005;184(3 Suppl):S112–4.
174. Cardosi RJ, Cox CS, Hoffman MS. Postoperative neuropathies after major pelvic surgery. Obstet Gynecol. 2002;100:240–4.
175. Kim S-H, Hyun S, Seung YL, Sung WP. Acetabular paralabral cyst as a rare cause of obturator neuropathy: a case report. Ann Rehabil Med. 2014;38(3):427–32.
176. Aydogmus S, Kelekci S, Aydogmus H, Ekmekci E, Secil Y, Ture S. Obturator nerve injury: an infrequent complication of TOT procedure. Case Rep Obstet Gynecol. 2014;2014:290382. doi:10.1155/2014/290382. Epub 2014 Sep 29.
177. Barrick EF. Entrapment of the obturator nerve in association with a fracture of the pelvic ring. A case report. J Bone Joint Surg Am. 1998;80(2):258–61.
178. Fricker RM, Troeger H, Pfeiffer KM. Obturator nerve palsy due to fixation of an acetabular reinforcement ring with transacetabular screws. A case report. J Bone Joint Surg Am. 1997;79(3):444–6.
179. Lavernia CJ, Cook CC, Hernandez RA, Sierra RJ, Rossi MD. Neurovascular injuries in acetabular reconstruction cage surgery: an anatomical study. J Arthroplasty. 2007;22(1):124–32.
180. Weale AE, Newman P, Ferguson IT, Bannister GC. Nerve injury after posterior and direct lateral approaches for hip replacement. A clinical and electrophysiological study. J Bone Joint Surg Br. 1996;78(6):899–902.
181. Yang KH, Han DY, Park HW, Park SJ. Intraarticular entrapment of the obturator nerve in acetabular fracture. J Orthop Trauma. 2001;15(5):361–3.
182. Harma M, Sel G, Açıkgöz B, Harma Mİ. Successful obturator nerve repairing: intraoperative sural nerve graft harvesting in endometrium cancer patient. Int J Surg Case Rep. 2014;5(6):345–6.

Osteoid Osteoma

183. Jaffe H. "Osteoid osteoma": a benign osteoblastic tumor composed of osteoid and atypical bone. Arch Surg. 1935;31:709–28.
184. Unni KK. Osteoid osteoma. In: Unni KK, editor. Dahlin's bone tumors: general aspects and data on 11,087 cases. 5th ed. Philadelphia: Lippincott Raven Publishers; 1996. p. 121–30.
185. Campanacci M. Osteoid osteoma. In: Campanacci M, editor. Bone and soft tissue tumours. Padova: Piccin Nuova Libraria S.p.A; 1999. p. 391–414.
186. Frassica FJ, Waltrip RL, Sponseller PD, Ma LD, McCarthy Jr EF. Clinicopathologic features and treatment of osteoid osteoma and osteoblastoma in children and adolescents. Orthop Clin North Am. 1996;27(3):559–74.
187. Szendroi M, Köllo K, Antal I, Lakatos J, Szoke G. Intraarticular osteoid osteoma: clinical features, imaging results, and comparison with extraarticular localization. J Rheumatol. 2004;31(5):957–64.
188. Randelli F, Favilla S, Banci L, D'ambrosi R, Pace F. Femoro acetabular impingement and osteoid osteoma: a strange and misleading association. ISHA 2013 meeting, Munich.
189. Banga K, Racano A, Ayeni OR, Deheshi B. Atypical hip pain: coexistence of femoroacetabular impingement (FAI) and osteoid osteoma. Knee Surg Sports Traumatol Arthrosc. 2014. [Epub ahead of print].
190. Gitelis S, Schajowicz F. Osteoid osteoma and osteoblastoma. Orthop Clin North Am. 1989;20(3):313–25.
191. Klein MH, Shankman S. Osteoid osteoma: radiologic and pathologic correlation. Skeletal Radiol. 1992;21(1):23–31.
192. Cassar-Pullicino VN, McCall IW, Wan S. Intra-articular osteoid osteoma. Clin Radiol. 1992;45:153–60.
193. Helms CA, Hattner RS, Vogler III JB. Osteoid osteoma: radionuclide diagnosis. Radiology. 1984;151(3):779–84.
194. Ryan PJ, Fogelman I. Bone SPECT in osteoid osteoma of the vertebral lamina. Clin Nucl Med. 1994;19(2):144–5.

195. Nogues P, Marti-Bonmati L, Aparisi F, Saborido MC, Garci J, Dosdá R. MR imaging assessment of juxta cortical edema in osteoid osteoma in 28 patients. Eur Radiol. 1998;8(2):236–8.
196. Gaeta M, Minutoli F, Pandolfo I, Vinci S, D'Andrea L, Blandino A. Magnetic resonance imaging findings of osteoid osteoma of the proximal femur. Eur Radiol. 2004;14(9):1582–9.
197. Scalici J, Jacquel A, Mukish P, Trouilloud P, Baulot E. Intra-articular osteoid osteoma of the hip misdiagnosed by MRI: an unusual cause of unexplained hip pain. Orthop Traumatol Surg Res. 2011;97(8):881–5. doi:10.1016/j.otsr.2011.05.015. Epub 2011 Nov 8.
198. Schnapauff D, Streitparth F, Jöhrens K, Wieners G, Collettini F, Hamm B, Gebauer B. CT-guided radiofrequency ablation of osteoid osteoma using a novel battery-powered drill. Skeletal Radiol. 2014.
199. Said HG, Abdulla Babaqi A, Abdelsalam E-AM. Hip arthroscopy for excision of osteoid osteoma of femoral neck. Arthrosc Tech. 2014;3(1):e145–8.
200. Ricci D, Grappiolo G, Franco M, Della RF. Case report: osteoid osteoma of the acetabulum treated with arthroscopy-assisted radiofrequency ablation. Clin Orthop Relat Res. 2013;471(5):1727–32. doi:10.1007/s11999-012-2772-y. Epub 2013 Jan 12.
201. de Los SO, Filomeno P, Rey R, Cúneo A. Acetabular osteoid osteoma excision by controlled hip dislocation: a case report. J Pediatr Orthop B. 2013;22(3):195–9. doi:10.1097/BPB.0b013e32835f57fc.
202. Tokis A, Tsakotos G, Demesticha T. Arthroscopic treatment of recurrent acetabulum osteoid osteoma. Knee Surg Sports Traumatol Arthrosc. 2014;22(4):871–3. doi:10.1007/s00167-013-2805-4. Epub 2013 Dec 18.
203. Shoji T, Yasunaga Y, Yamasaki T, Mori R, Hamanishi M, Shimose S, Ochi M. T2 mapping magnetic resonance imaging encourages an arthroscopic approach for osteoid osteoma in the acetabulum. Arthrosc Tech. 2014;3(2):e251–4. doi:10.1016/j.eats.2013.11.006. eCollection 2014.

Cruralgia

204. Nadler SF, Campagnolo DI, Tomaio AC, Stitik TP. High lumbar disc: diagnostic and treatment dilemma. Am J Phys Med Rehabil. 1998;77(6):538–44.
205. Kortelainen P, Puranen J, Koivisto E, Lähde S. Symptoms and signs of sciatica and their relation to the localization of the lumbar disc herniation. Spine (Phila Pa 1976). 1985;10(1):88–92.
206. Rubin DI. Epidemiology and risk factors for spine pain. Neurol Clin. 2007;25(2):353–71.
207. Wasserman S. Ueber ein neues Schenkelnervsymptom nebst Bemerkungn zur Diagnostik der Schenkelnerverkrankungen. Dtsch Z Nervenheilk. 1918;43:140–3.
208. Geraci MC, Alleva JT. Physical examination of the spine and its functional kinetic chain. In: Cole AJ, Herring SA, editors. The low back pain handbook. Philadelphia: Hanley & Belfus; 1996. p. 60.
209. Suri P, Hunter DJ, Katz JN, Li L, Rainville J. Bias in the physical examination of patients with lumbar radiculopathy. BMC Musculoskelet Disord. 2010;11:275.
210. Iversen T, Solberg TK, Romner B, Wilsgaard T, Nygaard Ø, Waterloo K, Brox JI, Ingebrigtsen T. Accuracy of physical examination for chronic lumbar radiculopathy. BMC Musculoskelet Disord. 2013;14:206.
211. Rainville J, Jouve C, Finno M, Limke J. Comparison of four tests of quadriceps strength in L3 or L4 radiculopathies. Spine (Phila Pa 1976). 2003;28(21):2466–71.
212. Hahne AJ, Ford JJ, McMeeken JM. Conservative management of lumbar disc herniation with associated radiculopathy: a systematic review. Spine (Phila Pa 1976). 2010;35(11):E488–504. doi:10.1097/BRS.0b013e3181cc3f56.
213. Postacchini F. Management of herniation of the lumbar disc. J Bone Joint Surg Br. 1999;81(4):567–76.

Buttock Claudication

214. Prince J, Smits M, Van Herwaarden J, Arntz J, Vonken E, et al. Endovascular treatment of internal iliac artery stenosis in patients with buttock claudication. PLoS One. 2013. doi:10.1371/journal.pone.0073331.
215. Chaer R, Faries S, Lin S, Dayal R, McKinsey JF, Kent K. Successful percutaneous treatment of gluteal claudication secondary to isolated bilateral hypogastric stenoses. J Vasc Surg. 2006;43:165–8.
216. Hodgson KJ, Sumner DS. Buttock claudication from isolated bilateral internal iliac arterial stenoses. J Vasc Surg. 1988;7:446–8.
217. Smith G, Train J, Mitty H, Jacobson J. Hip pain caused by buttock claudication. Relief of symptoms by transluminal angioplasty. Clin Orthop Relat Res. 1992;284:176–80. PubMed: 1395290.
218. Senechal Q, Auguste MC, Louail B, Lagneau P, Pernes JM. Relief of buttock claudication by percutaneous recanalization of an occluded superior gluteal artery. Cardiovasc Intervent Radiol. 2000;23:226–7.
219. Batt M, Baque J, Bouillanne PJ, Hassen-Khodja R, Haudebourg P. Percutaneous angioplasty of the superior gluteal artery for buttock claudication: a report of seven cases and literature review. J Vasc Surg. 2006;43:987–91.

Clinical Diagnosis of FAI: An Evidence-Based Approach to History and Physical Examination of the Hip

3

Aparna Viswanath and Vikas Khanduja

Contents

A. Viswanath, MBBS, BSc, MRCS • V. Khanduja, MA, MSc, FRCS, FRCS (Orth) (✉)
Department of Trauma & Orthopaedics, Addenbrooke's – Cambridge University Hospitals, Box 37, Hills Road, Cambridge CB2 0QQ, UK
e-mail: vk279@cam.ac.uk

Assessing the young adult hip can be challenging. It is not simply about finding a "square peg in a round hole" [1]; patients exhibit a spectrum of disorders. The first hurdle is characterising these symptoms to differentiate major structural abnormalities in the hip from extra-articular soft tissue problems. As many patients presenting with hip pain often have an active lifestyle, they may have concomitant pathologies, which may be coincidental findings or compensatory disorders. Ultimately the goal is to ascertain an aetiology or structural abnormality and select an appropriate treatment option.

3.1 Diagnosing Femoroacetabular Impingement

Femoroacetabular impingement (FAI) as a possible cause for "idiopathic" osteoarthritis of the hip was first described just over two decades ago by Ganz and co-workers in Switzerland [2–4]. Essentially it is the abutment of the femoral head-neck junction against the acetabular rim during the physiological range of movement of the hip joint. This mechanical process leads to progressive breakdown of the chondro-labral junction, which in turn may lead to osteoarthritis. The process may be as a result of abnormal morphology of the femoral head-neck junction (CAM lesion), acetabulum (pincer) or a combination of both.

O.R. Ayeni et al. (eds.), *Diagnosis and Management of Femoroacetabular Impingement*, DOI 10.1007/978-3-319-32000-7_3

There are, however, sceptics who don't believe that we have enough evidence to prove a causal effect [5]. There certainly is paucity of level I or II evidence to support the theory that FAI causes osteoarthritis. This extends to a lack of evidence to show a pathognomonic feature to aid in the diagnosis. Unlike many conditions in orthopaedics, the radiographic features associated with FAI are also seen in the asymptomatic population [6–8]. Therefore, diagnosing FAI relies on a good history and clinical examination along with radiological signs on plain radiographs and ideally an MRI to assess the articular cartilage and the labrum. In this chapter, the pertinent evidence that guides the initial assessment of the young adult with hip pain is highlighted.

3.2 Demographics

FAI is a condition that is pertinent in the young adult. It is considered that carefully selected patients younger than 55 may benefit from joint preservation surgery, and therefore it is important to be able to identify these individuals and hopefully circumvent the need for joint replacement surgery in the future [9].

At the other end of the spectrum, patients should be skeletally mature to warrant this diagnosis. Carsen et al. studied the radiological appearances of CAM deformities and showed that in the open physes group of patients, none had a femoral head-neck structural abnormality [10]. However, CAM-type lesions began to be apparent soon after physeal closure in some volunteers. This is further supported by a longitudinal study by Agricola et al. which shows that femoral head-neck junction flattening increased significantly ($p = 0.002$) over a 2-year period during physeal closure [11].

There have been few studies looking into the prevalence of FAI across different ethnic groups, and these studies have revealed that FAI is rare in the Japanese population [12, 13]. This is despite a radiologically proved mechanical abutment of the femoral head on the acetabular rim. Geographically FAI tends to be a disease of the Western world occurring in a skeletally mature population.

Activity levels have been strongly associated with FAI. A recent study compared semiprofessional footballers to amateur players and assimilated findings from a clinical examination and MRI study [14]. This showed significantly higher numbers of positive impingement in the semiprofessional group ($p = 0.048$) with a higher α angle also seen in this group ($p = 0.008$). A retrospective review of high-level athletes and recreational athletes also showed that the former were more likely to undergo bilateral surgery and at a younger age [15].

3.3 History

As with other disciplines, it is important to have a system when either taking a history or performing clinical examination. As stated previously, one of the main aims in taking a history is to be able to differentiate intra-articular causes of pain from extra-articular soft tissue problems. If we take this one step further, the painful hip may be characterised in layers [15]:

1. The osteochondral layer pertaining to the acetabulum, femoral head and the pelvis
2. Structural soft tissues such as the capsule, ligamentum teres, labrum and ligamentous complex
3. Core muscles of the hip and hemipelvis providing stability
4. Lower extremity structures which cross the hip joint or cause referred pain, e.g. lumbosacral plexus, lateral femoral cutaneous nerve and sciatic nerve

Bearing this in mind, questions posed should help us in identifying a predominant layer within which the abnormality lies.

3.3.1 Pain

This is a good starting point and follows a comprehensive format to taking a pain history. Without pain being a predominant feature, caution should be used in pursuing a diagnosis of FAI.

The site of the pain is often a deep-seated pain at the groin. In a study by Clohisy et al., 51 subjects were asked detailed questions with regard to their pain [16]. Eighty-eight percent of patients reported groin pain, and 67 % had lateral hip pain. These were the commonest sites for patients, who went on to be diagnosed with FAI, to report pain. It should be noted that few patients pointed to only one region of pain, but even in those who presented with buttock pain, most had corresponding groin pain (87 %). In another study looking at preoperative data from 301 subjects who underwent joint preservation surgery, 81 % reported deep groin pain [17]. Again, significant overlap with pain in other regions – including trochanteric, buttock and sacroiliac – was noted in 61 %, 52 % and 23 %, respectively. Pain may also be referred down the anterior thigh [18]. Another feature seen when asking about the site of pain is the "C sign" [19, 20]. The patient's hand forms a "C" with the thumb posterior and the fingers gripping deep into the anterior groin. It should not be mistaken for lateral hip pain as it indicates a deep groin pain.

In Clohisy's study [16], 65 % of patients described an insidious onset, with 21 % attributing pain from a traumatic event. As Byrd points out though, on close questioning even in those who recall a precipitating event, "the athlete will frequently recall prior non-specific symptoms of a groin strain" [21]. He goes on to state that many athletes presenting with hip pain may recount that even at a young age, they were not as flexible as their team-mates.

Pain is often sharp and stabbing in nature, although stiffness has been reported in 33 % of the patients [17]. Commonly, "deep intermittent discomfort during or after activity" is described on initial presentation [22]. Mechanical features such as catching, locking and popping may be featured and are often exacerbated by twisting, turning or pivoting movements. These associated symptoms often imply an intra-articular cause, but it should be noted that extra-articular snapping tendons might also cause similar features albeit in a different location. Byrd has also previously noted that snapping around the hip joint, either due to the iliotibial band or the iliopsoas tendon, is an asymptomatic coincidental finding in 10% of the population [23]. Generally, such symptoms can be attributed to layer 1 or 2 as described above. Deep flexion itself can be uncomfortable [21] and should be noted in the patient's history possibly as difficulty in getting out of a car and/or pain when sitting for prolonged periods. Byrd also states that as degenerative changes progress, pain may become more constant with activities and become less intermittent [21].

As well as the site, onset, character, radiation and severity of pain, one should ask about exacerbating movements or activities. In Clohisy's study [16], pain was activity related in 71 % of the hips, with running (69 %), pivoting (63 %) and walking (58 %) being most problematic. The most effective means of alleviating pain was rest (67 %) and frequent changing of position (52 %). He found that, even in his young cohort of patients (average age 35), many had substantial limitations in function and activity levels. Notably women also complain of posterior hip pain during sexual intercourse [22], and Yen and Kocher note that dyspareunia can be a problem for both men and women [24].

Needless to say, if features from the history are suggestive of lumbar spine pathology, then this should be investigated fully before undertaking hip surgery. That is not to say that the two pathologies cannot coexist. In fact ensuring that the predominant features are the primary problem can be difficult, for example, the pain of trochanteric bursitis can be most obvious, but ensuring that primary intra-articular hip pathology is not missed is crucial. Byrd noted that hip disorders can go undetected for many months before the source of symptoms is discovered. In his study he showed that 60 % of athletes were treated for another pathology for 7 months before it was recognised that the hip joint might be the problem [25]. In 2013, a study was published looking at those athletes who had previously undergone a tenotomy (either adductor or rectus abdominis) for long-standing groin pain [26]. Even in the 75 % of patients satisfied with their treatment, one-third had a clinically positive hip impingement test. Of the 25 % not satisfied, all had signs of hip impingement with almost half requiring arthroscopic surgery prior to participating in the study. This study clearly shows that athletic pubalgia can co-exist or mimic intra-articular hip pathology in a substantial number of cases.

Equally other causes for hip pain with very similar symptoms have been reported. A case study published this year shows that a malunited anterior inferior iliac spine fracture can mimic the symptoms of FAI [27]. Another study by Villar et al. shows that the fat pad present at the anterior head-neck junction of the hip joint might be a source of pain mimicking FAI if indeed the fat pad becomes entrapped [28].

3.3.2 Previous Hip Problems

A detailed history should be undertaken including hip problems as an infant or child. Dysplasia is not uncommon in the adult population and its treatment varies significantly from that of FAI, although the two usually co-exist. Childhood hip history should include previous hip surgery, hip trauma and risk factors for osteonecrosis [9]. Previous Legg-Calve-Perthes disease is also a recognised risk factor for FAI [29]. Another study looking at the role of genetics in FAI concluded that having a sibling with CAM-type lesion or pincer-type lesion leads to a 2.8- or 2.0-fold risk, respectively, of developing symptomatic FAI [30].

Slipped upper femoral epiphysis (SUFE) is another observed association with FAI [31]. In a recent case-control study, the lateral view femoral head-neck index (LVHNI) was measured to look for an SUFE-like deformity. The 96 hips treated for FAI had significantly higher LVHNI than the control group ($p<0.001$) [32]. They concluded that CAM-type cases are probably due to SUFE even if this was subclinical in adolescence. A recent MRI study looked at the slip-like morphology of the hips and concluded that SUFE is likely to be a risk factor for CAM-type FAI [33]. Not all studies agree, however, and another recent prospective study looking at preprofessional football players pre-physeal closure and post-physeal closure indicates that a subclinical SUFE is unlikely to be the cause of FAI [11]. Instead, the head-neck junction flattening seen soon after physeal closure is hypothesised to be due to high-impact loading activities during growth. Regardless of the actual aetiology, a good history should be taken assessing whether SUFE was previously diagnosed or treated or whether the patient had ever had a period of hip pain or limping in keeping with a missed diagnosis of SUFE.

Finally, the patient should be questioned on his/her occupation and the effect of the symptoms on their activities of daily living, recreational activities and their occupation. If the patient is indulging in sporting activities, then it is essential to ascertain the level at which the patient is involved in that particular sport and also the amount of time spent per week in sporting activities. The history is then concluded with a detailed past medical history and social and personal history. In the past medical history, specific focus should be laid upon any evidence of inflammatory arthropathy or hypermobility especially in females.

Having completed a thorough history, the examiner should have a good understanding of the onset of the patient's symptoms, pain profile, lifestyle and exacerbating factors and previous hip pathology. It should be possible to try and understand which layer the primary pathology lies in. A clinical examination may now be undertaken to confirm this.

3.4 Examination

The clinical examination is an important part of formulating a diagnosis. As shown in a cross-sectional study, an abnormal clinical examination correlates with increasing chondro-labral lesions seen on MRI [34]. Additionally, without a strong clinical suspicion of FAI, radiographic findings are insignificant as stated in multiple papers [5, 35, 36]. Byrd also stated that clinical examination has a high sensitivity (98 %) for localising intra-articular hip problems [37].

The general formula of the orthopaedic examination is "look, feel, move…special tests". Examining the young adult hip is no different, but each of these manoeuvres should be performed in five positions:

- Standing
- Seated
- Supine
- Lateral
- Prone

Each position of examination gives the examiner different information, which when amalgamated should guide the examiner as to the site of pathology.

3.4.1 Standing

It is best to start with the patient exposed from the waist down and in a standing position. Inspection will reveal general body habitus, previous scars, malalignment or asymmetry, pelvic tilt and limb length discrepancy.

Gait can also be assessed, again looking for symmetry, quickened stance phase (suggestive of pain on that side), swing through (showing hip ROM), foot progression angle (giving information on developmental torsion of the lower limb bones) and Trendelenburg (for abductor function). If the patient has previously mentioned snapping or popping, it may be pertinent to ask them to reproduce their symptoms now. If the snapping is around the greater trochanter, then it is most likely due to snapping of the tensor fascia lata over the greater trochanter [38], and if the snapping is in the groin, then it is most often due to a labral tear or the iliopsoas tendon snapping in the anterior aspect of the hip joint. Trendelenburg sign can also be elicited using single-leg stance and observation of the patient's pelvis (Fig. 3.1).

Thus far, the examination is similar to that of a standard hip examination. Prior to asking the patient to sit, it may be worth testing the patient's capability to deep squat. A pilot study of 76 patients showed that a positive test for deep squat was if maximal squat recreated the patient's groin pain or they were unable to perform the test due to pain [39]. A painful deep squat was also noted by Byrd as a relevant clinical finding [21]. A biomechanical study also showed that in deep flexion, the pelvis rotates posteriorly in those with CAM-type FAI to compensate for the bony abutment [40]. This study used an electromagnetic tracking device, and it is doubtful whether that level of pelvic posterior tilt could be appreciated by physical examination alone.

At this stage the patient should be assessed for signs of hypermobility as per Beighton's criteria [41].

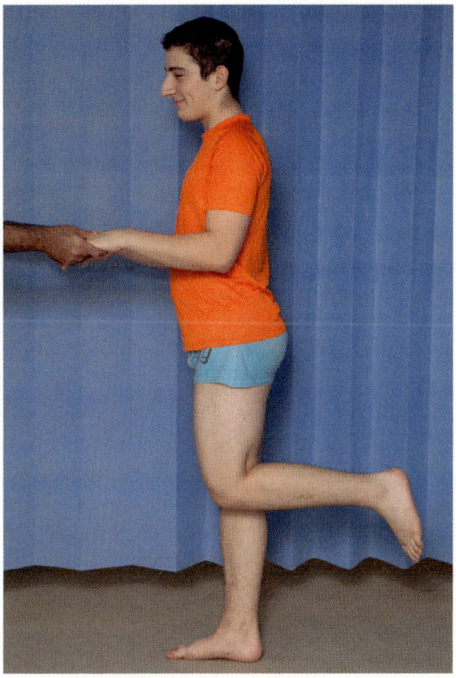

Fig. 3.1 Trendelenburg sign test

3.4.2 Seated

In the seated position, inspection of posture can provide information on the function of the core muscles. Listing to one side – suggestive of a neuromuscular condition – and pelvic tilt can also be appreciated in this posture. Again, asking the patient to stand up before lying down will show how comfortable they are with resisted hip extension. Passive internal and external rotation of both hips may be carried out with the patient in the seated position when the hips are flexed to 90° [42]. Strength of iliopsoas can be assessed in the seated position by asking the patient to raise their knee off the examination couch against resistance.

3.4.3 Supine

The majority of the clinical examination is performed in this position. Inspection forms the initial part of the examination, looking for resting rotation and limb length. An excessively externally rotated limb may point towards laxity of the anterior capsule [43]. For completeness, a brief

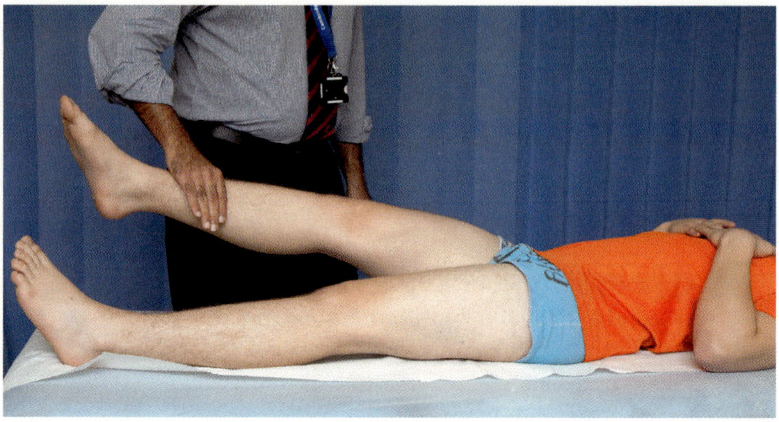

Fig. 3.2 Resisted straight leg raise

examination of myotomes and dermatomes can be undertaken here along with a straight leg raise.

Three studies have looked specifically at the diagnostic accuracy of clinical tests when examining the young adult hip [43–45].

Prior to moving the hip, bony and soft tissue palpation may be undertaken at this stage to look for tenderness and/or swellings. The sequence involves palpating the anterior superior iliac spine and inguinal canal and checking for a cough impulse at the hernia orifices, pubic symphysis, greater trochanter and ischial tuberosity. The adductors, abductors and iliopsoas and rectus are subsequently palpated for tenderness. It must be born in mind that tender soft tissues or tendinous insertion points may be a concomitant finding or an isolated one.

The logroll test involves internal rotation (IR) and external rotation (ER) of the resting extended hip. Although not sensitive, this is a specific test [21] and localises hip joint injuries by rolling the femoral head in relation to the acetabulum and isolating this from surrounding soft tissues. It is also a commonly performed test amongst musculoskeletal clinicians and has good inter-rater reliability [46]. Although thought to be specific, one study found that it so rarely produced a positive result; its usefulness in determining intra-articular pathology was questioned [46]. In another study, its positive predictive value was deemed to be low and there are no data available on its specificity [43].

The resisted straight leg raise (RSLR) test consists of hip flexion against resistance of the examiner with the fully extended leg in 30° or 45° of hip flexion whilst the patient lies supine (Fig. 3.2). In one meta-analysis, this test was described in 8 of 21 studies [43] and was noted to have a specificity of 0.9–1.0. Another study looked specifically at four pain provocation hip manoeuvres performed pre- and post-intra-articular fluoroscopically guided hip injection [47]. It showed that RSLR (also called the Stinchfield manoeuvre) was the most specific test for clinically localising pain arising from an intra-articular source, with a specificity of 0.32.

Thomas' test is a well-known test used predominantly to isolate the hip from any lumbar spine pathology and also to elicit fixed flexion deformity of the hip. This test involves the patient lying supine and being asked to bring both knees towards their chest. They are then asked to extend one leg fully, whilst the examiner places one hand under the patient's lumbar spine to identify lumbar lordosis. It can be used in the assessment of FAI to ensure pelvic tilt is not affecting the range of movement (ROM), but also may in itself be a sign of anterior impingement, as shown in one study used in a recent meta-analysis of diagnostic tests [43].

The range of movement (ROM) of the affected hip compared with the contralateral side is the most commonly performed test [46]. The inter-rater reliability of assessing ROM was studied by blinding nine independent examiners. To aid in their assessment, a goniometer was made available and proved that all examiners were within five degrees of each other when assessing flexion and within seven degrees of each other when assessing rotation [46]. Restricted flexion and restricted internal rotation in flexion are well established to be a common finding in patients with anterior FAI [2, 48, 49]. A cross-sectional study identified those asymptomatic adolescents with <10° IR with hips in 90° flexion [34]. They used age-matched controls, imaged the two groups and found that reduced ROM as described above has a high positive predictive value for anterior FAI. Clohisy et al. also reported that the average flexion in patients with symptomatic FAI is only 97° compared with 101° on the asymptomatic hip [16]. However, a study looking at 40 asymptomatic volunteers showed that the mean maximum midsagittal passive flexion, measured at the time of bony impingement, was 96°±6° [50]. Another study used 3D CT-based kinematic analysis to compare ROM in hips with FAI with anatomically normal hips [51]. They found a statistically significant decrease ($p<0.001$) in the amount of achievable flexion in FAI hips, with 105° compared with 122° in normal hips.

Flexion-adduction-internal rotation test or anterior impingement test is another special test used in 20 of 21 studies included in a meta-analysis of diagnostic hip tests [43]. It is performed with the patient supine. The examiner passively moves the patient's hip into 90° flexion and then applies adduction and finally internal rotation (Fig. 3.3a,b). It classically reproduces the patient's pain due to impingement of the anterior femoral head-neck junction on the acetabular margin. It has been stated that 88 % of patients with FAI will have a positive anterior impingement test. Variations on the flexion-adduction-internal rotation position (FADDIR) have been described, with the patient in the lateral recumbent position rather than supine and with flexion taken to the maximal degree prior to adduction and IR forces being applied. Overall, the FADDIR test has been reviewed in a recent meta-analysis [44] and shown to be one of only 2 of 11 provocation tests found to be eligible to be in their study criteria. This manoeuvre has been deemed to have clinical value in the diagnosis of FAI and anterior labral tears [21, 43, 44, 51]. It should, however, be noted that although the test has a high sensitivity, it has a low specificity, and therefore caution should be used with using this test only for a diagnosis of FAI [5].

Continuing on from the hip in flexion and IR, the hip may now be axially loaded in this position to elicit pain. This has been used to determine anterior labral tears, but in the meta-analysis by Tijssen et al. [43], it has no data available on its specificity and is noted to have a poor positive predictive value (PPV). Only 2 out of 21 studies utilised this test in their evaluation of the young adult hip.

Patrick's test is a commonly used test and describes the hip being taken into a flexed, fully abducted and externally rotated position (FABER), so the leg is in a "figure of four" position (Fig. 3.3c). It is useful in localising sacroiliac joint dysfunction. In a study by Maslowski et al., FABER was deemed to have a sensitivity of 0.82 with a PPV of 0.46 [47]. In this study, the test was considered positive if downward pressure on the abducted, externally rotated knee reproduced the patient's hip pain. Other examiners consider a positive result to be a decrease in ROM compared to the contralateral side; however this is likely to be due to a modification of Patrick's test where the buttock is not off the table. What is considered a positive result varies enormously between the papers using this test to identify either FAI or labral tears.

The Fitzgerald test, as described by Tijssen et al. [43], is when the hip is brought into acute flexion, external rotation and full abduction and is then extended with internal rotation and adduction. The patient lies supine. Extension with abduction and external rotation from the fully flexed, adducted and internally rotated position completes the test. Pain or a click is a positive result. Only one of the papers reviewed by Tijssen et al. [43] utilised this test, which showed a high sensitivity for detecting labral tears or FAI; however not one paper from the more recent meta-analysis used it [44].

A multitude of other positions have been described to try and reproduce hip pain, but few are reproducible and none have been adequately analysed to provide sensitivity, specificity and PPV.

3.4.4 Lateral

In the lateral position the patient can more completely be assessed for peritrochanteric disorders. Focal tenderness around the greater trochanter can point towards trochanteric bursitis and also the possibility of abductor tears or gluteus medius

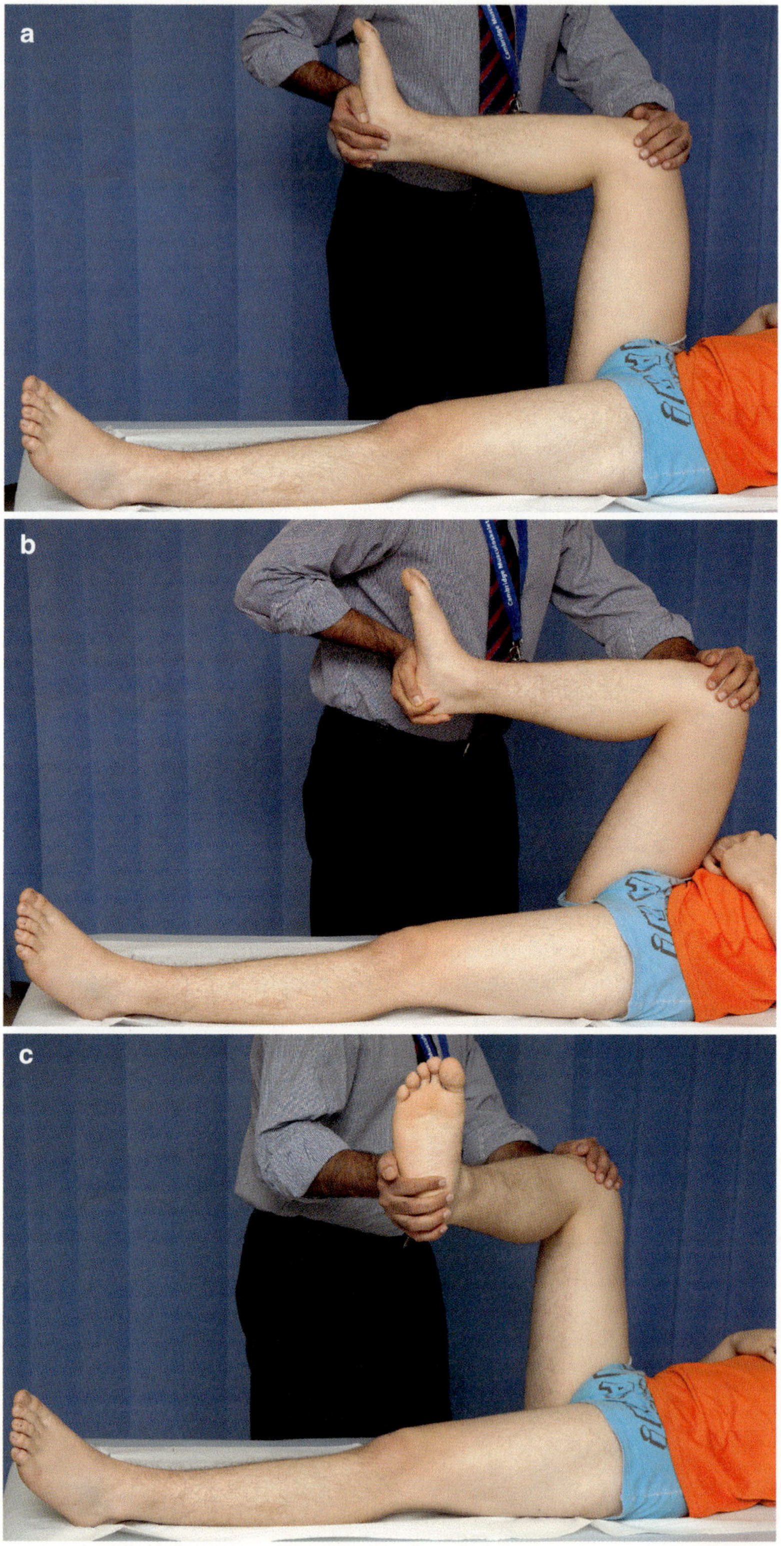

Fig. 3.3 (**a**, **b**) Faddir. (**c**) Faber testing

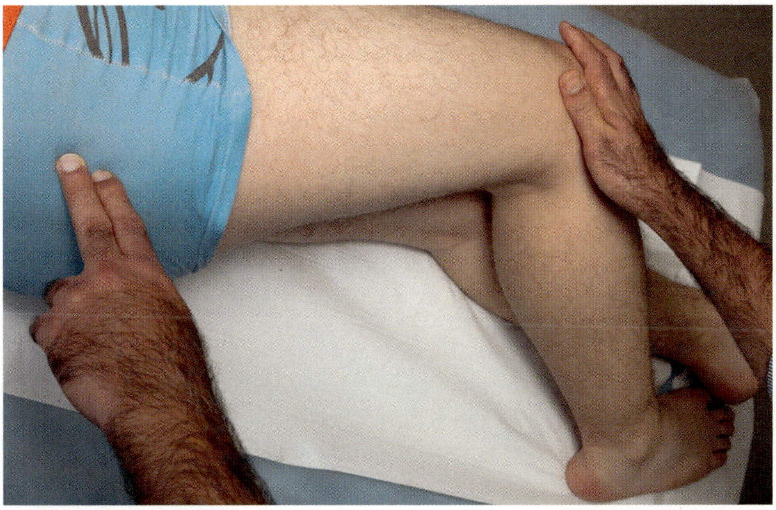

Fig. 3.4 Palpation of it band in lateral position

tendinopathy, which can accompany patients with FAI [52]. In addition, snapping hip may be elicited using Ober's test. This test was originally described in 1935 to elicit a tight IT band [53]. In this test, the patient lies in the lateral position with the affected limb upward. The examiner stands behind the patient and passively flexes the uppermost (affected) knee. The examiner then abducts and fully extends the hip with one hand whilst placing a hand over the trochanteric region. The examiner then passively adducts the extended hip to see if the knee adducts past the midline whilst feeling for a "snap" of the IT band over the greater trochanter (Fig. 3.4). This test is mostly useful for excluding other soft tissue causes of hip pain and is itself not a useful diagnostic test for either FAI or labral pathology.

In this position, asking the patient to abduct their hip against resistance can also test gluteal weakness. The results should be compared to the contralateral side. Some examiners find this easier with the patient supine.

3.4.5 Prone

The prone examination should be performed to evaluate posterior hip pain due to proximal hamstring syndrome, ischial bursitis or sciatic nerve irritation. This position also allows for a clinical assessment of femoral version with the use of the Craig test [54]. This test involves flexing the patient's knee to 90° whilst prone, with the examiner's hand on the greater trochanter. An assessment of the amount of internal rotation necessary to make the greater trochanter maximally prominent can be carried out, which provides an estimation of femoral anteversion or retroversion. Posterior impingement test may also be carried out in this position and involves extension of the affected hip with the examiner taking the hip into full abduction and external rotation. This test can also be carried out in the supine position if the examiner wishes. Pain implies a positive result [55]. This test has not been carried out frequently enough to provide values regarding its sensitivity or specificity.

3.5 Concluding the Examination

As with most other orthopaedic examinations, the history and clinical findings are taken together with plain radiographs in two views. There should be positive findings in all three basic elements in order to support a diagnosis of acetabular, labral or femoral pathology. Radiographic features, such as crossover sign or a high α angle, should not be taken as useful without correlating clinical features as studies have shown a high incidence of such findings in the asymptomatic population [35, 36]. Also, other investigations may be necessary to confirm the diagnosis such as MRI, MR arthrogram or fluoroscopically guided intra-articular injection to confirm that the symptoms are indeed intra-articular in origin.

Of the special tests for the examination of the young adult hip, the anterior impingement test and FABER test have been shown to have high sensitivity and reproducibility for establishing the diagnosis of FAI [43, 44, 57, 58], with a 96 % interobserver reliability of the impingement test.

Sceptics of FAI as a causative factor in osteoarthritis [5] are quick to point out the lack of good evidence to support either the aetiology or specificity of clinical findings, but this paucity of level I studies is likely due to the fact that 60 % of publications regarding FAI have been within the last 3 years [56]. Furthermore, clinical tests in many subspecialties have been found to have low specificity and sensitivity in their own right (e.g. special tests for shoulder examination), but when results are taken together, a reliable diagnosis can be made.

The direction currently taken for FAI is similar to previously described paths of other orthopaedic and sports medicine pathologies, but the time has come to define the condition and support its intervention with well-designed randomised trials [59].

Take-Home Points

1. FAI typically causes a deep groin stabbing or catching pain in the young, but skeletally mature, adult with an active lifestyle.
2. History often includes the intermittent nature of the pain as well as inability to tolerate low-seated positions for prolonged periods. Pain in activities, which require deep flexion and rotation, appears to be the hallmark. Mechanical symptoms like clicking and locking are frequently present.
3. Clinical examination can be variable, but a reduced ROM especially flexion in internal rotation with pain reproduced on flexion-adduction-internal rotation or reduction in flexion alone of the hip is a predominant feature of the condition.
4. Radiological features should not be taken in isolation without a supportive history and clinical examination. MR and CT scans are essential in defining morphology and assessing the articular cartilage and labrum, and intra-articular injections of local anaesthetic are frequently required to confirm diagnosis.
5. As a recently described condition, evidence is mounting daily to support the findings in FAI. The lack of good level I and II studies at present is likely to change as more patients are followed up post-procedure.

Key Evidence Related Sources

1. Hack K, Di Primio G, Rakhra K, Beaule PE. Prevalence of cam-type femoroacetabular impingement morphology in asymptomatic volunteers. J Bone Joint Surg Am. 2010;92(14):2436–44.
2. Clohisy JC, Knaus ER, Hunt DM, Lesher JM, Harris-Hayes M, Prather H. Clinical presentation of patients with symptomatic anterior hip impingement. Clin Orthop Relat Res. 2009;467:638–44.
3. Bedi A, Dolan M, Leunig M, Kelly BT. Static and dynamic mechanical causes of hip pain. Arthroscopy. 2011;27:235–51.
4. Tijssen M, van Cingel R, Willemsen L, de Visser E. Diagnostics of femoroacetabular impingement and labral pathology of the hip: a systematic review of the accuracy and validity of physical tests. Arthroscopy. 2012;28(6):860–71.
5. Reiman MP, Goode AP, Hegedus EJ, Cook CE, Wright AA. Diagnostic accuracy of clinical tests of the hip: a systematic review with meta-analysis. Br J Sports Med. 2013;47(14):893–902.

References

1. Reider B. Round hole, square peg. Am J Sports Med. 2014;42(4):789–92.
2. Ganz R, Parvizi J, Beck M, Leunig M, Notzli H, Siebenrock KA. Fem- oroacetabular impingement: a cause for osteoarthritis of the hip. Clin Orthop Relat Res. 2003;417:112–20.
3. Imam S, Khanduja V. Current concepts in the diagnosis and management of femoroacetabular impingement. Int Orthop. 2011;35(10):1427–35.
4. Khanduja V, Villar RN. Arthroscopic surgery of the hip current concepts and recent advances. J Bone Joint Surg Br. 2006;88(12):1557–66.
5. Rubin DA. Femoroacetabular impingement: fact, fiction, or fantasy? [Review]. AJR Am J Roentgenol. 2013;201(3):526–34.
6. Gosvig KK, Jacobsen S, Sonne-Holm S, Gebuhr P. The prevalence of cam-type deformity of the hip joint: a survey of 4151 subjects of the Copenhagen Osteoarthritis Study. Acta Radiol. 2008;49:436–41.
7. Hack K, Di Primio G, Rakhra K, Beaule PE. Prevalence of cam-type femoroacetabular impingement morphology in asymptomatic volunteers. J Bone Joint Surg Am. 2010;92(14):2436–44.
8. Kang AC, Gooding AJ, Coates MH, Goh TD, Armour P, Rietveld J. Computed tomography assessment of hip joints in asymptomatic individuals in relation to femoroacetabular impingement. Am J Sports Med. 2010;38(6):1160–5.
9. Clohisy JC, Keeney JA, Schoenecker PL. Preliminary assessment and treatment guidelines for hip disorders in young adults. Clin Orthop Relat Res. 2005;441: 168–79.
10. Carsen S, Moroz PJ, Rakhra K, Ward LM, Dunlap H, Hay JA, Willis RB, Beaule PE. The Otto Aufranc Award. On the etiology of the cam deformity: a cross-sectional pediatric MRI study. Clin Orthop Relat Res. 2014;472(2):430–6.
11. Agricola R, Heijboer MP, Ginai AZ, Roels P, Zadpoor AA, Verhaar JA, Weinans H, Waarsing JH. A cam deformity is gradually acquired during skeletal maturation in adolescent and young male soccer players: a prospective study with minimum 2-year follow-up. Am J Sports Med. 2014;42(4):798–806.
12. Yamamura M, Miki H, Nakamura N, Murai M, Yoshikawa H, Sugano N. Open-configuration MRI study of femoro-acetabular impingement. J Orthop Res. 2007;25:1582–8.
13. Takeyama A, Naito M, Shiramizu K, Kiyama T. Prevalence of femoroacetabular impingement in Asian patients with osteoarthritis of the hip. Int Orthop. 2009;33:1229–32.
14. Lahner M, Jahnke NL, Zirke S, Teske W, Vetter G, von Schulze Pellengahr C, Daniilidis K, Hagen M, von Engelhardt LV. The deviation of the mechanical leg axis correlates with an increased hip alpha angle and could be a predictor of femoroacetabular impingement. Int Orthop. 2014;38(1):19–25.
15. Nawabi DH, Bedi A, Tibor LM, Magennis E, Kelly BT. The demographic characteristics of high-level and recreational athletes undergoing hip arthroscopy for femoroacetabular impingement: a sports-specific analysis. [Review]. Arthroscopy. 2014;30(3):398–405.
16. Clohisy JC, Knaus ER, Hunt DM, Lesher JM, Harris-Hayes M, Prather H. Clinical presentation of patients with symptomatic anterior hip impingement. Clin Orthop Relat Res. 2009;467:638–44.
17. Philippon MJ, Maxwell RB, Johnston TL, Schenker M, Briggs KK. Clinical presentation of femoroacetabular impingement. Knee Surg Sports Traumatol Arthrosc. 2007;15:1041–7.
18. Bedi A, Dolan M, Leunig M, Kelly BT. Static and dynamic mechanical causes of hip pain. Arthroscopy. 2011;27:235–51.
19. Byrd JWT. Physical examination. In: Byrd JWT, editor. Operative hip arthroscopy. 2nd ed. New York: Springer; 2005. p. 36–50.
20. Byrd JWT. Evaluation of the hip: history and physical examination. North Am J Sports Phys Ther. 2007;2: 231–40.
21. Byrd JW. Femoroacetabular impingement in athletes: current concepts. Am J Sports Med. 2014;42(3):737–51.
22. Thomas GE, Palmer AJ, Andrade AJ, Pollard TC, Fary C, Singh PJ, O'Donnell J, Glyn-Jones S. Diagnosis and management of femoroacetabular impingement. Br J Gen Pract. 2013;63(612):e513–5.
23. Byrd JWT. Evaluation and management of the snapping iliopsoas tendon. Instr Course Lect. 2006;55: 347–55.
24. Yen YM, Kocher MS. Clinical and radiographic diagnosis of femoroacetabular impingement. J Pediatr Orthop. 2013;33 Suppl 1:S112–20.
25. Byrd JWT, Jones KS. Hip arthroscopy in athletes. Clin Sports Med. 2001;20(4):749–62.
26. Sansone M, Ahlden M, Jonasson P, Thomee R, Falk A, Sward L, Karlsson J. Can hip impingement be mistaken for tendon pain in the groin? A long-term follow-up of tenotomy for groin pain in athletes. Knee Surg Sports Traumatol Arthrosc. 2014;22(4):786–92.
27. Alhaneedi GA, Abdullah AS, Ghouri SI, Abuodeh Y, Al Dosari MM. Avulsion fracture of anterior inferior iliac spine complicated by hypertrophic malunion causing femoroacetabular impingement: case report. Int J Surg Case Rep. 2015;11:117–20.
28. Jayasekera N, Aprato A, Villar RN. Fat pad entrapment at the hip: a new diagnosis. PLoS One. 2014;9(2):e83503 [Electronic Resource].
29. Snow SW, Keret D, Scarangella S, Bowen JR. Anterior impingement of the femoral head: a late phenomenon of Legg- Calvé-Perthes' disease. J Pediatr Orthop. 1993;13(3):286–9.
30. Pollard TCB, Villar RN, Norton MR, Fern ED, Williams MR, Murray DW, Carr AJ. Genetic influences in the aetiology of femoroacetabular impingement: a sibling study. J Bone Joint Surg Br. 2010;92(2):209–16.
31. Fraitzl CR, Käfer W, Nelitz M, Reichel H. Radiological evidence of femoroacetabular impingement in mild

slipped capital femoral epiphysis: a mean follow-up of 14.4 years after pinning in situ. J Bone Joint Surg Br. 2007;89:1592–6.
32. Murgier J, Reina N, Cavaignac E, Espie A, Bayle-Iniguez X, Chiron P. The frequency of sequelae of slipped upper femoral epiphysis in cam-type femoroacetabular impingement. Bone Joint J. 2014;96-B(6):724–9.
33. Albers CE, Steppacher SD, Haefeli PC, Werlen S, Hanke MS, Siebenrock KA, Tannast M. Twelve percent of hips with a primary cam deformity exhibit a slip-like morphology resembling sequelae of slipped capital femoral epiphysis. Clin Orthop Relat Res. 2015;473(4):1212–23.
34. Yuan BJ, Bartelt RB, Levy BA, Bond JR, Trousdale RT, Sierra RJ. Decreased range of motion is associated with structural hip deformity in asymptomatic adolescent athletes. Am J Sports Med. 2013;41(7): 1519–25.
35. Zaltz I, Kelly BT, Hetsroni I, Bedi A. The crossover sign overestimates acetabular retroversion. Clin Orthop Relat Res. 2013;471(8):2463–70.
36. Fukushima K, Uchiyama K, Takahira N, Moriya M, Yamamoto T, Itoman M, Takaso M. Prevalence of radiographic findings of femoroacetabular impingement in the Japanese population. J Orthop Surg. 2014;9:25.
37. Byrd JWT, Jones KS. Diagnostic accuracy of clinical assessment, magnetic resonance imaging, magnetic resonance arthrography, and intra-articular injection in hip arthroscopy patients. Am J Sports Med. 2004;32:1668–74.
38. Ilizaliturri VM, et al. Endoscopic iliotibial band release for external snapping hip syndrome. Arthroscopy. 2006;22(5):505–10.
39. Ayeni O, Chu R, Hetaimish B, Nur L, Simunovic N, Farrokhyar F, Bedi A, Bhandari M. A painful squat test provides limited diagnostic utility in CAM-type femoroacetabular impingement. Knee Surg Sports Traumatol Arthrosc. 2014;22(4):806–11.
40. Van Houcke J, Pattyn C, Vanden Bossche L, Redant C, Maes JW, Audenaert EA. The pelvifemoral rhythm in cam-type femoroacetabular impingement. Clin Biomech. 2014;29(1):63–7.
41. Beighton P, Horan FT. Surgical aspects of the Ehlers-Danlos syndrome a survey of 100 cases. Br J Surg. 1969;56(4):255–9.
42. Martin HD, Kelly BT, Leunig M, Philippon MJ, Clohisy JC, Martin RL, Sekiya JK, Pietrobon R, Mohtadi NG, Sampson TG, Safran MR. The pattern and technique in the clinical evaluation of the adult hip: the common physical examination tests of hip specialists. Arthroscopy. 2010;26(2):161–72.
43. Tijssen M, van Cingel R, Willemsen L, de Visser E. Diagnostics of femoroacetabular impingement and labral pathology of the hip: a systematic review of the accuracy and validity of physical tests. Arthroscopy. 2012;28(6):860–71.
44. Reiman MP, Goode AP, Cook CE, Hölmich P, Thorborg K. Diagnostic accuracy of clinical tests for the diagnosis of hip femoroacetabular impingement/labral tear: a systematic review with meta-analysis. Br J Sports Med. 2015;49:811.
45. Reiman MP, Goode AP, Hegedus EJ, Cook CE, Wright AA. Diagnostic accuracy of clinical tests of the hip: a systematic review with meta-analysis. Br J Sports Med. 2013;47(14):893–902.
46. Ratzlaff C, Simatovic J, Wong H, Li L, Ezzat A, Langford D, Esdaile JM, Kennedy C, Embley P, Caves D, Hopkins T, Cibere J. Reliability of hip examination tests for femoroacetabular impingement. Arthritis Care Res. 2013;65(10):1690–6.
47. Maslowski E, et al. The diagnostic validity of hip provocation maneuvers to detect intra-articular hip pathology. PM R. 2010;2(3):174–81.
48. Beck M, Leunig M, Parvizi J, et al. Anterior femoroacetabular impingement: Part II. Midterm results of surgical treatment. Clin Orthop Relat Res. 2004;418:67–73.
49. Siebenrock KA, Schoeniger R, Ganz R. Anterior femoro-acetabular impingement due to acetabular retroversion. J Bone Joint Surg Am. 2003;85A:278–86.
50. Larkin B, van Holsbeeck M, Koueiter D, Zaltz I. What is the impingement-free range of motion of the asymptomatic hip in young adult males? Clin Orthop Relat Res. 2015;473(4):1284–8.
51. Kubiak-Langer M, Tannast M, Murphy SB, Siebenrock KA, Langlotz F. Range of motion in anterior femoroacetabular impingement. Clin Orthop Relat Res. 2007;458:117–24.
52. Khanduja V, Villar RN. Hip arthroscopy in the elite athlete. ISAKOS. 2013; Abstract presentation.
53. Ober FR. Back strain and sciatica. JAMA. 1935;1(04):1580–1.
54. Skendzel JG, Weber AE, Ross JR, Larson CM, Leunig M, Kelly BT, Bedi A. The approach to the evaluation and surgical treatment of mechanical hip pain in the young patient: AAOS exhibit selection. [Review]. J Bone Joint Surg Am. 2013;95(18):e133.
55. Philippon MJ, Stubbs AJ, Schenker ML, et al. Arthroscopic management of femoroacetabular impingement: osteoplasty technique and literature review. Am J Sports Med. 2007;35(9):1571–80.
56. Haddad FS, Konan S. Femoroacetabular impingement: not just a square peg in a round hole. Bone Joint J. 2013;95-B(10):1297–8.
57. Laborie LB, Lehmann TG, Engesaeter IO, Engesaeter LB, Rosendahl K. Is a positive femoroacetabular impingement test a common finding in healthy young adults? Clin Orthop Relat Res. 2013;471(7):2267–77.
58. Prather H, Harris-Hayes M, Hunt DM, Steger-May K, Mathew V, Clohisy JC. Reliability and agreement of hip range of motion and provocative physical examination tests in asymptomatic volunteers. PM R. 2010;2:888–95.
59. Reiman MP, Thorberg K. Femoroacetabular impingement surgery: are we moving too fast and too far beyond the evidence? Br J Sports Med. 2015;49: 782–4.

4 Evidence for the Utility of Imaging of FAI

Danny Arora and Daniel Burke Whelan

Contents

D. Arora, MD, FRCS(C)
D.B. Whelan, MD, MSc, FRCS(C) (✉)
Department of Orthopaedic Surgery,
University of Toronto Orthopaedic Sports Medicine,
Toronto, ON, Canada
e-mail: WhelanD@smh.ca

Femoroacetabular impingement (FAI) is an increasingly recognized cause and one of many accepted causes for labral pathology of the hip, specifically in the young, active adult [1–3]. There have been a few reports on the correlation of FAI and the development of osteoarthritis of the hip secondary to the bony impingement and subsequent chondrolabral damage [1, 4].

FAI often presents with clinical signs of intra-articular hip irritation secondary to labral pathology in patients with groin pain. During the physical examination, the physician can further characterize the groin pain and perform special hip impingement tests, such as the flexion, adduction, and internal rotation (FADDIR) test, which is the most sensitive physical examination test for FAI [5]. The mainstay of diagnosing FAI as a cause of intra-articular hip pain is, however, via radiographic imaging. All other adjuncts are used to confirm the diagnosis. Some authors believe that adding an intra-articular injection helps with the accuracy of the diagnosis [6, 7]. Nonetheless, the diagnosis of FAI is predominantly radiographic.

Despite recent advances in the diagnostic evaluation, obtaining an accurate diagnosis can prove to be challenging; therefore, it is essential to introduce standardized and consistent radiographic views as well as parameters for their interpretation that can serve as a foundation for accurate diagnosis, disease classification, prognostication, and surgical decision-making [8].

O.R. Ayeni et al. (eds.), *Diagnosis and Management of Femoroacetabular Impingement*,
DOI 10.1007/978-3-319-32000-7_4

4.1 What Radiographic Views to Order?

There are many different views that have been described to help visualize and quantify different parameters of hip alignment, morphology, and position. Clohisy et al. [8] outlined a systematic approach to radiographic evaluation of hip dysfunction in the adult patient. The most commonly employed views are an anteroposterior (AP) pelvic view [9, 10], a 45° or a 90° Dunn view [12, 13], a frog-leg lateral view [11, 14], and a false-profile view [14, 15]. To improve diagnostic accuracy and disease classification, radiographs must be obtained with use of the same standardized imaging protocol. The techniques for obtaining each view will be outlined below.

4.1.1 Anteroposterior Pelvic View

The AP pelvic view is taken with the patient supine with their legs internally rotated 15° (Fig. 4.1). The tube-to-film distance should be 120 cm with the tube oriented perpendicular to the table [8]. The beam is directed vertically to the midportion of the pelvis, specifically midway from the superior border of the symphysis pubis and a line connecting the anterior superior iliac spines (ASISs) [10]. Pelvic tilt, inclination, and rotation should be taken into account when analyzing this view. If the pelvic inclination is adequate, the coccyx should be directly in line with the symphysis pubis. Proper tilt is controlled by maintaining the distance between the tip of the coccyx and the superior border of the symphysis pubis at 1–2 cm [54]. Increased pelvic tilt or rotation has been shown to produce apparent retroversion in an anteverted hip [15]. Siebenrock et al. [15] published sex-specific values for pelvic tilt (referencing the distance between the superior aspect of the symphysis and the sacrococcygeal junction) and noted that an average distance of 32.3 mm was typical in men, as compared with 47.3 mm in women.

Recently, Pullen et al. [16] have shown variability in supine versus weight-bearing anteroposterior (AP) pelvic radiographs in their study of non-arthritic hips in adults with hip pain. They found significant variability with respect to pelvic tilt and radiographic measures of acetabular coverage, where the change from supine to weight bearing typically, but not uniformly, resulted in more posterior pelvic tilt and therefore decreased acetabular coverage. In the supine views, the anterior pelvic tilt was demonstrated, which resulted in increased acetabular coverage. This data brings into question the optimal position when obtaining an AP pelvic radiographic view.

4.1.2 45° or 90° Dunn Views

The 45° or 90° Dunn views are taken with the patient supine (Figs. 4.2 and 4.3). The affected leg is flexed 45° or 90° and abducted 20° with

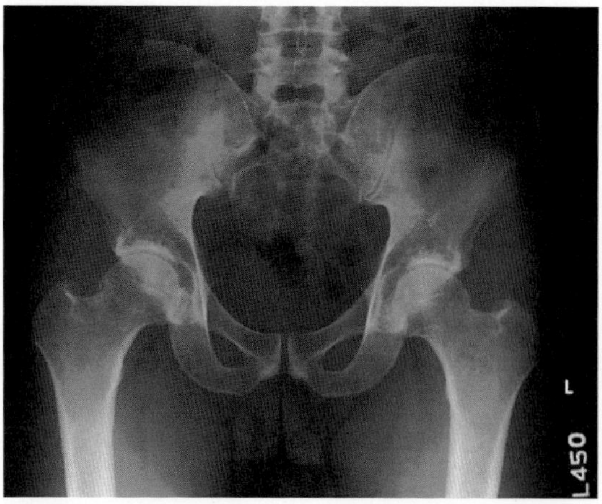

Fig. 4.1 AP view

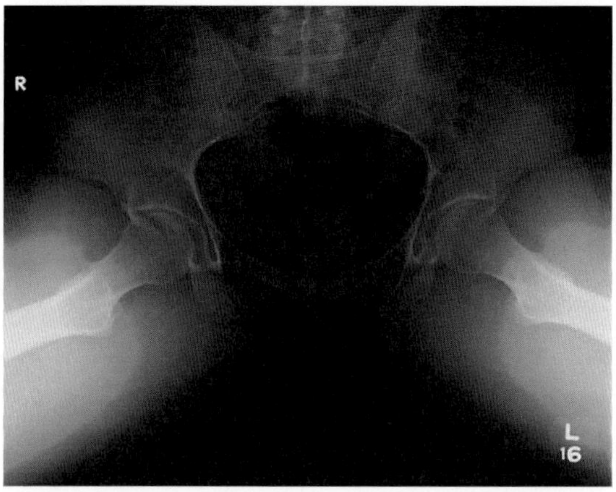

Fig. 4.2 45° Dunn view

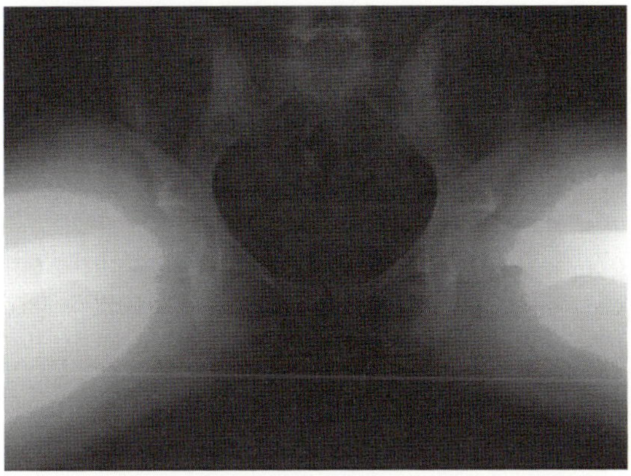

Fig. 4.3 90° Dunn view

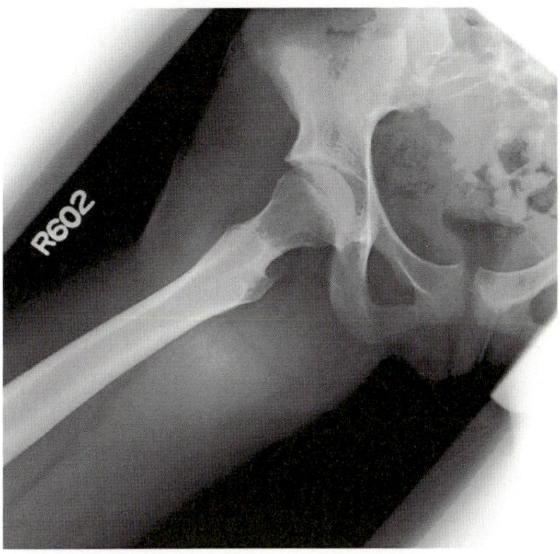

Fig. 4.4 Frog lateral view

neutral rotation. The beam is directed at a midpoint between the symphysis pubis and a line between the anterior superior iliac spines (ASISs). The tube-to-film distance should be about 100 cm perpendicular to the table [8]. The Dunn views are best used to appreciate head sphericity, head-neck junction, and offset [8].

4.1.3 Frog-Leg Lateral View

The frog-leg lateral view is taken with the patient supine, the affected limb flexed 30–40°, and the hip abducted 45° (Fig. 4.4). The heel of the affected limb should lean on the medial aspect of the con-

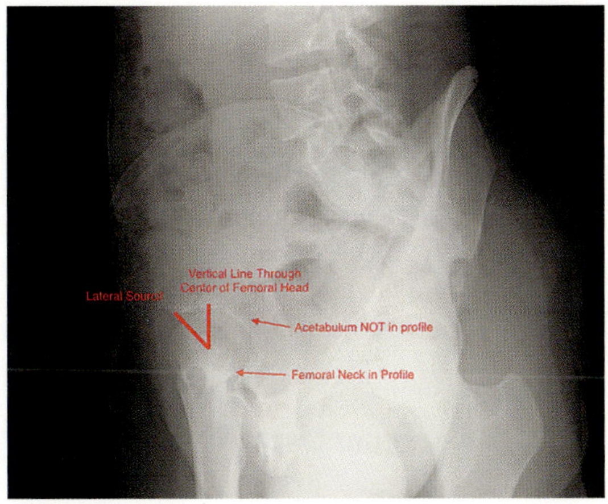

Fig. 4.5 False profile view

tralateral knee. The beam is directed at a midpoint between the symphysis pubis and a line between the anterior superior iliac spines (ASISs) with the tube-to-film distance of 100 cm [8]. The frog-leg lateral view also profiles the femoral head sphericity, the head-neck junction, and the offset, keeping in mind that the greater trochanter can obscure this specific zone. It is important to note that in this view, the lateral of the proximal femur is visualized but it is not a lateral of the acetabulum, hence the use of a false-profile view for better acetabular assessment.

4.1.4 False-Profile View

The false-profile view is taken with the patient in a standing position. The affected limb is against the cassette and the pelvis is rotated 65° in relation to the wall stand (Fig. 4.5). The foot on the affected side should be parallel to the cassette. The beam is centered over the femoral head with a tube-to-film distance of 100 cm [8]. In this view, anterior coverage of the femoral head is appreciated, as well as anterior or posterior acetabular wear [8].

4.2 What Radiographic Parameters to Assess?

Each of the above views provides specific information, from which many radiographic parameters are measured and used to establish the diagnosis of FAI. A systematic approach when interpreting each view should aid the surgeon in his/her decision-making. As a general rule, the AP pelvic view provides the most information on acetabular bony morphology. The Dunn and the frog-leg lateral views highlight the morphological differences of the proximal femur, whereas the false-profile lateral views provide important acetabular morphological information.

4.2.1 Acetabular Depth

The AP pelvic view is most helpful in obtaining a general sense of acetabular bony morphology. One can also get an appreciation of acetabular depth. Using this view, the hips can be classified as being globally "overcovered" or as having a "deep socket" if they fall into two general categories: "coxa profunda," [4] if the floor of the acetabular fossa lies at or medial to the ilioischial line (ICC = 0.02; range = −0.72–0.44) [17], or "protrusio acetabuli," if the femoral head sits medial to the ilioischial line (ICC = 0.10; range = −0.57–0.49) [17]. In a recent study, Nepple et al. [18] found that the presence of coxa profunda can be a normal finding and has a limited role in diagnosing pincer-type FAI. To further assess femoral head overcoverage, they recommend investigating the following parameters: crossover sign, posterior wall sign, lateral center-edge angle, anterior center-edge angle, and acetabular inclination. These parameters help to further distinguish global overcoverage from localized areas where the acetabular margin may be prominent.

4.2.2 Acetabular Inclination

The Tönnis angle [19] is used to calculate the degree of acetabular inclination. It represents the horizontal orientation of the weight-bearing zone of acetabulum on an AP pelvic radiograph. It is measured by calculating the angle between a horizontal line at the most inferior aspect of the sclerotic acetabular sourcil parallel to the teardrop line and a line extending to the most lateral edge of the sclerotic acetabular sourcil [19]. The normal range for this angle measurement is 0–10°. Values of >10° and <0° are considered to have increased and decreased inclination, respectively. In general, acetabuli with increased Tönnis angles are usually dysplastic and may be subject to structural instability, whereas those with decreased Tönnis angles are at risk for pincer-type femoroacetabular impingement [8] (ICC = 0.70; range = 0.48–0.83) [17].

4.2.3 Acetabular Coverage

The lateral center-edge angle (LCEA) of Wiberg [20] is the most common measure of acetabular coverage. Specifically, it is used to quantify the superolateral acetabular coverage and is best measured on an AP pelvic view. It is the angle between a line drawn perpendicular to the transverse axis of the pelvis and a line drawn from the center of the femoral head extending to the most superolateral point of the sclerotic acetabular sourcil (weight-bearing zone). An LCEA of <20° is considered as femoral head undercoverage or, traditionally, acetabular dysplasia [21–24]. An LCEA of >40° is found to be abnormal and defined as acetabular overcoverage or profunda, seen specifically in pincer-type FAI [21, 25–28]. When analyzing the reliability to interpret common radiographic findings of the adult hip by various observers, Carlisle et al. found that the LCEA was the most consistently assessed value between readers, with an excellent intra-rater observer (ICC = 0.88; range = 0.85–0.91) and interobserver value (ICC = 0.64; range = 0.52–0.75) [29].

On a false-profile lateral view, the anterior center-edge angle of Lequesne [14] is calculated to assess the anterior femoral head coverage. It is the angle between a vertical line through the center of the femoral head and a line extending to the most anterior portion of the sclerotic acetabular sourcil. An angle of <20° can be indicative of anterior undercoverage, seen in entities like dysplasia [8] (ICC = 0.38; range = 0.26–0.53) [29].

4.2.4 Acetabular Version

Acetabular version can also be investigated on the AP pelvic view. Acetabular anteversion is appreciated on the AP pelvic view, when the anterior portion of the anterior acetabular rim is superior and medial to the posterior rim and does not cross the posterior portion of the rim before reaching the lateral aspect of the sourcil. Less commonly, acetabular retroversion is seen when the anterior portion of the acetabular rim does cross the posterior portion of the rim before reaching the lateral edge of the sourcil. This has been described as the "crossover" sign [9] (ICC = 0.29; range = −0.25–0.59) [30]. True acetabular retroversion is characterized by global anterior overcoverage with corresponding posterior undercoverage and may result in isolated anterior impingement or combined anterior impingement with posterior coverage deficiency, leading to posterior instability. This morphology is different from focal cranial retroversion, which is characterized by localized overcoverage only at the cranial aspect of the acetabulum with normal posterior wall coverage. The presence of a posterior wall sign (the posterior wall of the acetabulum sits medial to the center of the femoral head [10]) (ICC = 0.20; range = −0.40–0.54) [17] and an ischial spine sign [31] (exaggerated size of the ischial spine projecting medial to the pelvic inlet (ilioischial line)) (ICC = 0.55; range = 0.20–0.74) [17] are radiographic findings on the AP pelvic radiograph that are suggestive of acetabular retroversion [31].

Zaltz et al. [32] demonstrated that acetabular retroversion remains difficult to identify and cannot be definitively diagnosed based on the presence of a "crossover" sign or ischial spine sign alone, even on a well-aligned pelvic radiograph with acceptable tilt and obliquity. Furthermore, Larson et al. [33] demonstrated in their CT-based study that the presence of a crossover sign (53 %; 95 % CI, 46–60 %) and a positive posterior wall sign (20 %; 95 % CI, 15–26 %) were frequent findings in a young asymptomatic cohort and may very well be a normal variant rather than pathologic.

4.2.5 Femoral Head Morphology

On AP and different lateral views, the femoral head sphericity and offset should be assessed. A Mose template [34] is a template, where concentric circles are used as reference for measuring head sphericity. As a rudimentary guideline, if the femoral epiphysis extends beyond the reference circle margin by >2 mm, the head is considered aspherical. If the femoral epiphysis does not extend beyond 2 mm, then the femoral head is considered spherical [34, 35]. Deviations in head sphericity may be observed not only in FAI but also in avascular necrosis (secondary to segmental collapse) and as sequelae of residual childhood hip conditions such as Legg-Calve-Perthes disease and slipped capital femoral epiphysis (SCFE).

4.2.6 Head-Neck Junction and Offset

On all the views, one can appreciate the femoral head-neck junction and analyze the relationship of the radius of curvature anteriorly versus posteriorly. Clohisy et al. [8] described that a head-neck junction is said to have symmetric concavity, when both the anterior and posterior concavities are symmetric. Otherwise, if the concavity at the anterior aspect of the head-neck junction has a radius of curvature that is greater than that at the posterior aspect of the head-neck junction, the hip is considered to have a moderate decrease in terms of head-neck offset. Finally, if the anterior aspect of the head-neck junction has a convexity, as opposed to a concavity, the head-neck junction is considered to have a prominence (i.e., a "CAM" lesion). Peelle et al. [36] calculated the head-neck offset ratio, which can be measured on lateral radiographs. It is the ratio of three lines: the first is through the center of the long axis of the femoral neck; the second is parallel to the first line, through the most anterior aspect of the femoral neck; the third line is parallel to the second line, through the most anterior aspect of the femoral head. The distance between the second and third line is then divided by the diameter of the femoral head, the normal being an absolute value of ≥9 mm or a ratio of the head diameter of ≥0.17 [37]. A ratio of <0.17 indicates that a CAM deformity is likely present [36] (ICC=0.86; range=0.76–0.92) [17].

Nötzli et al. [38] described the alpha angle, which is a measurement of femoral head-neck dysplasia, in other words, CAM-type impingement. Originally it was measured on magnetic resonance imaging (MRI) axial views, but can also be calculated on a lateral-type radiograph. It is calculated by measuring the angle between a line drawn from the center of the femoral head to the point of the anterolateral aspect of the head-neck junction where the contour of the femoral head loses its sphericity and the prominence starts (i.e., where the radius of the femoral head begins to increase beyond the radius found more centrally in the acetabulum where the head is more spherical). Originally, the reported average value was 42° (range=33–48°) in normal controls (ICC=0.84; range=0.72–.091) [17], compared with 74° (range=55–95°) in patients with symptomatic FAI [38–40]. Several threshold values have been suggested to describe when the alpha angle indicates a pathologic entity that may benefit from surgery [8, 41–43]. The most widely accepted threshold angle is 55° and is considered to be indicative of CAM impingement [25] (ICC=0.19; range=−0.43–0.54) [17]. Inter- and intra-rater reliability with FAI parameters measured on conventional radiographs is reportedly poor in several studies [8, 29, 44]. Lohan et al. [45] found in their retrospective analysis of MR arthrographic studies that the alpha angle measurement was statistically of no value in suggesting the presence or absence of CAM-type FAI with an up to 30 % of the mean value intra-observer variability between the first and second alpha angle measurements for each of their 78 subjects (mean sensitivity=39,3 %; mean specificity=70.1 %).

4.2.7 Degree of Osteoarthritis (OA)

The Tönnis OA grade can be used to quantify the degree of OA in the impinging hip and can be seen on all views. The scale ranges from 0, which is normal (no signs of OA), to 1, which is mild (increased sclerosis, slight joint space narrowing, no or slight loss of head sphericity), to 2, which is moderate (small cysts, moderate joint space narrowing, and loss of head sphericity), to 3, which is severe (large cysts, severe joint space narrowing, and loss of head sphericity) [19] (Table 4.1).

Table 4.1 Tönnis osteoarthritis grading scale

Grade	Characteristics
0 – Normal	Absence of signs of OA
1 – Mild	Increased sclerosis Slight joint space narrowing No or slight loss of head sphericity
2 – Moderate	Small cysts Moderate joint space narrowing Loss of head sphericity
3 – Severe	Large cysts Severe joint space narrowing Loss of head sphericity

4.3 Additional Imaging

4.3.1 Fluoroscopy

Intraoperative fluoroscopy has been advocated by many and proven to be extremely valuable. It is an essential tool to direct osteochondroplasty intraoperatively. It aids in quantifying the location, configuration, and extent of the CAM lesion prior to the resection and in judging the adequacy of the resection thereafter. Unfortunately, it is the senior author's experience that the same concept does not often apply for pincer lesions, as a true AP radiograph can be difficult to replicate fluoroscopically on the operating table.

Larson and Wulf [46] described a reproducible and systematic intraoperative fluoroscopic evaluation of the hip for the management of CAM and pincer deformities during arthroscopic treatment of FAI. Ross et al. [47] found that their six (6) intraoperative fluoroscopic views allowed further confirmation of bony resection and helped avoid inadequate resections with resultant impingement. They stated that their intraoperative fluoroscopic views are reproducible and could prove to be critical in the absence of a preoperative 3D CT scan.

Although recent studies have demonstrated that fluoroscopy-assisted hip arthroscopy entails safe levels of radiation [48, 49], some may argue that our fluoroscopic views – in addition to preoperative radiographs and CT – may generate summative doses of radiation that could be avoided. Budd et al. [48] determined on 50 consecutive hip arthroscopies that the mean total fluoroscopy time was 1.10 min and the mean dose area product value was 297.2 $cGycm^2$ and concluded that a low maximum dose of radiation was achieved and supports its safe use. Gaymer et al. [49] calculated the maximal theoretical risk to a fetus on 166 hip arthroscopies in women of childbearing age. They found that the maximal theoretical dose was 2.99 mGy to the fetus, which places the procedure as low-risk category.

4.3.2 Computed Tomography (CT)

The diagnosis and treatment of CAM-type FAI rely on the radiographic identification of deformity and correction of the 3-dimensional (3D) asphericity and loss of offset at the femoral head-neck junction, respectively. Advanced imaging allows for a 3D understanding of the correction needed, but does not necessarily facilitate the intraoperative localization in the absence of navigated instrumentation [38]. Although a considerable ionizing radiation exposure risk is to be taken into account, high-resolution computed tomography (CT) has allowed for increased precision and better definition of osseous morphology of the hip.

4.3.3 Magnetic Resonance Imaging (MRI)

Magnetic resonance imaging (MRI) is the preferred modality for the investigation of intra-articular hip pathology [50]. Several studies have demonstrated evidence of MR findings in acetabular labra in asymptomatic volunteers. In 200 asymptomatic hips, Lecouvert et al. [51] found a homogenous low-intensity signal in 44 % of labra, which seemed to decrease significantly with age. Conversely, they also found that the frequency of heterogeneous signal intensities increased with age in 42 % of cases. Cotten et al. [52] later showed in 52 asymptomatic hips that intralabral regions of intermediate or high signal intensity were found in 57 % of hips. Abe et al. [53] detected similar findings, where in 56 % of their labral segments of 71 asymptomatic hips, homogenous low signal intensity was detected.

Although the demonstration of labral abnormality on an MRI is not essential to the diagnosis of FAI, it does likely indicate the sequelae of the condition in those who have intra-articular hip pain and findings on other imaging modalities consistent with impingement.

Mintz et al. [54] found a sensitivity of 96 %, a specificity of 33 %, and an overall accuracy of 94 % for the detection of labral tears at 1.5 T. Sundberg et al. [55] found comparable results for the detection of labral tears comparing 3-T non-arthrographic with 1.5-T arthrographic techniques. Nowadays, non-contrast MRI is suboptimal for evaluating cartilage and labrum; however, with the development of stronger magnet MRs, this evaluation is improving. It still remains that an MR of the hip, which is a small field of view focus, is more sensitive than an MR of the pelvis, which has a larger field of view.

Magnetic resonance arthrography (MRA) has emerged as the optimal modality for evaluating labrum and cartilage. Compared with hip arthroscopy as gold standard, direct MRA is reported to have sensitivity of 63–100 %, specificity of 44–100 %, and accuracy values of 65–96 % [56–59]. For the detection of labral tears, the interobserver reliability has been reported to be moderate [55–59]. Byrd et al. [5] found in a comparative study between MRI and direct MRA that the clinical assessment can accurately determine the existence of intra-articular hip pathology but is often poor at defining its etiology. An MRI variably shows intra-articular damage with a 42 % false-negative rate. An MRA is found to be more sensitive, but with doubling false-positive interpretation rates. Both studies demonstrated poor reliability in assessing articular damage, but when identified, these studies were 100 % specific. Toomayan et al. [57] found in their sensitivity evaluation of acetabular labral tears in 51 hips that conventional MRI with large field of view was only 8 % sensitive, while conventional MRI with small field of view was only 25 % sensitive in detecting labral tears. In contrast, MRA with small field of view was 92 % sensitive in detecting acetabular labral tears. This study highlighted the importance of both small field of view and intra-articular contrast material in the accurate diagnosis of labral abnormalities.

4.4 The Interobserver and Intra-observer Reliability

The interobserver and intra-observer reliabilities of radiographic hip measurements are quite variable in the literature. Clohisy et al. [60] reported poor agreement among 6 hip surgeons. More recent studies have shown more promising results [9, 61]. Mast et al. [61] found an interobserver reliability varying between 0.45 and 0.97 and an intra-observer reliability ranging from 0.55 to 1.0 for common hip measurements. Ayeni et al. [17] recently showed a low reliability between radiologists and orthopedic surgeons in diagnosing FAI pathology on radiographs using standard hip measurements. There was however, a higher interobserver reliability within each specialty ranging from fair to good (ICC = 0.59–0.74 and ICC = 0.70–0.72, respectively). Orthopedic surgeons had the highest interobserver reliability when identifying pistol grip deformities (ICC = 0.81) or abnormal alpha angles (ICC = 0.81). These large ranges of interobserver results have pushed for an increased use in advanced imaging with computed tomography (CT) scans and added 3-dimensional (3D) reconstructive views, as well as magnetic resonance imaging (MRI).

4.5 Cost-Utility of Imaging for FAI

The use of imaging is essential in the operative treatment of FAI; however, time and cost of all the diagnostic testing have not been extensively investigated. Kahlenberg et al. [62] studied the average number of health-care providers seen, as well as the average number of diagnostic imaging tests ordered on 78 patients, and then calculated the average total amount spent per patient prior to diagnosis of FAI. They calculated the minimum cost of diagnosis (AP pelvic and lateral hip radiographs and an MRI, including a visit to an orthopedic surgeon) to be US$ 690.62 and the average total amount spent per patient in their cohort US$ 2,456.97, which amounts to US$ 1,766.35 higher than the calculated minimum cost. They also found that the average duration between onset of symptoms and diagnosis of a labral tear was 32.0 months. It is important for all health-care professionals to recognize and appropriately manage or refer these patients, not only to lower cost but more so to avoid the loss of economic productivity on a societal level.

Conclusion

The association between the radiographic findings of femoroacetabular impingement, the correction thereof, and the impact of diagnosis and treatment of the condition on long-term function and prognosis still remain uncertain. Further investigations are required to better define and quantify the diagnostic criteria and thresholds for intervention.

Take-Home Points

1. FAI remains predominantly a radiographic diagnosis in symptomatic patients, which justifies the need for imaging in order to appropriately assess the severity and location of lesions associated with FAI.
2. The essential radiograph for the diagnosis of pincer-type FAI is the AP pelvis on which the center-edge angle and cross-over sign can be assessed. Both these parameters have exhibited moderate intra- and interobserver reliability, as well as acceptable sensitivity and specificity.
3. A radiograph for the diagnosis of CAM-type FAI is the Dunn lateral view, on which the alpha angle can be assessed. This parameter has demonstrated good intra-and interobserver

reliability, as well as good sensitivity and specificity.

4. Computed tomography (CT) (especially 3D reconstructions) can help further define bony morphology around the hip and better characterize and confirm FAI subtypes and surgical indications. Concerns regarding increased radiation exposure with CT have led to improvements in the technique.
5. Magnetic resonance imaging (MRI) (with or without arthrography, MRA) is a useful adjunct to plain radiographs and CT in assessing the sequelae of FAI, specifically edema patterns, cartilage, and labral lesions.

Key Evidence Related Sources

1. Byrd JW, Jones KS. Diagnostic accuracy of clinical assessment, magnetic resonance imaging, magnetic resonance arthrography, and intra-articular injection in hip arthroscopy patients. Am J Sports Med. 2004;32(7):1668–74.
2. Clohisy JC, Carlisle JC, Beaule PE, et al. A systematic approach to the plain radiographic evaluation of the young adult hip. J Bone Joint Surg Am. 2008;90 Suppl 4:47–66.
3. Ayeni RO, Chan K, Whelan DB, Gandhi R, Williams D, Harish S, Choudur H, Chiavaras MM, Karlsson J, Bhandari M. Diagnosing femoroacetabular impingement from plain radiographs: do radiologists and orthopaedic surgeons differ? Orthop J Sports Med. 2014;2:7.
4. Tannast M, Siebenrock KA, Anderson SE. Femoroacetabular impingement: radiographic diagnosis – what the radiologist should know. AJR Am J Roentgenol. 2007;188(6):1540–52.
5. Zaltz I, Kelly BT, Hetsroni I, Bedi A. The crossover sign overestimates acetabular retroversion. Clin Orthop Relat Res. 2013;471(8):2463–70.

References

1. Ganz R, Parvizi J, Beck M, Leunig M, Notzli H, Siebenrock KA. Femoroacetabular impingement: a cause for osteoarthritis of the hip. Clin Orthop Relat Res. 2003;417:112–20.
2. McCarthy JC, Noble PC, Schuck MR, Wright J, Lee J. The Otto E. Aufranc Award: the role of labral lesions to development of early degenerative hip disease. Clin Orthop Relat Res. 2001;393:25–37.
3. Philippon MJ, Briggs KK, Yen YM, Kuppersmith DA. Outcomes following hip arthroscopy for femoroacetabular impingement with associated chondrolabral dysfunction: minimum two-year follow-up. J Bone Joint Surg Br. 2009;91(1):16–23.
4. Beck M, Kalhor M, Leunig M, Ganz R. Hip morphology influences the pattern of damage to the acetabular cartilage: femoroacetabular impingement as a cause of early osteoarthritis of the hip. J Bone Joint Surg Br. 2005;87(7):1012–8.
5. Byrd JW. Physical examination. In: Operative hip arthroscopy. New York: Springer; 2005. p. 36–50.
6. Parvizi J, Leunig M, Ganz R. Femoroacetabular impingement. J Am Acad Orthop Surg. 2007;15(9):561–70.
7. Byrd JW, Jones KS. Diagnostic accuracy of clinical assessment, magnetic resonance imaging, magnetic resonance arthrography, and intra-articular injection in hip arthroscopy patients. Am J Sports Med. 2004;32(7):1668–74.
8. Clohisy JC, Carlisle JC, Beaule PE, et al. A systematic approach to the plain radiographic evaluation of the young adult hip. J Bone Joint Surg Am. 2008;90 Suppl 4:47–66.
9. Jamali AA, Mladenov K, Meyer DC, et al. Anteroposterior pelvic radiographs to assess acetabular retroversion: high validity of the "cross-over-sign.". J Orthop Res. 2007;25:758–65.
10. Reynolds D, Lucas J, Klaue K. Retroversion of the acetabulum: a cause of hip pain. J Bone Joint Surg Br. 1999;81(2):281–8.
11. Dunn DM. Anteversion of the neck of the femur; a method of measurement. J Bone Joint Surg Br. 1952;34:181–6.
12. Meyer DC, Beck M, Ellis T, Ganz R, Leunig M. Comparison of six radiographic projections to assess femoral head/neck asphericity. Clin Orthop Relat Res. 2006;445:181–5.
13. Clohisy JC, Nunley RM, Otto RJ, Schoenecker PL. The frog-leg lateral radiograph accurately visualized hip cam impingement abnormalities. Clin Orthop Relat Res. 2007;462:115–21.
14. Lequesne M, de Seze. False profile of the pelvis. A new radiographic incidence for the study of the hip. Its use in dysplasias and different coxopathies. Rev Rhum Mal Osteoartic. 1961;28:643–52. French.
15. Siebenrock KA, Kalbermatten DF, Ganz R. Effect of pelvic tilt on acetabular retroversion: a study of pelves from cadavers. Clin Orthop Relat Res. 2003;407:241–8.

16. Pullen W, Henebry A, Gaskill T. Variability of acetabular coverage between supine and weight-bearing pelvic radiographs. Am J Sports Med. 2014;42(11):2643.
17. Ayeni RO, Chan K, Whelan DB, Gandhi R, Williams D, Harish S, Choudur H, Chiavaras MM, Karlsson J, Bhandari M. Diagnosing femoroacetabular impingement from plain radiographs: do radiologists and orthopaedic surgeons differ? Orthop J Sports Med. 2014;2:7.
18. Nepple JJ, Lehmann CL, Ross JR, Schoenecker PL, Clohisy JC. Coxa profunda is not a radiographic parameter for diagnosing pincer-type femoroacetabular impingement. J Bone Joint Surg Am. 2013;95(5):417–23.
19. Tönnis D. Congenital dysplasia and dislocation of the Hip in children and adults. Heidelberg/Germany: Springer; 1987.
20. Wiberg G. Studies on dysplastic acetabula and congenital subluxation of the hip: with special reference to the complication of osteoarthritis. Acta Chir Scand Suppl. 1939;58:7–38.
21. Monazzam S, Bomar JD, Cidambi K, Kruk P, Hosalkar H. Lateral center-edge angle on conventional radiography and computed tomography. Clin Orthop Relat Res. 2013;471(7):2233–7.
22. Murphy SB, Ganz R, Muller ME. The prognosis in untreated dysplasia of the hip: a study of radiographic factors that predict the outcome. J Bone Joint Surg Am. 1995;77:985–9.
23. Murphy SB, Kijewski PK, Millis MB, Harless A. Acetabular dysplasia in the adolescent and young adult. Clin Orthop Relat Res. 1990;261:214–23.
24. Werner CM, Ramseier LE, Ruckstuhl T, Stromberg J, Copeland CE, Turen CH, Rufibach K, Bouaicha S. Normal values of Wiberg's lateral center-edge angle and Lequesne's acetabular index: a coxometric update. Skeletal Radiol. 2012;41:1273–8.
25. Tannast M, Siebenrock KA, Anderson SE. Femoroacetabular impingement: radiographic diagnosis – what the radiologist should know. AJR Am J Roentgenol. 2007;188(6):1540–52.
26. Colvin AC, Koehler SM, Bird J. Can the change in center-edge angle during pincer trimming be reliably predicted? Clin Orthop Relat Res. 2011;469:1071–4.
27. Kutty S, Schneider P, Faris P, Kiefer G, Frizzell B, Park R, Powell JN. Reliability and predictability of the centre-edge angle in the assessment of pincer femoroacetabular impingement. Int Orthop. 2012;36:505–10.
28. Philippon MJ, Wolff AB, Briggs KK, Zehms CT, Kuppersmith DA. Acetabular rim reduction for the treatment of Femoroacetabular impingement correlates with preoperative and postoperative center-edge angle. Arthroscopy. 2010;26:757–61.
29. Carlisle JC, Zebala LP, Shia DS, et al. Reliability of various observers in determining common radiographic parameters of adult hip structural anatomy. Iowa Orthop J. 2011;31:52–8.
30. Anderson LA, Peters CL, Park BB, Stoddard GJ, Erickson JA, Crim JR. Acetabular cartilage delamination in femoroacetabular impingement: risk factors and magnetic resonance imaging diagnosis. J Bone Joint Surg Am. 2009;91(2):305–13.
31. Kalberer F, Sierra RJ, Madan SS, Ganz R, Leunig M. Ischial spine projection into the pelvis: a new sign for acetabular retroversion. Clin Orthop Relat Res. 2008;466(3):677–83.
32. Zaltz I, Kelly BT, Hetsroni I, Bedi A. The cross-over sign overestimates acetabular retroversion. Clin Orthop Relat Res. 2013;471(8):2463–70.
33. Larson CM, Moreau-Gaudry A, Kelly BT, Byrd JW, Tonetti J, Lavallee S, Chabanas L, Barrier G, Bedi A. Are normal hips being labeled as pathologic? A CT-based method for defining normal acetabular coverage. Clin Orthop Relat Res. 2015;473(4):1247–54.
34. Mose K. Methods of measuring in Legg-Calvé-Perthes disease with special regard to the prognosis. Clin Orthop Relat Res. 1980;150:103–9.
35. Weinstein SL. Legg-Calvé-Perthes disease. In: Morrissy RT, editor. Lovell and Winter's pediatric orthopaedics. 3rd ed. Philadelphia: Lippincott; 1990. p. 867–8.
36. Peelle MW, Della Rocca GJ, Maloney WJ, Curry MC, Clohisy JC. Acetabular and femoral radiographic abnormalities associated with labral tears. Clin Orthop Relat Res. 2005;441:327–33.
37. Maheshwari AV, Malik A, Dorr LD. Impingement of the native hip joint. J Bone Joint Surg Am. 2007;89:2508–18.
38. Notzli HP, Wyss TF, Stoecklin CH, Schmid MR, Treiber K, Hodler J. The contour of the femoral head-neck junction as a predictor for the risk of anterior impingement. J Bone Joint Surg Br. 2002;84(4):556–60.
39. Beaule PE, Zaragoza E, Motamedi K, Copelan N, Dorey FJ. Three-dimensional computed tomography of the hip in the assessment of femoroacetabular impingement. J Orthop Res. 2005;23(6):1286–92.
40. Johnston TL, Schenker ML, Briggs KK, Philippon MJ. Relationship between offset angle alpha and hip chondral injury in femoroacetabular impingement. Arthroscopy. 2008;24(6):669–75.
41. Allen D, Beaule PE, Ramadan O, Doucette S. Prevalence of associated deformities and hip pain in patients with cam-type femoroacetabular impingement. J Bone Joint Surg Br. 2009;91(5):589–94.
42. Gosvig KK, Jacobsen S, Palm H, Sonne-Holm S, Magnusson E. A new radiological index for assessing asphericity of the femoral head in cam impingement. J Bone Joint Surg Br. 2007;89(10):1309–16.
43. Tannast M, Siebenrock KA. Conventional radiographs to assess femoroacetabular impingement. Instr Course Lect. 2009;58:203–12.
44. Nouh MR, Schweitzer ME, Rybak L, Cohen J. Femoroacetabular impingement: can the alpha angle be estimated? AJR Am J Roentgenol. 2008;190(5):1260–2.
45. Lohan DG, Seeger LL, Motamedi K, Hame S, Sayre J. Cam-type FAI: is the alpha angle the best

MR arthrography has to offer? Skeletal Radiol. 2010;39(2):203–4.
46. Larson CM, Wulf CA. Intraoperative fluoroscopy for evaluation of bony resection during arthroscopic management of femoroacetabular impingement in the supine position. Arthroscopy. 2009;25(10): 1183–92.
47. Ross JR, Bedi A, Stone RM, Sibilsky Enselman E, Leunig M, Kelly BT, Larson CM. Intraoperative fluoroscopic imaging to treat cam deformities: correlation with 3-dimensional computed tomography. Am J Sports Med. 2014;42(6):1370–6.
48. Budd H, Patchava A, Khanduja V. Establishing the radiation risk from fluoroscopic-assisted arthroscopic surgery of the hip. Int Orthop. 2012;36(9):1803–6.
49. Gaymer CE, Achten J, Auckett R, Cooper L, Griffin D. Fluoroscopic radiation exposure during hip arthroscopy. Arthroscopy. 2013;29(5):870–3.
50. Beaule PE, Zaragoza E, Copelan N. Magnetic resonance imaging with gadolinium arthrography to assess acetabular cartilage delamination: a report of four cases. J Bone Joint Surg Am. 2004;86-A:2294–8.
51. Lecouvet FE, VandeBerg BC, Melghem J, et al. MR imaging of the acetabular labrum: variations in 200 asymptomatic hips. Am J Roentgenol. 1996;167:1025–8.
52. Cotten A, Boutry N, Demondion X, et al. Acetabular labrum: MRI in asymptomatic volunteers. J Comput Assist Tomogr. 1998;22:1–7.q.
53. Abe I, Harada Y, Oinuma K, Kamikawa K, Kitahara H, Morita F, Moriya H. Acetabular labrum: abnormal findings at MR imaging in asymptomatic hips. Radiology. 2000;216(2):576–81.
54. Mintz DN, Hooper T, Connell D, et al. Magnetic resonance imaging of the hip: detection of labral and chondral abnormalities using noncontrast imaging. Arthroscopy. 2005;21:385–93.
55. Sundberg TP, Toomayan GA, Major NM. Evaluation of the acetabular labrum at 3.0-T MR imaging compared with 1.5-T MR arthrography: preliminary experience. Radiology. 2006;238:706–11.
56. Chan YS, Lien LC, Hsu HL, Wan YL, Lee MS, Hsu KY, Shih CH. Evaluating hip labral tears using magnetic resonance arthrography: a prospective study comparing hip arthroscopy and magnetic resonance arthrography diagnosis. Arthroscopy. 2005;21:1250.
57. Toomayan GA, Holman WR, Major NM, Kozlowicz SM, Vail TP. Sensitivity of MR arthrography in the evaluation of acetabular labral tears. AJR Am J Roentgenol. 2006;186:449–53.
58. Freedman BA, Potter BK, Dinauer PA, Giuliani JR, Kuklo TR, Murphy KP. Prognostic value of magnetic resonance arthrography for Czerny stage II and III acetabular labral tears. Arthroscopy. 2006;22:742–7.
59. Keeney JA, Peelle MW, Jackson J, et al. Magnetic resonance arthrography versus arthroscopy in the evaluation of articular hip pathology. Clin Orthop Relat Res. 2004;(429):163–9.
60. Clohisy JC, Carlisle JC, Trousdale R, et al. Radiographic evaluation of the hip has limited reliability. Clin Orthop Relat Res. 2009;467(3): 666–75.
61. Mast NH, Impellizzeri F, Keller S, Leunig M. Reliability and agreement of measures used in radiographic evaluation of the adult hip. Clin Orthop Relat Res. 2011;469:188–99.
62. Kahlenberg CA, Han B, Patel RM, Deshmane PP, Terry MA. Time and cost of diagnosis for symptomatic femoracetabular impingement. Orthop J Sports Med. 2014;2(3):2325967114523916.

Pathophysiology of Femoroacetabular Impingement (FAI)

5

Gavin C.A. Wood, Hamad Alshahrani, and Michel Taylor

Contents

G.C.A. Wood, MBChB, FRCS Edin, FRCSC (✉)
M. Taylor, MD
Clinical Fellow, Queens University,
Kingston, ON, Canada
e-mail: orthowood@gmail.com

H. Alshahrani, SBOS, MD
Clinical Fellow, Division of Orthopedic Surgery,
Queens University, Kingston, ON, Canada

Department of Orthopaedic Surgery,
King Fahad Specialist Hospital, Queens University,
Dammam, Saudi Arabia

5.1 Introduction

The abnormal functional changes and pathology that are associated with FAI of the hip must be considered in a continuum as with any other disease process. The understanding of a pathological condition leads to appropriate intervention and treatment to prevent further pathology or damage and opens the doors for prevention. In this chapter we will examine the evidence surrounding the pathophysiology of FAI and where more research is needed. Only by appreciating the etiology of this condition can we hope to be even more effective in treating it and its sequelae.

5.2 Background

Ganz was formally recognized for introducing the concept of FAI with CAM, pincer, and combined models of abnormal hip morphology [1–3]. Goodman, Murray, Solomon, and Harris [4–8]

O.R. Ayeni et al. (eds.), *Diagnosis and Management of Femoroacetabular Impingement*,
DOI 10.1007/978-3-319-32000-7_5

had all previously described morphologic abnormalities leading to osteoarthritis before Ganz and Stulberg described that abnormal morphology of the hip leads to hip pain and subsequent arthritis in children with Legg-Calve-Perthes (LCP) disease [9]. The abnormal morphologies of the hip joint seen in LCP, developmental dysplasia of hip (DDH), and slipped upper femoral epiphyses (SUFE, also known as slipped capital femoral epiphysis, or SCFE) have been recognized as causing hip problems in the young and leading to secondary osteoarthritis in early adulthood [7, 9–12]. Surgical corrections of these deformities through various types of osteotomies have been shown to improve clinical symptoms and function and delay the onset of hip osteoarthritis. High joint reaction forces combined with an incongruent hip joint and abnormal biomechanics lead to pain, restricted range of motion, and accelerated cartilage damage [4, 5, 13]. The pathophysiological underlining DDH is currently best understood where prevention or early recognition can provide the best outcome when treatment is applied [14].

This leaves certain questions: Why do certain patients develop hip pain at an early age with no obvious hip joint abnormality or previous injury?

Similarly why do certain patients develop osteoarthritis of the hip in early adulthood as opposed to in their more senior years?

The description of FAI by Ganz recognized the more subtle abnormal morphology of the hip leading to impingement and specific patterns of soft tissue damage [3]. The various anatomical morphologies of hip shapes could be considered along a spectrum, with DDH being at one end of that spectrum and CAM pincer-type impingement at the other with the most biomechanically efficient hip being somewhere in the middle. Although the etiology of hip osteoarthritis is multifactorial [7, 11, 12] and FAI is only one factor, by understanding its pathophysiology, we can potentially monitor at risk patients. Subsequently surgical correction of the deformity at an earlier stage in the pathological process could potentially delay the onset of degenerative changes.

5.3 Definition of FAI

FAI is a clinical diagnosis with distinct radiographical features where an underlining pathologic mechanical deformity combined with repetitive movements such as flexion and/or rotation causes hip pain and restricted hip motion (145). It occurs due to repetitive impingement or collision of soft tissues between the proximal femur and acetabular rim (2,13,68). It can occur during normal movements of the hip when large structural abnormalities are present or in normal-shaped hip joints when engaging in supraphysiologic movements. Those patients without abnormal morphology but with some laxity or excessive demands of the hip particularly in high impact with flexion and internal rotation may lead to symptoms of FAI [15, 16]. Once soft intra-articular damage is present, it becomes a pathological entity and pain ensues.

Since the description of FAI and treatment, results have shown improved pain and hip function with surgical intervention [17], (124-130), and further analysis has revealed different patterns of soft tissue damage. CAM impingement is due to a lack of offset at the femoral head-neck junction. Femoral head asphericity combined with a normal acetabulum produces a pattern of damage at the anterosuperior acetabulum usually centered at the 1 o'clock position (Fig. 5.1), with separation at the chondrolabral junction and subsequent delamination of cartilage from the under-

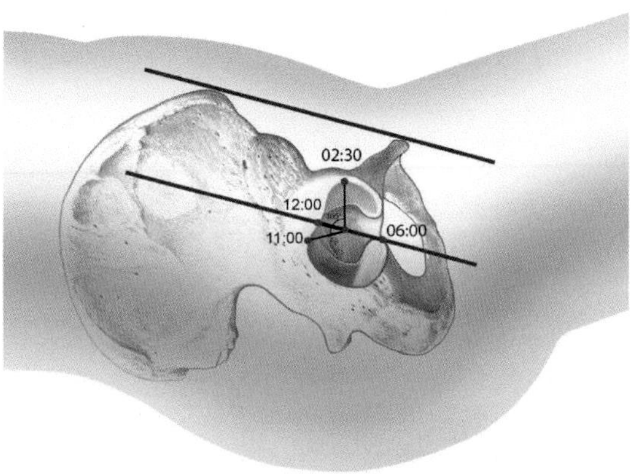

Fig. 5.1 Clock face representation of acetabulum

lying bony acetabulum. This occurs due to the compression and shear force of the CAM sliding into the anterosuperior acetabulum during flexion (71). The labrum and cartilage are stretched and pushed outward and inward, respectively, causing separation and an undersurface tear of the labrum with delamination, however with relative sparing of labral integrity (13,72,21,79,80). Posteroinferior labral damage and ossification are due to a contra coup lesion and stem from impingement and leverage causing posterior wall damage (2,28,81). Johnston et al. (15) studied the relationship between the size of CAM-type lesions, as quantified by the radiographic alpha angle (12), and the presence of cartilage damage, labral injury, and changes in range of motion. A higher alpha angle was associated with chondral defects of the acetabular rim and full-thickness delamination of the acetabular cartilage. In addition, patients with detachment of the base of the labrum had a higher mean alpha angle of greater than 57°.

Pincer-type deformity is due to a deep socket and overcoverage of the femoral head by the acetabular rim. During flexion, the labrum is compressed between the femoral neck and acetabular rim. The zone of maximal damage seen is between 11 and 1 o'clock with a circumferential narrow band of injury to the labrum (Fig. 5.1). A focal rim lesion, or cephalad retroversion of the acetabulum, is a distinct dynamic mechanical cause of FAI that is more common in females (2,3,74), which leads to repetitive contact stresses between a normal femoral neck and an abnormal area of focal acetabular overcoverage.

These pathological findings occur secondary to relative or absolute retroversion of the acetabulum anterosuperiorly and more normal anteversion inferomedially. Focal rim lesions (Fig. 5.2) need to be distinguished from global overcoverage and impingement, which can result from coxa profunda, coxa protrusio, true acetabular retroversion (20,75,76), or even iatrogenic overcorrection after periacetabular osteotomy (77,78).

In contrast to CAM-induced injury, pincer impingement lesions typically induce primary, intra-substance labral injury and are often less reparable. Heterotopic bone ossification can occur due to microtrauma at the base of the labrum, which induces bone growth; the cartilage damage depth is much less than that which is seen with the CAM lesion and posteroinferior acetabular cartilage lesion often seen as cartilage fibrillation. In later stages, the bone formation cannot be distinguished from the native bone, and the labrum may be absent on imaging (80,82). This overgrowth of rim fractures can exacerbate pincer impingement. Overall, a focal rim lesion results in relatively limited chondral damage as compared with the deep chondral injury and delamination that are associated with CAM-type impingement (2,13,21). A mixed type of impingement will give variations on the above patterns [16].

Sufficient evidence has established that impingement occurs with these typical and predictable patterns of injury. That the more severe hip deformities lead to greater joint damage [18]. That not addressing the morphological abnormality and only treating the soft tissue problem has shown inferior results [19–40]. These observations have established the importance of abnormal morphology as the cause and effect of the pathophysiology of FAI.

5.4 What Predisposes to FAI?

FAI is a clinical diagnosis related to abnormal morphology of the hip and most often is of an insidious nature. Patients without these morphological abnormalities are less likely to develop symptoms unless an injury has occurred. Approximately 90 % of patients with labral pathology have underlying structural abnormalities in the morphology of the hip [41–44]. The nature of the development of these abnormal bony morphologies is currently not fully understood. Knowing and understanding the pathophysiology is an integral part in the successful treatment, and while the exact mechanism of primary FAI is still under debate, there are several recognized primary causes.

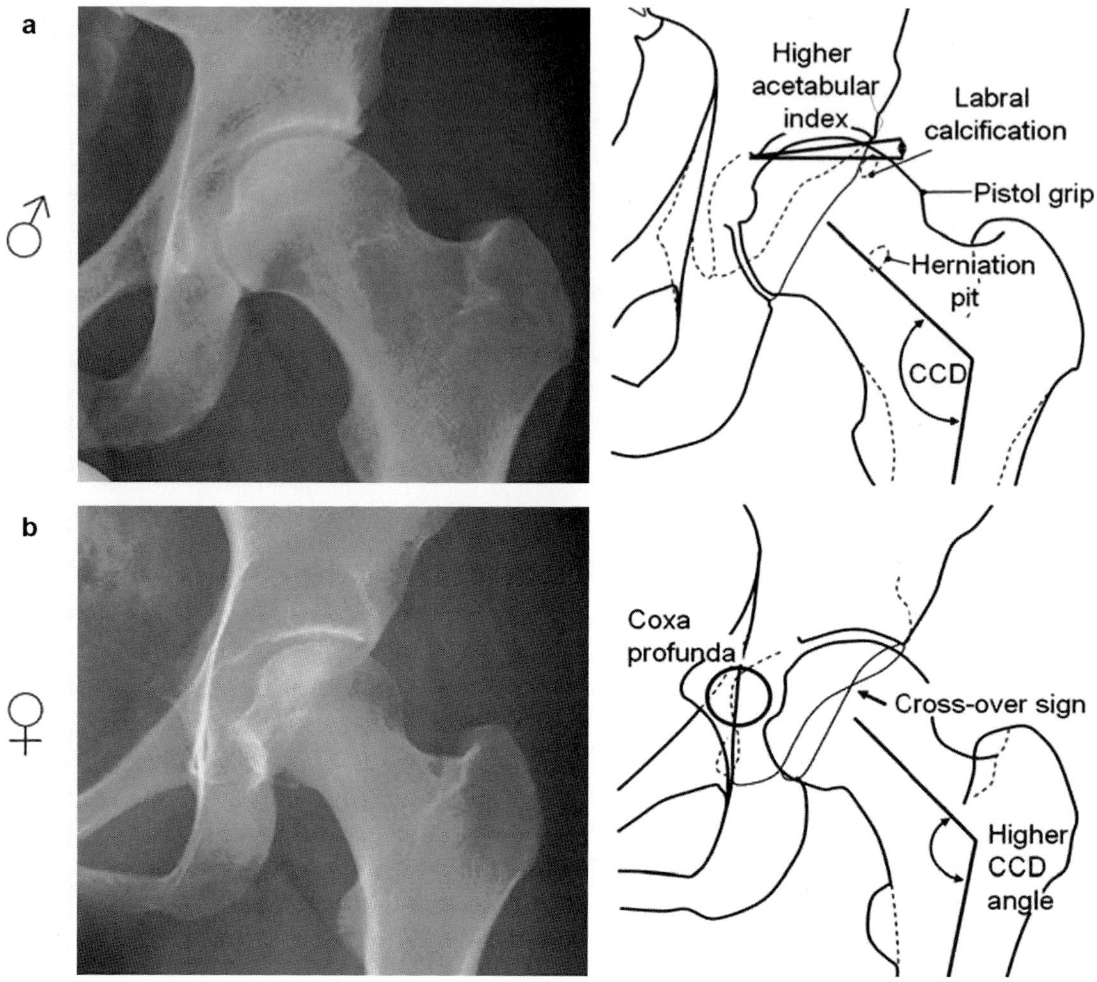

Fig. 5.2 Predominant morphologic differences of the proximal femur and acetabulum when comparing males to females. Males (**a**) show a predominance of femoral-sided findings, whereas females (**b**) show more acetabular-sided findings

5.5 Primary

5.5.1 Race

Hoaglund and Steinbach (89) report racial differences in the prevalence of hip OA with Caucasians (3–6 %) having a higher prevalence than East Indians, Blacks, Hong Kong Chinese, and Native Americans (all <1 %). Other anatomic studies of the proximal femur have shown structural differences between Caucasian and Asian hips (90,92), specifically differences in femoral anteversion and head sphericity (90,91), with Caucasian hip joints indicating a "barrel-shaped" femoral head (90). There was also a tendency toward slightly larger femoral head diameters in caucasian females (mean, 4.3 cm) compared with Chinese females (mean, 4.0 cm) (90). Dudda et al. (92) compared radiographs of Chinese and Caucasian women without osteoarthritis and found that Caucasian women had a higher prevalence of femoral head asphericity, in addition to a higher prevalence of acetabular overcoverage. Studies in Japan have shown that most hip OA cases are due to developmental dysplasia of the hip [45, 46]. The prevalence of FAI was low 0.6 % and acetabular retroversion was more likely the cause of non-dysplastic hips [47, 48]. In contrast in Denmark Gosvig concluded high-risk OA due to deep socket and pistol grip deformity similar to that reported by Hoaglund [45, 49]. This evidence can in part explain the racial differences of hip shape and the development of OA.

5.5.2 Sex

Identifying sex-specific disease patterns is important to improving diagnostic and treatment algorithms. An accurate understanding of differences in FAI disease patterns between males and females may improve sex-dependent diagnostic criteria. CAM-type FAI previously has been described as a problem in young males, while pincer-type FAI has been noted as most common in middle-aged females (3,2).

The prevalence of CAM-type deformity in asymptomatic volunteers is reportedly between 14 and 24 %, with males being more affected than females by a ratio of 3.8:1 (93,94). Females have a higher incidence of coxa profunda, positive crossover sign, and increased Sharpe angles (95) (Fig. 5.2). All are consistent with the findings showing a higher prevalence of deep acetabular socket in women but a higher prevalence of pistol grip deformity in men.

Studies have shown that females had significantly smaller alpha angles but increased anteversion compared with men with symptomatic FAI (97,98), reporting only 34 % (compared with 72 % of males) having a maximum alpha angle of >60°. Internal rotation in flexion was greater in females indicating that diagnostic criteria for males and females are different (96).

5.5.3 Genetics

Pollard and colleagues evaluated the siblings of patients undergoing treatment for idiopathic FAI and compared them to a cohort of spouses of both the siblings and patients. Their study found that siblings of patients treated for a CAM-type FAI have a relative risk of 2.8 of also having a CAM-type deformity (99). This risk was highest (3.2; range, 1.9–5.4) in brothers of male patients and lowest (1.9; range, 0.8–4.9) in sisters of female patients (Table 5.1). The authors went on to state that deformities contributing to FAI are "determined at conception or that there is a genetic predisposition to abnormal development or subclinical hip disease before skeletal maturity" (99). Further, they add, "the high prevalence of CAM deformity in the siblings in the absence of clinical features and OA suggests that the deformity is a primary, not secondary, phenomenon" (99). Their conclusion may not explain the low risk in sisters of female patients and that activity level in highly active families and sex differences may play a part. Some evidence exists that race, sex, and genetics may partly explain that FAI development is established prior to birth; it may also be due to cultural differences and how we live our daily lives impacts the development of our hip. Further studies looking at different ethnic groups living in the same culture may answer this question.

5.5.4 Reactive Forces

Initially following the establishment of FAI, some proposed the CAM and pincer lesions were simply bony growths resulting or adapting from bony impingement perhaps as a protective mechanism from further damage. The likelihood of bony changes occurring beyond physeal closure is low as previously described; certainly calcification of the labrum and bony rim developments can result

Table 5.1 Summary of morphological classification for each hip in the sibling and control groups

Morphological classification							
Group	Gender	Number	Hips	Normal (%)	Pure CAM (%)	Mixed (%)	Pure pincer (%)
Control	Male	39	78	53 (*67.9*)	12 (*15.4*)	2 (*2.6*)	11 (*14.1*)
	Female	38	76	55 (*72.4*)	5 (*6.6*)	4 (*5.3*)	12 (*15.8*)
Siblings	Male	54	108	41 (*38.0*)	33 (*30.6*)	16 (*14.8*)	18 (*16.7*)
	Female	42	84	42 (*50.0*)	15 (*17.9*)	5 (*6.0*)	22 (*26.2*)

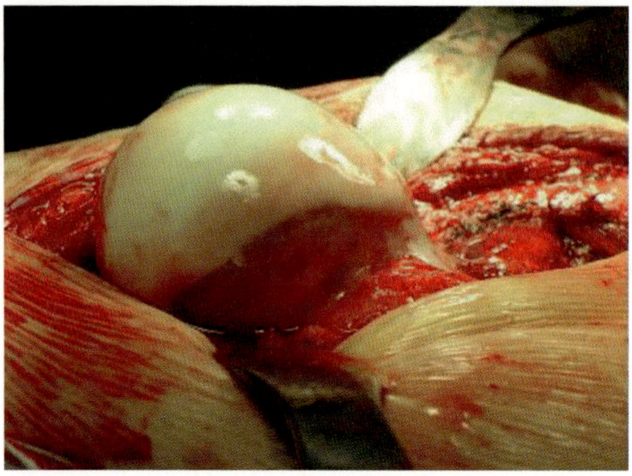

Fig. 5.3 Normal hyaline cartilage of CAM lesion

from Pincer impingement but they don't grow beyond the boundary of the labrum. Unlike osteophytes, the CAM lesions do not appear to have the potential for growth or recurrence following resection. In contrast evidence of recorticalization of the bone in the first 2 years following CAM resection has been shown [37, 38]. Histological analysis of cartilage overlying the CAM and pincer lesions reveals normal hyaline cartilage and hyaline cartilage is unable to form after skeletal maturation (Fig. 5.3). If CAM lesions were a result of the impingement process, they would continue to enlarge with time and would consist of fibrocartilage as opposed to hyaline cartilage. There is no correlation with age and the degree of deformity or severity of alpha angles, loss of anterior offset, or other radiographic measurements [50]. The reactive changes that are seen with age and deformity are osteoarthritic changes and will be explored further when looking at the evidence of whether FAI leads to OA.

In contrast the physiological stresses that occur on the hip during childhood and the potential for remodeling are more likely. The level of sporting activity in childhood through running and climbing and perhaps more so in such sports requiring flexion and internal rotation has been linked to FAI. One study showed a higher prevalence of CAM deformity in adolescents involved in high impact activity during skeletal maturation [51] (101). There have been multiple reports describing the relationship between vigorous sporting activity in young people and the prevalence of CAM deformities of the proximal femur (100,101).

One theory to explain the higher prevalence of CAM deformity in athletes is that vigorous sporting activity during development of the proximal femur may lead to abnormal or altered development of the capital femoral physis (102). Epiphyseal extension toward the femoral neck is 12–15 % greater throughout the entire cranial hemisphere in young elite basketball players versus age-matched controls. Although the control hips showed an increase in epiphyseal extension as they progressed through physeal closure, epiphyseal extension in basketball players was markedly increased before physeal closure (102). If morphological changes do occur due to stresses through sports, it is before skeletal maturation and would most likely occur during hormonal changes when the bone is prone to softening and remodeling through the growth plate. Carter et al. found that the location of the CAM lesion associated with symptomatic FAI in skeletally immature patients occurs in close proximity to the level of the proximal femoral physis. With maturation, the origin of the CAM lesion becomes further away from the physis, presumably as additional growth occurs after the inciting event. This suggests that the growth plate—or more specifically, repetitive microtrauma to it—may play a causal role in the pathogenesis of CAM-type FAI [52]. Philippon et al. showed an association between age and alpha angle in the skeletally immature patient. The increase in alpha angle with age in this active population corroborates the theory of a developmental characteristic to CAM-type FAI [53]. When the open femoral physis is submitted to high stresses in competitive sports as the adolescent grows, it may be prone to development of a CAM deformity.

5.5.5 Slipped Capital Femoral Epiphysis (SCFE)

Slipped capital femoral epiphysis is one of the leading theories as to the cause of the CAM lesion. The resultant head slips posteriorly and leads to loss of the anterior offset at the head-neck junction. Similarly a CAM lesion is the loss of asphericity of the femoral head mainly anteriorly or anterolaterally on the femoral head-neck junction with loss of head-neck offset in this region.

SCFE typically occurs in teenagers before the growth physes fuse with symptomatic children with detectable slips requiring surgery. Severe slips fixed in situ have been a source of impingement with reports of femoral osteotomies being required to correct and alleviate such impingement. A higher prevalence of SCFE is seen in males more than females. The presentation of such children and their level of symptoms vary and it is recognized that many mild slips could and can go undetected.

Goodman previously described SCFE as a posterior angulated head-neck tilt, translation of the femoral head with loss of anterior offset between head and neck that can result in an asphericity as the head slips and moves posteriorly [6] (Fig. 5.4).

The radiographic measurements that assess head-neck tilt, anterior offset ratio (AOR), and alpha angle are described (Fig. 5.4). Abnormal alpha angles in these individuals indicate the loss of the head-neck junction or asphericity of the femoral head. Loss of AOR depicts the translation of the femoral head on the neck. Head-neck tilt describes the angle of the femoral head in relationship to the angle of the neck. The occurrence of abnormal values in all three of these measurements would reflect a femoral head position as depicted and explained by Goodman consistent with SCFE. In contrast an abnormal alpha angle and AOR but with normal head-neck tilt would depict a translated but not tilted femoral head—a shape or abnormality that may not be consistent with SCFE. The same radiographic appearances described by Goodman are found in CAM lesions and were also more prevalent in the male population. The prevalence of abnormal radiographic measurements as defined for SCFE was found in up to 70 % of patients [50, 54]. These measurements and their severity showed no correlation with age indicat-

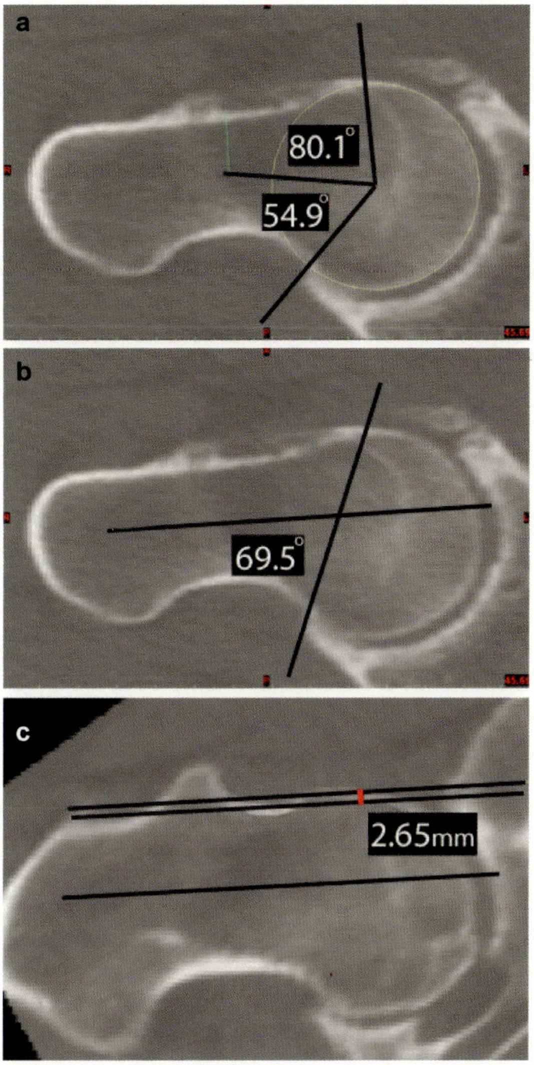

Fig. 5.4 Method of measuring the alpha and beta angles. (**a**) A *line* is drawn from the center of the femoral neck at its narrowest point to the center of the femoral head. To determine the alpha angle, the angle is measured between the *first line* and a *second line* drawn from the center of the femoral head to the anterior loss of sphericity. Beta angle measures the angle between *line 1* and a line drawn from the center of the femoral head to the posterior head-neck junction. (**b**) Head-neck tilt. *Line 1* was drawn down the long axis of the femoral neck, though not necessarily through the center of the femoral head. The tilt is the angle between the first line and a second drawn from anterior loss of sphericity to posterior head-neck junction. (**c**) Anterior offset. The first line is *line 1* from head-neck tilt. *Line 2* is drawn parallel to *line 1* along the anterior cortex of the femoral neck, and *line 3* is drawn along the anterior cortex of the femoral head. The AO is the perpendicular distance between *lines 2 and 3*

ing it was a static deformity that did not deteriorate with time [50, 54].

FAI is not detected until symptoms start and similar to SCFE could reflect the subtle nature of the disease process that preceded the onset of symptoms. The pathology goes undetected and it is for this reason it has been proposed that subclinical SCFE, not acute enough to come to medical attention, is a major contributor to the development of CAM-type FAI. A study looking at asymptomatic children who underwent radiographs and CT scans performed for other reasons revealed no evidence of abnormal morphology of the hip indicative of CAM deformity until approximately age 10–12 years [55]. Beaule in a MRI study assessment of asymptomatic pediatric patients pre- and post-physeal closure concluded CAM deformity likely develops during physeal closure and is associated with increased activity levels [56]. The coincidental timing of these changes prior to physeal closure corresponds to the age that SCFE occurs and perhaps why most patients suffering the discomfort of FAI are seen in their late teens, 20s, and 30s. A counter argument against SCFE as a cause of FAI, are reports that patients with CAM deformity do not show orientational growth plate disturbances found in SCFE [57, 58]. Failure of the beta angle to change with the increased alpha angle may refute the evidence for the capital physes slipping to be a causative factor in CAM pathology [59]. Others propose that SCFE is a cause with the osteocartilaginous bump a result of an extended physis as a result of a SCFE or similar type injury.

5.5.6 Global Acetabular Overcoverage: Protrusio and Coxa Profunda

Pincer-type impingement is seen when a deep socket provides functional overcoverage on a well-centered femoral head. Focal pincer lesions involve bony overhang of the anterosuperior acetabulum, often due to acetabular retroversion. Classic radiographic findings of a crossover sign, ischial spine sign, and sometimes a posterior wall sign (indicating posterior wall insufficiency) are detected on an anteroposterior (AP) pelvis projection. In contrast, a deep socket causes global pincer impingement, with relative global overcoverage of the femoral head. Generally accepted as a medialization of the acetabulum, there are various radiographic criteria that have been used to define acetabular protrusio. A center-edge angle (CEA) of Wiberg greater than 40° is considered diagnostic of protrusio (Fig. 5.5) (103,105,106). In contrast, coxa profunda is considered a less severe form of global pincer impingement with

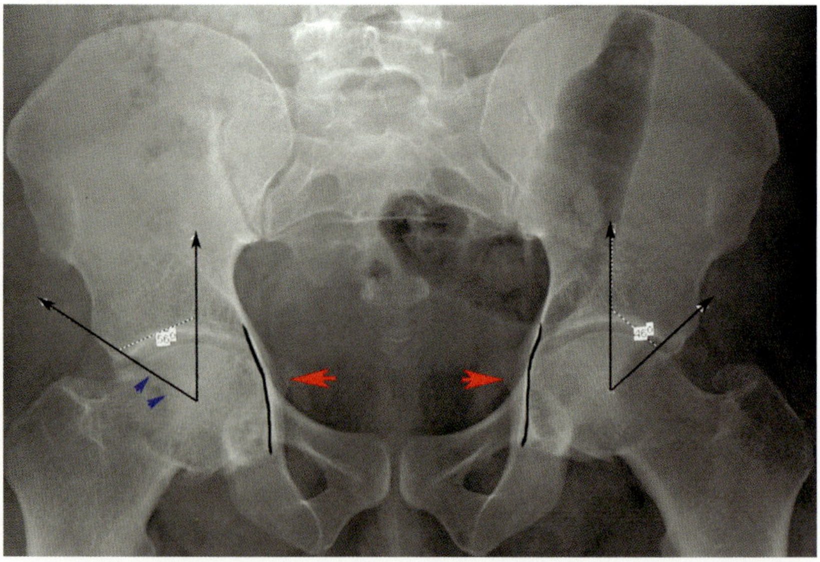

Fig. 5.5 AP pelvis radiograph showing right protrusion acetabuli with CEA of 56° and CAM morphology of proximal femur. The left hip has a CEA of 46° and CAM morphology. The *red arrows* indicate bilateral ischial spine signs. No crossover signs are seen. The *blue arrows* indicate the margin of the CAM deformity with a possible impaction defect from mechanical FAI

the medial acetabular wall overlapping or medial to the ilioischial line (104). Moreover, global pincer impingement (whether protrusio or profunda) has a prominent posterior wall lateral to the femoral head center (104). Any of these acetabular dysmorphisms may coexist with acetabular retroversion and/or CAM morphology. In some cases, the softening of bonc due to underlining hormonal or metabolic causes is thought to lead to this deformity. It is for those reasons patients can develop pincer impingement through time after skeletal maturity. Similarly acetabular overcoverage can be functional due to hyperlordosis at the lumbosacral junction leading to anterior pelvic tilt [60, 61]. If not functional, most likely genetic and must be assessed for posterior wall deficiency. Like DDH, this is most likely a developmental problem that may stem from intrauterine and the first years of life. All radiographic assessments must be done in at least two planes as subtleties of radiographic findings can be due to more than one abnormality or patient position. The complexity of these deformities that can coexist has led many to using 3 Dimensional CT reconstruction images to evaluate the painful hip.

5.6 Secondary Causes of FAI

5.6.1 FAI Following Surgical Intervention

Periacetabular osteotomies provide a temporary surgical solution for the treatment of symptomatic acetabular dysplasia and have shown good functional, clinical, and radiographical outcomes (139,141) and good preservation of the hip joint at 10 (136) and 20 years (143). However, several studies, which include retrospective reviews and case series, have described the occurrence of impingement symptomatology such as pain and range of motion restriction following periacetabular osteotomies (PAO) (136-143).

In conditions of hip dysplasia, there is a lack of femoral head-neck offset with a deformed, aspherical femoral head but this is usually compensated by decreased anterior acetabular coverage. However, after surgical correction is achieved with the osteotomy, an iatrogenic pincer-type impingement can be created, and with the asphericity of the femoral head, this can lead to combined-type impingement causing anterior impingement. This has been noted to be as high as 30–48 % postoperatively (136,139). Myers et al. in 1999 describe five cases of "secondary impingement syndrome" following periacetabular osteotomy (137). All their patients presented with groin pain and symptoms of anterior impingement and reduced range of motion in flexion, adduction, and internal rotation. MR arthrograms confirmed labral injury and chondral damage in the involved hips.

Preoperative asphericity of the femoral head is protected by under coverage of the acetabulum. Following reorientation, relative overcoverage produces anterior impingement (144).

Albers et al. describe the concept of "optimal acetabular orientation" which was introduced in order to maximize the final position of the acetabulum at reorientation in order to minimize the problem of overcorrection and retroversion (144). The authors use six radiographic parameters such as femoral coverage, anterior coverage, posterior coverage, lateral center edge angle, acetabular index, and extrusion index and consider reorientation optimal if at least 4/6 of these parameters are within an acceptable range. The same researchers performed a retrospective study to determine whether proper acetabular reorientation with periacetabular osteotomy and a spherical femoral head would improve hip 10-year survivorship or slow the progression of osteoarthritis. They reviewed 147 patients who underwent 165 periacetabular osteotomies and divided these patients into two groups: proper orientation and spherical femoral head vs. improper reorientation and aspherical head with a minimal follow-up of 10 years. They found that proper reorientation with a spherical femoral head increased survivorship and decreased the progression of osteoarthritis.

5.6.2 Femoral Neck Fractures and FAI

Ganz et al. were the first to describe FAI secondary to malunion and bony overgrowth following surgical fixation of proximal femur fractures

(107). They postulated that malreduction and malunion following surgical reduction and fixation could lead to abnormal morphology of the femoral head-neck junction such as varus malunion, shortening, retroversion, and decreased femoral head-neck offset resulting in abnormal hip mechanics and impingement (108-111). Since their original description, this concept has been supported by several reports and case series (108,109,114).

Eighty-five percent of elderly patients (>85 years) who had undergone surgical fixation with multiple cancellous screws or sliding hip screw construct for femoral neck fractures had radiographic evidence of CAM-type FAI (109), significantly higher than the 1–17 % reported in the asymptomatic general population (112,45). They also found that 86 % of Garden type III and IV fractures showed evidence of CAM-type FAI while only 72 % of Garden I and II fractures. Whether the radiographic changes are the result of the surgical fixation and malunion or due to changes in the proximal femoral head-neck offset seen with aging is unclear (113) and previous reports have described a high incidence of CAM impingement in patients over 50 years who were undergoing hip resurfacing arthroplasty [50] (114).

In contrast, another study compared hip fracture in patients under 50 years of age who were treated with reduction and internal fixation with population-based controls (135). Radiographic signs of impingement and degenerative arthritis were analyzed and the authors found that 75 % of hips treated with internal fixation had at least one sign indicative of impingement versus 17 % in the general population (112,45). These findings would seem to contradict previous reports that have suggested that femoral head-neck abnormalities are a consequence of advanced age (113) rather than fracture malunion. Furthermore, 22 hips (31 %) had radiographic evidence of degenerative arthritis at final follow-up as judged by their Tonnis score and again displaced subcapital B-3 fractures were most likely to display arthritic changes. Interestingly, 94 % of hips without any radiographic signs of impingement also did not have signs of arthritis at last follow-up (109).

Eijer et al. reported 9 patients with a mean age of 33 years who had sustained a femoral neck fracture and experienced subsequent pain, gait disruption, and decreased range of motion especially in flexion, adduction, and internal rotation with positive impingement test in the affected hip (108). Radiographs and intraoperative assessment showed insufficient fracture reduction and malunion in all patients. The authors stated that femoral head retroversion and varus malalignment lead to anterior and anterolateral impingement, respectively. Intraoperatively, anterior labral damage and acetabular cartilage lesions, similar to those seen with FAI, were seen in all patients with an abnormal femoral head-neck contour.

In contrast, some authors have suggested that the impingement and the radiographical changes seen postoperatively in patients with femoral neck fractures were the cause of the nonunion or malunion rather than the effect (115). Regardless, a proximal femur fracture and subsequent malreduction and/or malunion appear to increase the risk of developing radiographical and clinical signs of CAM-type impingement. The cause and effect between these postoperative radiographical findings and the subsequent development of hip arthritis remain unclear. These findings however do support the importance of initial anatomic reduction in both the AP and axial planes and stable fixation when dealing with proximal femoral fractures (111,116). The results also highlight the importance of close monitoring and early postoperative detection when treating a patient who has suffered a similar type fracture with subsequent malunion. Surgical intervention may facilitate hip preservation, in this specific patient population, preventing possible FAI symptomatology and its sequelae.

5.6.3 FAI and the "Pathological CAM Lesion"

FAI symptomatology and radiographic changes can also be caused by pathological lesions. Several case reports and series have been published describing classical FAI symptomatology resulting from both benign and malignant lesions in the proximal femur (117-122). The patients are typically young active adults who present with pain and progressive decrease in hip range of motion (117). The widened and dysplastic femoral head and neck create a mechanical block leading to abnormal contact between the proximal femur and acetabular rim, limiting the range of motion and leading to the typical FAI presentation of pain, positive impingement and FABER test, and decreased flexion, adduction, and internal rotation. The changes seen on the femoral side are often associated with acetabular labral tears and cysts with signs of progressive arthritic changes.

Tripathy et al. describe the case of a 23-year-old soccer player who presented with FAI symptoms secondary to an intra-articular chondrosarcoma of the femoral head (117). The patient presented with groin pain and demonstrated limited hip flexion; adduction and internal rotation and these movements also reproduced his pain. Radiographs and MRI showed a lytic lesion on the anteroinferior aspect of the femoral head and no evidence of acetabular chondrolabral pathology. Open excisional biopsy was performed and pathology confirmed intermediate grade malignant chondrosarcoma with tumor free margins. Postoperatively, the symptoms of impingement had resolved and the patient had returned to full physical and sporting activity with full range of motion at 6 months.

Similar case reports of osteochondromas, osteoid osteoma, multiple hereditary exostosis, and synovial chondromatosis causing similar FAI symptoms and chondrolabral damage have been described (123,132-134,119,120,122).

Hussain et al. also published the case of a young adult who presented with symptoms suggestive of FAI caused by a solitary osteochondroma of the greater trochanter (118). Plain radiographs and MRI showed a calcified mass adjacent to the greater trochanter on the involved side with communicating medullary canal. Imaging also showed a bony bump on the anterosuperior aspect of the femoral neck as well as degenerative changes on the acetabular side and a positive crossover sign. Through a posterior lateral approach, an excisional biopsy was performed and pathology confirmed the lesion to be an osteochondroma. Postoperatively, he continued to complain of anterior groin pain associated with hip flexion, adduction, and internal rotation, and seven months following the initial procedure, the patient underwent hip arthroscopy with labral debridement and repair and osteochondroplasty with complete resolution of symptoms. This would suggest that the standard CAM lesion and acetabular retroversion were the likely underlying cause of the mechanical impingement symptoms rather than osteochondroma per se.

Benign and malignant lesions of the proximal femur can lead to mechanical and pain symptoms typical of femoroacetabular impingement by creating anatomical abnormalities consistent with CAM lesions. There have yet to be described cases of acetabular or pelvic lesions recreating pincer-type lesions. Although infrequent, these "pathological CAM lesions" and their associated symptomatology and the resolution of symptoms following excision reinforce the reality of the CAM lesion as a unique entity leading to FAI symptoms. Whether or not these patients are at increased risk of developing hip osteoarthritis in the future has yet to be seen.

5.6.4 Legg-Calve-Perthes (LCP)

LCP is a disease of young (4–10 years) children who present with osteonecrosis of the femoral capital epiphysis, which inevitably heals but can lead to varying degrees of hip abnormality. The morphologic alterations occur on both the acetabular and femoral side. The femoral side typically has a short neck, trochanteric overgrowth, and a large flattened head with resultant femoral retroversion and coxa vara, coxa magna, and coxa breva. The acetabular side often becomes flattened and retroverted but with insufficient femoral head coverage and can lead to combinations of CAM and pincer impingement and in severe cases trochanteric impingement [62–66]. The Stulberg classification was a predictor of hip pathology in later life with Class I predicting a better prognosis than Class IV where patients often develop hip problems in their second decade and early osteoarthritis [67–69]. There is no doubt that LCP leads to abnormal hip biomechanics and in severe cases secondary osteoarthritis and is a form of FAI but unlikely to be the cause of the subtle abnormalities we consider in a previously described normal hip.

5.6.5 Does FAI and Sequelae Lead to Osteoarthritis (OA)?

OA of the hip can occur secondary to many etiological factors, e.g., LCP, DDH, and SCFE. It is often seen that patients can develop OA of the hip without any discernable causative factor and it is those patients that FAI has been proposed as the etiology of early adulthood arthritis [3]. The resultant chondral and labral lesions progress to degenerative joint disease with Ganz arguing that more than 90 % of OA is attributed to this pathological process [1–3]. It follows that damage such as chondral delamination and labral tears will progress over time.

5.7 Cartilage Response

The response of cartilage to overload and shear injury can be progressive and follows a somewhat predictable path. In overload, superficial layers of articular cartilage respond with matrix degradation. Hashimoto et al. have reported the metabolic activity levels in the articular cartilage of human subjects with femoroacetabular impingement (87). Articular cartilage obtained from the impingement zone (anterolateral head-neck junction) of hips with femoroacetabular impingement expressed markedly elevated levels of most chemokines and degradative enzymes, but not of the pro-inflammatory cytokine IL-1b, compared with normal articular cartilage (Fig. 5.6). Cartilage specimens from hips with femoroacetabular impingement also expressed significantly higher levels of certain chemokines and other markers (IL-8, CCL3L1, ADAMTS-4, and ACAN) compared with articular cartilage

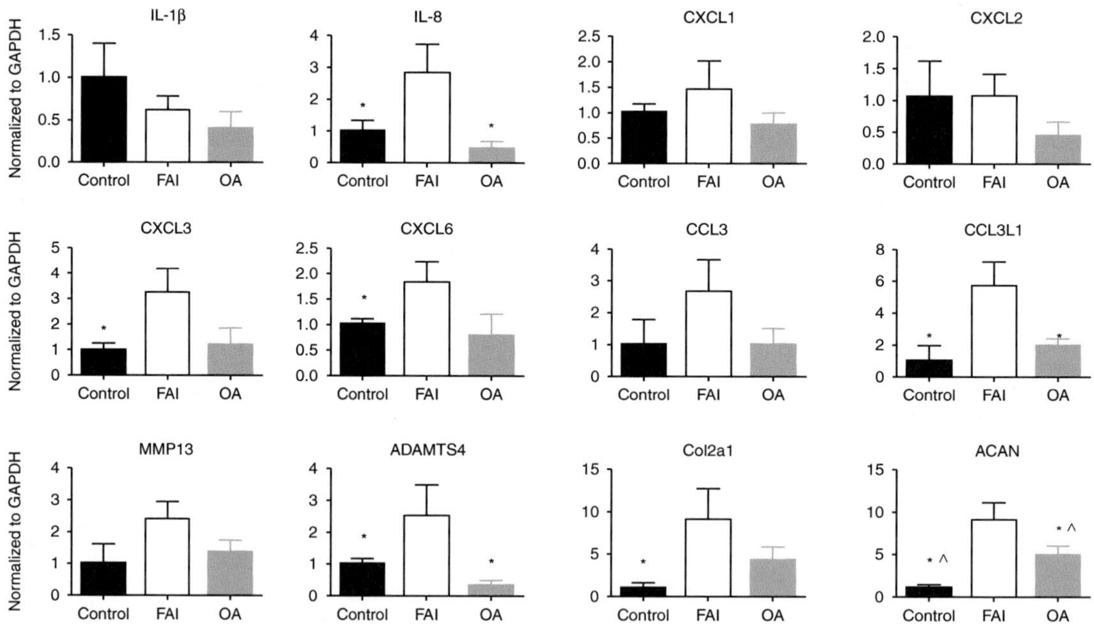

Fig. 5.6 Normalized mRNA expression of selected cytokine and chemokine, matrix-degrading, and structural matrix genes in articular cartilage samples obtained from hips with femoroacetabular impingement (*FAI*) and end-stage osteoarthritis (*OA*) compared with controls. Except for IL-1b and CXCL2, the expression of all genes was higher in hips with FAI compared with controls and hips with OA. Significant differences between two or more categories were observed for IL-8, CXCL3, CXCL6, CCL3L1, ADAMTS-4, COL2A1, and ACAN, indicating that the cartilage in hips with FAI was metabolically more active than the cartilage in hips with OA and controls. The data are expressed as the mean and the standard error of the mean relative to the mean expression of the control specimens. $^*P<0.05$ compared with hips with FAI. $P<0.05$ between controls and hips with OA

from hips with end-stage osteoarthritis. In the comparison among different stages of articular cartilage degradation, the cleavage/thinning stage was the most metabolically active. Importantly, there was a trend toward decreased expression of matrix protein genes (COL2A1 and ACAN) in end-stage osteoarthritis (OA) compared with femoroacetabular impingement, although this decrease was significant only for ACAN. Analysis of these tissues suggests that the mechanical disease of femoroacetabular impingement causes localized articular cartilage alterations that are consistent with early osteoarthritic degeneration. Specifically, articular cartilage in the femoroacetabular impingement zone had high metabolic activity, both catabolic and anabolic, that commonly preceded radiographic evidence of osteoarthritis.

The early pathophysiology of hip osteoarthritis is being established but much is still not understood, and limited information exists regarding the biologic cascade that mediates osteoarthritis in the human hip. Nevertheless, previous work suggests that early changes after injury to articular cartilage include hypertrophy, collagen deformation, proteoglycan depletion, and mild inflammation (83-85). These events are reversible, as chondrocytes can degrade damaged molecules and increase matrix production (86). Thus, both anabolism and catabolism are increased in early osteoarthritis, with the balance moving toward catabolism with disease progression (88). These previous observations are consistent with the data from the hips with femoroacetabular impingement and osteoarthritis in the present study (Fig. 5.6). The samples from hips with femoroacetabular impingement demonstrated higher metabolic activity involving inflammatory chemokine (IL 8 and CCL3L1), matrix-degrading (ADAMTS-4), and extracellular matrix (ACAN) genes compared with hips with end-stage osteoarthritis. The decrease in matrix protein gene expression in hips with end-stage osteoarthritis may indicate a loss of anabolic activity and an imbalance favoring catabolism.

Studies looking at clinical outcomes following surgical correction for FAI have consistently demonstrated positive outcomes [70, 71], and interestingly, these studies also found that early osteoarthritis or advanced chondral damage has inferior results [70, 71]. Many more level III and IV studies have shown similar findings in surgical outcomes [72, 73]. The counterargument is that the outcomes were poor due to a different disease process with joint damage having already been established. Currently, without sufficient long-term follow-up or randomized studies to include nonoperative treatment, we cannot be certain of the cause and effect relationship between FAI and OA. For this reason many studies are now looking at cross-sectional cohorts and populations in an attempt to find a relationship between FAI and OA. Studies in elderly patients with established OA that then look for evidence of FAI are fraught with issues of causal ambiguity as the impingement lesions seen can occur secondary to degenerative changes and it is hard to differentiate from premorbid impingement lesions from secondary arthritic changes [74]. Patients under 55 years of age with established OA undergoing hip resurfacing showed a high prevalence of FAI but again we don't know how much of the changes seen are secondary to the arthritic process [50]. Studies have examined the asymptomatic contralateral hip of patients with opposite hip degenerative changes looking for abnormal morphology and compared those results with controls. The risk of developing OA in the contralateral hip has been estimated between 5.5 and 8.3 % compared with 3 % in the control group after adjusting for age sex and BMI [75]. Longitudinal studies that begin prior to the onset of the disease process are best in order to determine the cause and effect relationship between FAI and osteoarthritis. Two such Dutch studies involving over 1500 patients aged 45–85 years and followed by 5 and 6 years with no or minimal OA at the start point found that increasing abnormalities of alpha angle and loss of offset consistent with FAI conferred increased risks of developing OA from 25 to 62 % compared with less than 2 % with more normal morphology [76].

This raises the question as to what is actually abnormal morphology. The alpha angle is widely used and confers a measurement of asphericity of the femoral head and loss of offset. The Chingford study was a robust longitudinal study of 1003 healthy women with radiographs at baseline and 19 years later. The morphology of those requiring total hip arthroplasty (THA) was compared to those who did not undergo THA and the alpha angles were measured. The median alpha angle of those who needed THA versus those who did not was 62.4 and 45.8, respectively. They also found that an alpha angle greater than 65° leads to an increased odds ratio of developing OA by 2.7 compared with an angle under 65 [77]. In one study as in others, there are patients who despite evidence of FAI have not developed OA or the need for THA. Epidemiological studies reported so far are mainly based on limited imaging such as AP radiographs that have some limitations in delineating anterior CAM lesions or accurate assessment of pincer lesions.

5.8 The Future

Studies examining the postoperative outcomes of FAI correction have shown significant improvements in clinical symptoms in short and midterm follow-up. These studies have also correlated over and under correction with poor functional outcomes [71].

This leads to the questions: What are we correcting and what is abnormal and what is normal?

The answer may not be so obvious. Charnley from his concept of total hip arthroplasty has led us to believe the hip is a ball and socket joint. In reality, in the native hip, this is likely not the case. Various shapes of hip joint exist but it is safe to acknowledge that both the femoral head and the acetabulum are more ellipsoid in shape rather than spherical [78]. The relationship between the two is likely more complex than a simple ball and socket joint with a center of rotation. While the hip joint enables flexion, extension, rotation, and the translation, the influence of the surrounding soft tissues including the capsule, ligamentum teres, and muscles is not fully understood. Rylander has looked at in vivo motion capture analysis of patients pre- and post-FAI surgery during level walking and found improved sagittal range of motion of the hip [79]. Kennedy has looked at gait analysis of FAI patients against controls and showed differences in hip and pelvic range of motion and hip with improved abduction compared to controls during level gait and deep squat [80]. These studies are small and few in number and gait analysis has been identified as a future measurement tool that needs refined [81].

The future of FAI requires more biomechanical studies and gait analysis while incorporating accurate pre- and postoperative data. The capturing of the angles and offsets and morphological shape changing that is corrected through surgeries and correlation with gait analysis should give greater clarification of the pathophysiology. Comparing and contrasting normal type hips with longitudinal data would be valuable and may establish there's more to FAI surgery than correcting the alpha angle.

Take-Home Points

1. Clinical FAI is the result of a combination of factors that combine activity with aberrant morphology.
2. Predisposing factors for FAI include: pediatric hip disease, gender, ethnicity, genetics and activity during hip maturation.
3. Secondary causes of FAI include: hip fracture malunion, iatrogenic surgical intervention.
4. Once clinically evident, FAI may initiate the process of joint degeneration starting with damage to intra articular structures (cartilage and labrum).

Key Evidence Related Sources

1. Ganz R, Gill TJ, Gautier E, Ganz K, Krugel N, Berlemann U. Surgical dislocation of the adult hip a technique with full access to the femoral head and acetabulum without the risk of avascular necrosis. J Bone Joint Surg Br. 2001;83(8):1119–24.
2. McCarthy JC, Noble PC, Schuck MR, Wright J, Lee J. The Otto E. Aufranc Award: The role of labral lesions to development of early degenerative hip disease. Clin Orthop Relat Res. 2001;393:25–37.
3. Kassarjian A, Yoon LS, Belzile E, Connolly SA, Millis MB, Palmer WE. Triad of MR arthrographic findings in patients with cam-type femoroacetabular impingement. Radiology. 2005;236(2):588–92.
4. Wenger DE, Kendell KR, Miner MR, Trousdale RT. Acetabular labral tears rarely occur in the absence of bony abnormalities. Clin Orthop Relat Res. 2004;426:145–50
5. Ng VY, Arora N, Best TM, Pan X, Ellis TJ. Efficacy of surgery for femoroacetabular impingement: a systematic review. Am J Sports Med. 2010;38(11):2337–45.

References

1. Ganz R, Gill TJ, Gautier E, Ganz K, Krugel N, Berlemann U. Surgical dislocation of the adult hip a technique with full access to the femoral head and acetabulum without the risk of avascular necrosis. J Bone Joint Surg Br. 2001;83(8):1119–24.
2. Ganz R, Leunig M, Leunig-Ganz K, Harris WH. The etiology of osteoarthritis of the hip: an integrated mechanical concept. Clin Orthop Relat Res. 2008;466(2):264–72.
3. Ganz R, Parvizi J, Beck M, Leunig M, Notzli H, Siebenrock KA. Femoroacetabular impingement: a cause for osteoarthritis of the hip. Clin Orthop Relat Res. 2003;417:112–20.
4. Murray RO. The aetiology of primary osteoarthritis of the hip. Br J Radiol. 1965;38:810–24.
5. Solomon L. Patterns of osteoarthritis of the hip. J Bone Joint Surg Br. 1976;58(2):176–83.
6. Goodman DA, Feighan JE, Smith AD, Latimer B, Buly RL, Cooperman DR. Subclinical slipped capital femoral epiphysis. Relationship to osteoarthrosis of the hip. J Bone Joint Surg Am. 1997; 79(10):1489–97.
7. Harris WH. Etiology of osteoarthritis of the hip. Clin Orthop Relat Res. 1986;213:20–33.
8. Harris WH, Bourne RB, Oh I. Intra-articular acetabular labrum: a possible etiological factor in certain cases of osteoarthritis of the hip. J Bone Joint Surg Am. 1979;61(4):510–4.
9. Stulberg SD, Cordell LD, Harris WH, et al., editors. Unrecognized childhood hip disease: a major cause of idiopathic osteoarthriti of hip. Proceedings of the third meeting of the Hip Society. Saint Louis: The CV Mosby Company; 1975.
10. Bombelli R. Osteoarthritis of the hip: pathogenesis and consequent therapy. Berlin: Springer; 1976.
11. Elmslie RC. Aetiological factors in osteoarthritis of hip. Br Med J. 1933;1:1–3.
12. Reginster JY. The prevalence and burden of arthritis. Rheumatology. 2002;41(Supp 1):3–6.
13. Murphy SB, Kijewski PK, Millis MB, Harless A. Acetabular dysplasia in the adolescent and young adult. Clin Orthop Relat Res. 1990;261:214–23.
14. Price CT, Ramo BA. Prevention of hip dysplasia in children and adults. Orthop Clin North Am. 2012;43(3):269–79.
15. Anderson SE, Siebenrock KA, Tannast M. Femoroacetabular impingement: evidence of an established hip abnormality. Radiology. 2010;257(1): 8–13.
16. Beck M, Kalhor M, Leunig M, Ganz R. Hip morphology influences the pattern of damage to the acetabular cartilage: femoroacetabular impingement as a cause of early osteoarthritis of the hip. J Bone Joint Surg Br. 2005;87(7):1012–8.
17. Naal FD, Miozzari HH, Wyss TF, Notzli HP. Surgical hip dislocation for the treatment of femoroacetabular impingement in high-level athletes. Am J Sports Med. 2011;39(3):544–50.
18. Johnston TL, Schenker ML, Briggs KK, Philippon MJ. Relationship between offset angle alpha and hip chondral injury in femoroacetabular impingement. Arthroscopy. 2008;24(6):669–75.
19. McCarthy JC, Noble PC, Schuck MR, Wright J, Lee J. The Otto E. Aufranc Award: The role of labral lesions

to development of early degenerative hip disease. Clin Orthop Relat Res. 2001;393:25–37.
20. Farjo LA, Glick JM, Sampson TG. Hip arthroscopy for acetabular labral tears. Arthroscopy. 1999;15(2):132–7.
21. Eriksson E, Arvidsson I, Arvidsson H. Diagnostic and operative arthroscopy of the hip. Orthopedics. 1986;9(2):169–76.
22. O'Leary JA, Berend K, Vail TP. The relationship between diagnosis and outcome in arthroscopy of the hip. Arthroscopy. 2001;17(2):181–8.
23. Peters CL, Erickson JA, Anderson L, Anderson AA, Weiss J. Hip-preserving surgery: understanding complex pathomorphology. J Bone Joint Surg Am. 2009;91 Suppl 6:42–58.
24. Beck M, Leunig M, Parvizi J, Boutier V, Wyss D, Ganz R. Anterior femoroacetabular impingement: part II. Midterm results of surgical treatment. Clin Orthop Relat Res. 2004;418:67–73.
25. Bardakos NV, Vasconcelos JC, Villar RN. Early outcome of hip arthroscopy for femoroacetabular impingement: the role of femoral osteoplasty in symptomatic improvement. J Bone Joint Surg Br. 2008;90(12):1570–5.
26. Bardakos NV, Villar RN. Predictors of progression of osteoarthritis in femoroacetabular impingement: a radiological study with a minimum of ten years follow-up. J Bone Joint Surg Br. 2009;91(2):162–9.
27. Beaule PE, Le Duff MJ, Zaragoza E. Quality of life following femoral head-neck osteochondroplasty for femoroacetabular impingement. J Bone Joint Surg Am. 2007;89(4):773–9.
28. Bizzini M, Notzli HP, Maffiuletti NA. Femoroacetabular impingement in professional ice hockey players: a case series of 5 athletes after open surgical decompression of the hip. Am J Sports Med. 2007;35(11):1955–9.
29. Brunner A, Horisberger M, Herzog RF. Sports and recreation activity of patients with femoroacetabular impingement before and after arthroscopic osteoplasty. Am J Sports Med. 2009;37(5):917–22.
30. Leunig M, Beaule PE, Ganz R. The concept of femoroacetabular impingement: current status and future perspectives. Clin Orthop Relat Res. 2009;467(3):616–22.
31. Lincoln M, Johnston K, Muldoon M, Santore R. Combined arthroscopic and modified open approach for cam femoroacetabular impingement: a preliminary experience. Arthroscopy. 2009;25(4):392–9.
32. Peters CL, Schabel K, Anderson L, Erickson J. Open treatment of femoroacetabular impingement is associated with clinical improvement and low complication rate at short-term followup. Clin Orthop Relat Res. 2010;468(2):504–10.
33. Philippon MJ, Briggs KK, Yen YM, Kuppersmith DA. Outcomes following hip arthroscopy for femoroacetabular impingement with associated chondrolabral dysfunction: minimum two-year follow-up. J Bone Joint Surg Br. 2009;91(1):16–23.
34. Philippon MJ, Stubbs AJ, Schenker ML, Maxwell RB, Ganz R, Leunig M. Arthroscopic management of femoroacetabular impingement: osteoplasty technique and literature review. Am J Sports Med. 2007;35(9):1571–80.
35. Ribas M, Ledesma R, Cardenas C, Marin-Pena O, Toro J, Caceres E. Clinical results after anterior mini-open approach for femoroacetabular impingement in early degenerative stage. Hip Int. 2010;20 Suppl 7:S36–42.
36. Ribas M, Marin-Pena OR, Regenbrecht B, De La Torre B, Vilarrubias JM. Hip osteoplasty by an anterior minimally invasive approach for active patients with femoroacetabular impingement. Hip Int. 2007;17(2):91–8.
37. Mardones R, Lara J, Donndorff A, Barnes S, Stuart MJ, Glick J, et al. Surgical correction of "cam-type" femoroacetabular impingement: a cadaveric comparison of open versus arthroscopic debridement. Arthroscopy. 2009;25(2):175–82.
38. Mardones RM, Gonzalez C, Chen Q, Zobitz M, Kaufman KR, Trousdale RT. Surgical treatment of femoroacetabular impingement: evaluation of the effect of the size of the resection. J Bone Joint Surg Am. 2005;87(2):273–9.
39. Yun HH, Shon WY, Yun JY. Treatment of femoroacetabular impingement with surgical dislocation. Clin Orthop Surg. 2009;1(3):146–54.
40. Bedi A, Kelly BT. Femoroacetabular impingement. J Bone Joint Surg Am. 2013;95(1):82–92.
41. Byers PD, Contepomi CA, Farkas TA. A post mortem study of the hip joint. Including the prevalence of the features of the right side. Ann Rheum Dis. 1970;29(1):15–31.
42. Hase T, Ueo T. Acetabular labral tear: arthroscopic diagnosis and treatment. Arthroscopy. 1999;15(2): 138–41.
43. Kassarjian A, Yoon LS, Belzile E, Connolly SA, Millis MB, Palmer WE. Triad of MR arthrographic findings in patients with cam-type femoroacetabular impingement. Radiology. 2005;236(2):588–92.
44. Wenger DE, Kendell KR, Miner MR, Trousdale RT. Acetabular labral tears rarely occur in the absence of bony abnormalities. Clin Orthop Relat Res. 2004;426:145–50.
45. Hoaglund FT, Shiba R, Newberg AH, Leung KY. Diseases of the hip. A comparative study of Japanese Oriental and American white patients. J Bone Joint Surg Am. 1985;67(9):1376–83.
46. Nakamura S, Ninomiya S, Nakamura T. Primary osteoarthritis of the hip joint in Japan. Clin Orthop Relat Res. 1989;241:190–6.
47. Fukushima K, Uchiyama K, Takahira N, Moriya M, Yamamoto T, Itoman M, et al. Prevalence of radiographic findings of femoroacetabular impingement in the Japanese population. J Orthop Surg Res. 2014;9:25.
48. Takeyama A, Naito M, Shiramizu K, Kiyama T. Prevalence of femoroacetabular impingement in

Asian patients with osteoarthritis of the hip. Int Orthop. 2009;33(5):1229–32.
49. Gosvig KK, Jacobsen S, Sonne-Holm S, Palm H, Troelsen A. Prevalence of malformations of the hip joint and their relationship to sex, groin pain, and risk of osteoarthritis: a population-based survey. J Bone Joint Surg Am. 2010;92(5):1162–9.
50. Giles AE, Corneman NA, Bhachu S, Rudan JF, Ellis RE, Grant H, et al. Shared morphology of slipped capital femoral epiphysis and femoroacetabular impingement in early-onset arthritis. Orthopedics. 2013;36(11):e1365–70.
51. Kapron AL, Anderson AE, Aoki SK, Phillips LG, Petron DJ, Toth R, et al. Radiographic prevalence of femoroacetabular impingement in collegiate football players: AAOS exhibit selection. J Bone Joint Surg Am. 2011;93(19):e111(1–10).
52. Carter CW, Bixby S, Yen YM, Nasreddine AY, Kocher MS. The relationship between cam lesion and physis in skeletally immature patients. J Pediatr Orthop. 2014;34(6):579–84.
53. Philippon MJ, Ejnisman L, Ellis HB, Briggs KK. Outcomes 2 to 5 years following hip arthroscopy for femoroacetabular impingement in the patient aged 11 to 16 years. Arthroscopy. 2012;28(9):1255–61.
54. Hack K, Di Primio G, Rakhra K, Beaule PE. Prevalence of cam-type femoroacetabular impingement morphology in asymptomatic volunteers. J Bone Joint Surg Am. 2010;92(14):2436–44.
55. Monazzam S, Bomar JD, Dwek JR, Hosalkar HS, Pennock AT. Development and prevalence of femoroacetabular impingement-associated morphology in a paediatric and adolescent population: a CT study of 225 patients. Bone Joint J. 2013;95-B(5):598–604.
56. Carsen S, Moroz PJ, Rakhra K, Ward LM, Dunlap H, Hay JA, et al. The Otto Aufranc Award. On the etiology of the cam deformity: a cross-sectional pediatric MRI study. Clin Orthop Relat Res. 2014;472(2):430–6.
57. Leunig M, Beck M, Woo A, Dora C, Kerboull M, Ganz R. Acetabular rim degeneration: a constant finding in the aged hip. Clin Orthop Relat Res. 2003;413:201–7.
58. Siebenrock KA, Wahab KH, Werlen S, Kalhor M, Leunig M, Ganz R. Abnormal extension of the femoral head epiphysis as a cause of cam impingement. Clin Orthop Relat Res. 2004;418:54–60.
59. Beaule PE, Zaragoza E, Motamedi K, Copelan N, Dorey FJ. Three-dimensional computed tomography of the hip in the assessment of femoroacetabular impingement. J Orthop Res Off Publ Orthop Res Soc. 2005;23(6):1286–92.
60. Gebhart JJ, Streit JJ, Bedi A, Bush-Joseph CA, Nho SJ, Salata MJ. Correlation of pelvic incidence with cam and pincer lesions. Am J Sports Med. 2014;42(11):2649–53.
61. Lazennec JY, Riwan A, Gravez F, Rousseau MA, Mora N, Gorin M, et al. Hip spine relationships: application to total hip arthroplasty. Hip Int. 2007;17 Suppl 5:S91–104.
62. Eijer H, Podeszwa DA, Ganz R, Leunig M. Evaluation and treatment of young adults with femoro-acetabular impingement secondary to Perthes' disease. Hip Int. 2006;16(4):273–80.
63. Ganz R, Huff TW, Leunig M. Extended retinacular soft tissue flap for intra-articular hip surgery: Surgical technique, indications and results of application. Instr Course Lect. 2009;58:241–55.
64. Quain S, Catterall A. Hinge abduction of the hip. Diagnosis and treatment. J Bone Joint Surg Br. 1986;68(1):61–4.
65. Snow SW, Keret D, Scarangella S, Bowen JR. Anterior impingement of the femoral head: a late phenomenon of Legg-Calve-Perthes' disease. J Pediatr Orthop. 1993;13(3):286–9.
66. Wenger DR, Kishan S, Pring ME. Impingement and childhood hip disease. J Pediatr Orthop B. 2006;15(4):233–43.
67. Stulberg SD, Cooperman DR, Wallensten R. The natural history of Legg-Calve-Perthes disease. J Bone Joint Surg Am. 1981;63(7):1095–108.
68. Herring JA, Kim HT, Browne R. Legg-Calve-Perthes disease. Part II: prospective multicenter study of the effect of treatment on outcome. J Bone Joint Surg Am. 2004;86-A(10):2121–34.
69. Larson AN, Sucato DJ, Herring JA, Adolfsen SE, Kelly DM, Martus JE, et al. A prospective multicenter study of Legg-Calve-Perthes disease: functional and radiographic outcomes of nonoperative treatment at a mean follow-up of twenty years. J Bone Joint Surg Am. 2012;94(7):584–92.
70. Bedi A, Chen N, Robertson W, Kelly BT. The management of labral tears and femoroacetabular impingement of the hip in the young, active patient. Arthroscopy. 2008;24(10):1135–45.
71. Clohisy JC, St John LC, Schutz AL. Surgical treatment of femoroacetabular impingement: a systematic review of the literature. Clin Orthop Relat Res. 2010;468(2):555–64.
72. Ng VY, Arora N, Best TM, Pan X, Ellis TJ. Efficacy of surgery for femoroacetabular impingement: a systematic review. Am J Sports Med. 2010;38(11):2337–45.
73. Matsuda DK, Carlisle JC, Arthurs SC, Wierks CH, Philippon MJ. Comparative systematic review of the open dislocation, mini-open, and arthroscopic surgeries for femoroacetabular impingement. Arthroscopy. 2011;27(2):252–69.
74. Resnick D, Niwayama G. Degenerative disease of extraspinal locations. In: Resnick D, editor. Diagnosis of bone and joint disorders. Philadelphia: WB Saunders; 1981. p. 1322–35.
75. Doherty M, Courtney P, Doherty S, Jenkins W, Maciewicz RA, Muir K, et al. Nonspherical femoral head shape (pistol grip deformity), neck shaft angle, and risk of hip osteoarthritis: a case-control study. Arthritis Rheum. 2008;58(10):3172–82.
76. Sankar WN, Nevitt M, Parvizi J, Felson DT, Agricola R, Leunig M. Femoroacetabular impingement: defining the condition and its role in the pathophysiology of osteoarthritis. J Am Acad Orthop Surg. 2013;21 Suppl 1:S7–15.

77. Nicholls AS, Kiran A, Pollard TC, Hart DJ, Arden CP, Spector T, et al. The association between hip morphology parameters and nineteen-year risk of end-stage osteoarthritis of the hip: a nested case-control study. Arthritis Rheum. 2011;63(11):3392–400.
78. Rasquinha BJ, Sayani J, Rudan JF, Wood GC, Ellis RE. Articular surface remodeling of the hip after periacetabular osteotomy. Int J Comput Assist Radiol Surg. 2012;7(2):241–8.
79. Rylander JH, Shu B, Andriacchi TP, Safran MR. Preoperative and postoperative sagittal plane hip kinematics in patients with femoroacetabular impingement during level walking. Am J Sports Med. 2011;39(Suppl):36S–42.
80. Kennedy MJ, Lamontagne M, Beaule PE. Femoroacetabular impingement alters hip and pelvic biomechanics during gait Walking biomechanics of FAI. Gait Posture. 2009;30(1):41–4.
81. Alradwan HK, Hamel-Smith M, Ayeni OM. Gait and lower extremity kinematic analysis as an outcome measure after femoroacetabular impingement surgery. Arthroscopy. 2015;31(2):339–44.

Evidence-Based Approach to the Nonoperative Management of FAI

6

Nolan S. Horner, Austin E. MacDonald,
Michael Catapano, Darren de SA,
Olufemi R. Ayeni, and Ryan Williams

Contents

N.S. Horner • A.E. MacDonald, MD(Cand)
M. Catapano
Michael G. DeGroote School of Medicine, McMaster University, 1280 Main St W, Hamilton, ON, Canada
e-mail: nolan.horner@medportal.ca

D. de SA, MD
Division of Orthopaedic Surgery, Department of Surgery, McMaster University, Hamilton, Ontario, Canada

O.R. Ayeni, MD, MSc, FRCSC (✉)
Division of Orthopaedic Surgery, Department of Surgery, McMaster University Medical Centre, Hamilton, ON, Canada
e-mail: ayenif@mcmaster.ca

R. Williams
Division of Physical Medicine and Rehabilitation, Department of Medicine, McMaster University, Hamilton, Ontario, Canada
e-mail: ryan.williams@medportal.ca

6.1 Rationale/Introduction

This chapter examines the gamete of non-operative treatment options for the management of femoroacetabular impingement (FAI). Developing an evidence-based approach is made difficult by the virtue of the lack of high-quality literature comparing each option with specific outcome measures. Often, the deformities associated with FAI are structural/mechanical in nature, and elucidating true benefits from nonoperative interventions that fail to address this remains a challenge [13]. Nonoperative approaches are targeted at mitigating the severity of symptomatology, although it is not known if they can be sufficient treatments for long-term relief of symptoms. Not only are there few peer-reviewed studies examining the efficacy of nonoperative treatment [6, 47], but there also exist few studies that evaluate outcomes such as return to sport/physical activity and other patient-important outcomes after nonoperative treatment [6, 47].

O.R. Ayeni et al. (eds.), *Diagnosis and Management of Femoroacetabular Impingement*,
DOI 10.1007/978-3-319-32000-7_6

Studying nonoperative management of FAI is more difficult than studying surgical outcomes, where preoperative and postoperative outcomes can be quantified using biomechanical dimensions as well as patient-completed questionnaires. In contrast, quantifying nonoperative outcomes must be completed using only patient-completed questionnaires as currently there are no objective markers to determine treatment efficacy, and as such it is more difficult to obtain statistical significance using these measures. Additionally, describing and quantifying the "amount" of physiotherapy a patient receives is generally not done in a uniform fashion [23]. This makes comparing studies, or even comparing patients within studies, difficult. Further complicating this picture is that young, active patients tend to prefer definitive surgical options, which could skew both nonoperative management and surgical treatment studies due to possible inclusion bias [23].

Nevertheless, many studies that examine clinical outcomes of patients with FAI recommend a trial of nonoperative management [6, 23]. The reasoning for this is that many patients improve enough to potentially avoid the risks of surgical intervention [14, 23]. This becomes even more important in a health-care system where resources are limited.

Though lacking large, randomized data to support such claim, Emara et al. [14] suggest that one potential benefit for nonoperative approaches remains in its ability to potentially delay or avoid surgical intervention. As well, it is widely believed that together with activity modification, nonoperative management can achieve good early results – and be potentially on par with either arthroscopic or open surgical management [14].

A systematic review of literature pertaining to nonoperative management of FAI, conducted by Wall et al., found five primary research studies that outlined or evaluated nonoperative treatment. Of these five primary research articles, three reported favorable outcomes. Sixty-five percent of all of the studies in this review indicated that nonoperative treatment as initial management was appropriate, with physical therapy and activity modification being the most common nonoperative treatments mentioned (in 48 % and 81 % of studies, respectively). They do warn to interpret the results with caution as the studies they reviewed were often of low-level clinical research and had a limited number of patients [45].

As alluded to earlier, the morphological abnormalities associated with FAI pose a challenge to manage via conservative means. Due to several pain generators and complex pathology in the majority of patients, nonoperative treatments often inadequately address these issues in patients. However, most patients try nonoperative treatment in the hopes of avoiding surgery or mitigating symptoms before resorting to operative intervention. The current evidence published on the multitude of different nonoperative treatments will be discussed here, with specific importance stressed on the evidence-based aspects.

6.2 Physiotherapy and Activity Modification

Physiotherapy and activity modification have been proposed as alternative nonoperative methods for managing FAI. Activity modification involves instructing patients to limit their activities to within their pain-free range of motion, to discontinue sport, to perform any activities of daily living with minimal friction, and/or to rest [14, 23, 42].

The goals of physiotherapy in the management of FAI can be to increase the pain-free range of motion (ROM) of the hip, to optimize the balance between muscle strength and length, and to reduce anterior femoral glide [14, 23]. In the literature discussing physiotherapy, there are discrepancies as to the recommended approaches for managing FAI. Many studies emphasize muscle strengthening (core, hip flexor, gluteus maximus) as the key component of physiotherapy [28, 35, 42]. Other literature also recommends that physiotherapy include stretches to address hip flexor and other generalized hip muscle tightness [22, 31]. Of note, however, few studies do exist suggesting that stretching may increase passive ROM and consequently worsen symptoms [15, 32].

The use of physiotherapy and activity modification as a modality to increase pain-free range of motion and, subsequently, return to sport has been controversial due to contradicting results of their efficacy. Within the four studies published reporting outcomes after using varying aspects of physiotherapy and activity modification, two found positive results, whereas two others found strikingly opposite results.

Using a stepwise treatment protocol, Hunt et al. [23] found that 11 of 18 patients progressed to eventual surgical intervention without demonstrating any temporary relief or increase of function despite active therapy and decreased activity. In keeping with these findings, 9 of 9 patients with radiographically confirmed FAI studied by Jager et al. continued to experience significant pain and hip dysfunction after a mean follow-up of 16.2 months after both consistent physiotherapy and NSAID use [25]. Although both of these studies reported limited to no efficacy for physiotherapy or activity modification, studies by Feely and Emara show applicability as selective patients obtain appreciable improvement. In the eight National Football League players treated by Feely et al., all eight players with FAI were able to return to play without a surgical intervention; however, there were limited outcomes reported pertaining to pain, ROM, or function [16]. Similarly, Emara et al. demonstrated a positive effect on patient-reported pain with a VAS score decrease from 6 to 2 and a functional increase with HHS of 91 compared to a baseline of 72 in 37 patients with "mild" FAI (alpha angle <60°) treated with both physiotherapy and activity modification over a 25–28-month period [14]. Pain reduction and increase in function were appreciable in most patients, as only 10 continued to have noticeable pain, of which only four opted for a surgical intervention [14].

Despite the contradicting evidence on the utility of physiotherapy and activity modification for FAI, these modalities are generally viewed as harmless, making the possibility of occasional positive outcomes attractive. Due to its non invasive nature and possibility of a good treatment response, 81 % and 48 % of narrative reviews and discussion articles recommend trials of activity modification and physiotherapy, respectively, prior to surgical interventions [45].

Current data from the literature suggests that the management of FAI using physiotherapy and/or activity modification approaches is beneficial for some patients. In some cases, these treatment options may be sufficient to allow athletes to return to sport; however, the current literature lacks evidence-based recommendations on specific activity modifications that can be made by athletes hoping to return to sport. Also, determining the extent of benefit to patients is limited by the quality of the current literature. Due to this, it is difficult to conclude to what extent a patient's improvement can be attributed to physiotherapy or activity modification, as each study uses varying nonsurgical management.

6.3 Nonsteroidal Anti-inflammatory Drugs (NSAIDs)

Many studies that examine nonoperative management of FAI mention the use of NSAIDs [6, 14, 47] and advocate for their use in the nonoperative treatment of FAI. Many of these studies, however, do not focus on NSAID management alone [6, 14, 47] nor do they often describe the dosage or type of NSAID used [6, 47]. This makes it extremely difficult to determine the sole efficacy of NSAIDs as the usefulness seen is confounded by the use of other nonoperative treatments and an inability to determine a dose effect or minimum needed dose.

One study, Emara et al. [14], used diclofenac as part of their nonoperative management program for FAI. They used a dose of 50 mg, twice a day, in combination with avoiding excessive physical activity for 2–4 weeks. This was only the first stage in a four-stage nonoperative management program that also involved physiotherapy, determining a safe ROM to avoid FAI pain, and modification of activities of daily living. While dosing was provided in this case, it was not the only intervention implemented which makes it difficult to determine the beneficial effects of NSAID use. There are also potential issues with patient compliance with medication, given the well-known side effects of NSAID medication (e.g., gastrointestinal ulcer and bleeding).

Although the use of NSAIDs has been supported in multiple studies, none discuss it as a sole intervention, but more as an adjuvant to other nonoperative treatments. As part of a regime, NSAIDs are expected to decrease inflammatory-mediated pain and increase pain-free ROM allowing patients to tolerate symptoms or increase the efficacy of other treatment protocols. However, studies have failed to comment on the associated risks of prolonged NSAID use including hypertension, renal issues, and gastric ulcers which become an important risk given the age and comorbidities of many patients with FAI.

6.4 General Exercise

Exercise in general, be it cardiovascular, strengthening, resistance, etc., is another area to be considered in the nonoperative management of FAI. While physiotherapy and manual therapy are mentioned above and are similar, exercise programs should be considered as well. Often, patients who are being treated for FAI are young and active [6, 34], so exercise programs must be recognized as important in the nonoperative management of FAI.

Due to the mechanical nature of FAI pain, return to physical activity too quickly can reproduce symptoms of impingement. Loudon and Reiman [34] outline an exercise program to allow long-distance runners to return to running after nonoperative therapy. They suggest that, in addition to facility-based rehabilitation (i.e., physiotherapy, athletic therapy), the athlete should not be allowed to run until they have painless hip motion. The athlete should continue to be active but should avoid activities that involve flexion and internal rotation of the hip. Swimming and walking are suggested. When returning to running, they should implement this gradually and should build in appropriate warm-ups and rest. Wright and Hegedus [47] describe an exercise program that combines physiotherapy and home exercise which allowed the patient to improve "95 %" in their pain and functionality from their initial visit.

As previously commented by Hunt et al. and Wall et al. [23, 45], these studies both agree that there is limited data on the subject of exercise in this setting and that more research, including randomized control trials, need to be undertaken to have more clarity on the issue.

6.5 Osteopathic, Chiropractic, Massage, and Manual Therapy

A systematic review of the literature on nonoperative treatment for FAI found that only 2 % (1 article) of the articles recommended osteopathy and chiropractic treatment [45]. Furthermore, to the best of the authors' knowledge, there exists no experimental data on the results obtained from osteopathic or chiropractic treatment of FAI. Chakraverty and Snelling suggest that osteopathic treatment may be effective in symptom control, but it may not be as useful in preventing the recurrence of symptoms [10]. That being said the authors do not specify what osteopathic methods would be useful in the symptom management of FAI and do acknowledge that strong flexing mobilization maneuvers often used by osteopaths may cause further labral injury [10]. Emary suggests that the role of chiropractors in FAI management lies in the diagnosis and timely referral of a patient to an orthopedic surgeon for appropriate treatment given that a chiropractor who attempts to treat the patient through stretching, manipulating, or mobilizing the hip may actually worsen the symptoms [15]. Indeed Clohisy et al. reported in their study that chiropractors represented 5 % of the 220 health-care professionals seen by patients with hip pain later diagnosed to be FAI prior to referral to an orthopedic surgeon [11]. In summary, the usefulness of osteopathic and chiropractic treatment in the management of FAI is unclear, and further clinical evidence is required prior to any recommendation for or against their approaches.

Bizzini et al. mentioned in their paper that massage therapy was useful in temporarily reducing symptoms in five professional ice hockey players diagnosed with FAI. However, all ultimately progressed to requiring surgical management [7]. To the best of the authors' knowledge, there is no other literature that presents primary data on massage and manual therapy in the management of FAI, and therefore, no informed conclusion can be reached on its effectiveness or lack thereof. In keeping, the applicability as a primary intervention does not appear substantiated; however, it may be useful in combination with more active therapies.

Additionally, as with several other musculoskeletal entities, many patients experience associated issues due to compensatory adaptations to function with their illness. These compensatory measures result in additional issues and pain that are not directly caused by the bony deformity of their FAI, but may be amenable to the discussed therapies.

6.6 Intra-articular Injections

6.6.1 Introduction to Intra-articular Injections

Intra-articular injections have become routine practice for several different musculoskeletal entities; however, their utility and efficacy for FAI remain debatable. Little high-quality evidence has been published, testing the efficacy of intra-articular hip injections to support or refute the use of injections such as hyaluronic acid (HA) or corticosteroid. As such, the decision to implement this is often left to individual physicians and their discussions with patients.

Although a lack of high-level evidence exists, 10 % of review articles published support the use of intra-articular injection of corticosteroids, and none comment on the use of HA based upon the authors' own clinical experience and opinion [45]. Despite the limited evidence, the possibility of injectates acting as a "bridging" agent to allow patients to function at relatively high levels until surgery or in combination with other nonoperative treatments remains attractive. In addition to this, intra-articular injections allow for local treatments which mitigate systemic side effects compared with oral medications and perhaps are an appealing avenue for patients who are not surgical candidates.

6.6.2 Theory

HA is a naturally synthesized glycosaminoglycan produced by host synovial cells, fibroblasts, and chondrocytes and secreted into the synovial fluid. As a major component of articular cartilage, it assists in inhibiting articular erosion [2] and maintaining smooth joint movement [8]. Therefore, theoretically, HA supplementation assists in maintaining articular cartilage and smooth joint movement. The predisposition to osteoarthritis in patients with FAI may be amenable to HA supplementation as it is expected to help prevent the erosion of articular cartilage [46]. More importantly for FAI, the enhanced viscosity and elastic nature of synovial fluid with HA supplementation [5] decrease stress and friction within the joint [18]. These decreased stress and friction translate to decreased pressure on the acetabulum and femoral head which assists in limiting progression of cartilage degradation and bony formation [5]. Ultimately, this may – at least theoretically – lead to less impingement and pain.

Secondary effects of HA include reduction of synovial inflammation [21, 36] and analgesic activity [19, 43] within the joint. As previously demonstrated, an inflammatory reaction is initiated due to the improper bone-to-bone contact resulting in synovial inflammation cascaded by inflammatory cytokines, free radicals, and proteolytic enzymes [5, 20]. In this setting there is impaired HA function in the joint [5, 20]. HA supplementation is suggested to reduce synovial inflammation by reducing the synthesis of inflammatory cytokines and indirectly reducing pain by breaking the inflammatory cascade. As well HA supplementation appears to decrease the synthesis of bradykinin and substance P and inhibit nocireceptors directly which assist in pain modification [17, 19, 43]. Based on this mechanism, the clinician may consider this option as part of his or her armamentarium.

Corticosteroid primarily addresses the inflammatory aspect of FAI, reducing pain and inflammation; however, it is not believed to have a disease-modifying effect. The mechanism of action of corticosteroids is complex, but ultimately has both an anti-inflammatory and immunosuppressive effect 3–10 days after injection [12, 26, 39]. Corticosteroids inhibit accumulation of inflammatory cells, phagocytosis, production of neutrophil superoxide, metalloprotease, and metalloprotease activator and prevent the synthesis and secretion of several inflammatory mediators such as prostaglandin and leukotrienes [26, 39]. Elimination of inflammatory mediators and general decrease in inflammation typically result in pain relief which allows increased function due to reduction of secondary pain inhibition of movement [12, 26, 39]. However, the use of corticosteroids has its limits, with evidence suggesting that one should limit injections to once every 3 months and no more than 3 a year to keep adverse effects minimal [9, 38]. With the majority of corticosteroid injections, there is local anesthetic introduced into the joint as well to increase the diagnostic applicability of the injection. The conventional belief is that intra-articular pain generators should be temporary relieved for the duration of the anesthetic action [4]. This allows physicians to better understand where the source of pain is and whether there is truly an intra-articular lesion that needs to be addressed.

6.6.3 Evidence-Based Medicine

Currently there has been a single level IV study focused on the effectiveness of intra-articular HA injections for FAI performed by Abate el al. [1]. This study focuses on using a visual analog score (VAS), Harris Hip Score (HHS), Lequesne index, and anti-inflammatory consumption at 6 and 12 months to determine if HA injections at baseline and 40 days, with the same dosing schedule at 6 months, were efficacious in 23 hips with FAI. Of note, VAS decreased from 6.7 ± 1.3 to 3.7 ± 1.8 to 1.7 ± 1.8 after 6 and 12 months, respectively. As well there was statistically significant improvement in HHS, Lequesne index, and anti-inflammatory consumption [1]. Globally, HA seems to be a promising nonoperative treatment as it was effective in their patient population with no long-term adverse effects. However, more supporting evidence needs to become available before the use of HA becomes a routine nonoperative treatment for FAI [1].

Similarly, there is a lack of research about the efficacy of corticosteroid to determine its usefulness in patients with FAI. Currently, there has been one level IV study looking at 54 patients with MRI-confirmed CAM or pincer lesions treated with intra-articular corticosteroid injections. Patients were injected with corticosteroid plus local anesthetic and tested at baseline, postinjection during the anesthetic period, and 14 days and 6 weeks postinjection. Postinjection scores during the anesthetic period decreased significantly from baseline; however, only 20 patients (37 %) and three patients (6 %) reported a clinically significant decrease in pain at 14 days and 6 weeks, respectively [30]. In contrast, a case series with three patients has shown variable positive results with intra-articular injections. However, these patients also used a variety of nonoperative treatments without any control group to determine the effect of confounders. As such, it is difficult to determine the specific effect of cortisone [40]. Current evidence is inconclusive for the use of corticosteroid for extended relief; however, there appears to be potential for diagnostic use and short-term relief.

It has been previously discussed that depending on the associated pathology and type of FAI, certain interventions, HA and corticosteroid, should have a larger or diminished effect. Despite the biological plausibility associated with these theories, there exists no clinical trial evaluating whether there is a difference in efficacy depending upon the variation of FAI. As with the majority of evidence relating to intra-articular injections for FAI, more information needs to be gathered to generate helpful clinical practice guidelines.

Although corticosteroid has yet to produce results that would make it routine practice for nonoperative treatment of FAI, some surgeons continue to use it solely based upon its diagnostic ability [3]. The majority of orthopedic surgeons treating FAI have yet to accept this protocol; however, recently there has been evidence to demonstrate its utility. Ayeni et al. have shown that a negative response to intra-articular injections with anesthetic seems to predict a higher likelihood of having a negative result from surgery with a negative likelihood ratio of 0.57 [4]. In contrast, significant pain relief after injection does not appear to predict good surgical results (1.15 positive likelihood ratio). Previous research demonstrates that diagnostic intra-articular hip injections are most commonly positive in patients with chondral damage with the severity of FAI and labral pathology not influencing pain relief [29]. This may lead us to believe that those without chondral damage and a negative diagnostic injection would be best treated with initial trial of nonoperative treatment.

Although intra-articular injections are considered benign inventions, there is a low risk of complications. Most studies quote a risk of 1 in 10,000 to a 1 in 200,000 risk of local bleeding, local nerve irritation, and allergic reaction to injectates or intra-articular injections [24]. All complications, excluding intra-articular infections, have been found to be self-limiting and resolve without the necessity for intervention. However septic arthritis has an associated morbidity which requires specific attention by the patient and physician. Additionally, there has been discussion of increased risk of infection if subsequent operative management is undertaken within a short time frame (less than 3 months). This has yet to be proven with recent evidence demonstrating no association between intra-articular injectates of corticosteroid and postoperative infections [37].

It has not escaped notice that there exists no conclusive evidence on the recommended doses of either corticosteroid or HA to inject.

6.6.4 Injection Technique

Intra-articular hip injections are performed under ultrasound or fluoroscopic guidance to ensure that important neurovascular structures are avoided and confirm intra-articular placement of injectate. Although both methods allow for confirmation of intra-articular placement [41, 44] which accounts for the unreliability of needle tip placement seen using a landmark-based approach [33], ultrasound guidance has become the preferred method over fluoroscopic guided injections despite being technician dependent. Ultrasound has become the preferred method most notably for its ability to allow an anterior approach which avoids chondral damage and has no associated radiation [44].

Under sterile conditions the patient is placed in the supine position with the hip flat and in neutral. Using ultrasound guidance, the patient is scanned starting at the inguinal crease with a curvilinear probe in an oblique position. Visualization of the femoral artery (and nerve) ensures its protection. The probe is then advanced inferiorly until the acetabulum and femoral head are identified, at which point the probe is rotated 90° to show the femoral head and neck junction in profile. It is in this head-neck junction or anterior recess where injectate is administered. The anterior recess remains the easiest access point as it avoids vital structures and avoids damage to the articular cartilage done by needle scuffing of the chondral surface. Using an in-plane technique, a spinal needle is advanced into the joint and injectates can be delivered under direct visualization. The physical examination is repeated postinjection to assess efficacy [27].

Conclusion

The applicability of nonoperative management in the treatment of FAI remains debatable due to limited evidence and a limited ability to address the bony deformities which cause FAI. The most promising interventions continue to be intra-articular injections, specifically those with hyaluronic acid, which have the most biological plausibility to reduce pain and bone-to-bone contact. Results after intra-articular injections of corticosteroid have not been as promising, though they remain widely employed as a diagnostic procedure to determine the proportion of pain generated by intra-articular sources. Beyond these interventions, only physiotherapy with activity modification has been considered as an option for FAI due to its non invasive manner and potential for benefit. Many authors agree with the suggestion of adjuncts to one or a combination of the therapies previously mentioned. These adjuncts include oral NSAID use, exercise, and osteopathic, chiropractic, massage, and manual therapy.

Despite the debate of its efficacy, the applicability of nonoperative management in an algorithm for the treatment of FAI cannot be refuted due to the limited side-effect profile and the chronic and non-progressing nature of FAI which often does not require urgent surgical treatment. Most authors suggest exhausting or trialing several different nonoperative measures before resorting to operative management. Currently, these modalities allow patients to work within and expand their pain-free ROM with the hope of increasing functionality as well as relieving pain.

Take-Home Points

1. Non operative management is an important consideration for the management of FAI but evidence is limited for the best regime.
2. A combined approach using oral NSAIDS, activity modification, physical therapy, and injections is the best strategy based on current evidence.
3. Non operative modalities should be catered to the patients capabilities, function and pain levels.
4. Current evidence is limited on specific strategies but emerging research will clarify best treatment options.

Key Evidence Related Sources

1. Ayeni OR, Farrokhyar F, Crouch S, Chan K, Sprague S, Bhandari M. Pre-operative intra-articular hip injection as a predictor of short-term outcome following arthroscopic management of femoroacetabular impingement. Knee Surg Sports Traumatol Arthrosc. 2014;22:801–5.
2. Clohisy JC, Knaus ER, Hunt DM, Lesher JM, Harris Hayes M, Prather H. Clinical presentation of patients with symptomatic anterior hip impingement. Clin Orthop Relat Res. 2009;467(3):638–44.
3. Hunt D, Prather H, Harris Hayes M, Clohisy JC. Clinical outcomes analysis of conservative and surgical treatment of patients with clinical indications of prearthritic, intra-articular hip disorders. PM R. 2012;4(7):479–87
4. Wall PD, Fernandez M, Griffin DR, Foster NE. Nonoperative treatment for femoroacetabular impingement: a systematic review of the literature. PM R. 2013;5(5):418–26

References

1. Abate M, Scuccimarra T, Vanni D, Pantalone A, Salini V. Femoroacetabular impingement: is hyaluronic acid effective? Knee Surg Sports Traumatol Arthrosc. 2014;22:889–92.
2. Axe JM, Snyder-Mackler L, Axe MJ. The role of viscosupplementation. Sports Med Arthrosc. 2013;21:18–22.
3. Ayeni OR, Belzile EL, Musahl V, Naudie D, Crouch S, Sprague S, Bhandari M. Results of the PeRception of femOroaCetabular impingement by Surgeons Survey (PROCESS). Knee Surg Sports Traumatol Arthrosc. 2014;22:906–10.
4. Ayeni OR, Farrokhyar F, Crouch S, Chan K, Sprague S, Bhandari M. Pre-operative intra-articular hip injection as a predictor of short-term outcome following arthroscopic management of femoroacetabular impingement. Knee Surg Sports Traumatol Arthrosc. 2014;22:801–5.
5. Balazs EA, Denlinger JL. Viscosupplementation: a new concept in the treatment of osteoarthritis. J Rheumatol Suppl. 1993;39:3–9.

6. Bedi A, Kelly BT. Femoroacetabular Impingement. J Bone Joint Surg Am. 2013;95(1):82–92.
7. Bizzini M, Notzil HP, Maffiuletti NA. Femoroacetabular impingement in professional Ice hockey players: a case series of 5 athletes after open surgical decompression of the hip. Am J Sports Med. 2007;35(11):1955–9.
8. Brockmeier SF, Shaffer BS. Viscosupplementation therapy for osteoarthritis. Sports Med Arthrosc. 2006;14:155–62.
9. Caldwell JR. Intra-articular corticosteroids. Guide to selection and indications for use. Drugs. 1996;52:507–14.
10. Chakraverty JK, Snelling NJ. Anterior hip pain – have you considered femoroacetabular impingement? Int J Osteopat Med. 2012;15:22–7.
11. Clohisy JC, Knaus ER, Hunt DM, Lesher JM, Harris Hayes M, Prather H. Clinical presentation of patients with symptomatic anterior hip impingement. Clin Orthop Relat Res. 2009;467(3):638–44.
12. Creamer P. Intra-articular corticosteroid treatment in osteoarthritis. Curr Opin Rheumatol. 1999;11: 417–21.
13. Dolan MM, Heyworth BE, Bedi A, Duke G, Kelly BT. CT reveals a high incidence of osseous abnormalities in hips with labral tears. Clin Orthop Relat Res. 2011;469(3):831–8. Epub 2010 Oct 1.
14. Emara K, Samir W, el Motasem H, Ghafar KA. Conservative treatment for mild femoroacetabular impingement. J Orthop Surg (Hong Kong). 2011;19(1):41–5.
15. Emary P. Femoroacetabular impingement syndrome: a narrative review for the chiropractor. J Can Chiropr Assoc. 2010;54(3):164–76.
16. Feeley BT, Powell JW, Muller MS, Barnes RP, Warren RF, Kelly BT. Hip injuries and labral tears in the national football league. Am J Sports Med. 2008;36(11):2187–95.
17. Ghosh P. The role of hyaluronic acid (hyaluronan) in health and disease: interactions with cells, cartilage and components of synovial fluid. Clin Exp Rheumatol. 1994;12:75–82.
18. Goa KL, Benfield P. Hyaluronic acid. A review of its pharmacology and use as a surgical aid in ophthalmology, and its therapeutic potential in joint disease and wound healing. Drugs. 1994;47:536–66.
19. Gomis A, Miralles A, Schmidt RF, Belmonte C. Intra-articular injections of hyaluronan solutions of different elastoviscosity reduce nociceptive nerve activity in a model of osteoarthritic knee joint of the guinea pig. Osteoarthritis Cartilage. 2009;17:798–804.
20. Greenwald RA. Oxygen radicals, inflammation, and arthritis: pathophysiological considerations and implications for treatment. Semin Arthritis Rheum. 1991;20:219–40 [PubMed].
21. Guidolin DD, Ronchetti IP, Lini E, Guerra D, Frizziero L. Morphological analysis of articular cartilage biopsies from a randomized, clinical study comparing the effects of 500–730 kDa sodium hyaluronate (Hyalgan) and methylprednisolone acetate on primary osteoarthritis of the knee. Osteoarthritis Cartilage. 2001;9:371–81.
22. Hart E, Metkar U, Rebello G, Grottkau B. Femoroacetabular impingement in adolescents and young adults. Orthop Nurs. 2009;28(3):117–24.
23. Hunt D, Prather H, Harris Hayes M, Clohisy JC. Clinical outcomes analysis of conservative and surgical treatment of patients with clinical indications of prearthritic, intra-articular hip disorders. PM R. 2012;4(7):479–87.
24. Hunter JA, Blyth TH. A risk-benefit assessment of intra-articular corticosteroids in rheumatic disorders. Drug Saf. 1999;21(5):353–65.
25. Jager M, Wild A, Westhoff B, Krauspe R. Femoroacetabular impingement caused by a femoral osseous head-neck bump deformity: clinical, radiological, and experimental results. J Orthop Sci. 2004;9(3):256–63.
26. Jessar RA, Ganzell MA, Ragan C. The action of hydrocortisone in synovial inflammation. J Clin Invest. 1953;32:480–2.
27. Kantarci F, Ozbayrak M, Gulsen F, Gencturk M, Botanlioglu H, Mihmanli I. Ultrasound-guided injection for MR arthrography of the hip: comparison of two different techniques. Skeletal Radiol. 2013;42:37–42.
28. Kaplan K, Shah M, Youm T. Femoroacetabular impingement: diagnosis and treatment. Bull NYU Hosp Jt Dis. 2010;68(2):70–5.
29. Kivlan BR, Martin RL, Sekiya JK. Response to diagnostic injection in patients with femoroacetabular impingement, labral tears, chondral lesions, and extra-articular pathology. Arthroscopy. 2011;27.
30. Krych AJ, Griffith TB, Hudgens JL, Kuzma SA, Sierra RL, Levy BA. Limited therapeutic benefits of intra-articular cortisone injection for patients with femoro-acetabular impingement and labral tear. Knee Surg Sports Traumatol Arthrosc. 2014;22: 750–5.
31. Kuhlman G, Domb B. Hip impingement: identifying and treating a common cause of hip pain. Am Fam Physician. 2009;80(12):1429–34.
32. Lavigne M, Parvizi J, Beck M, Siebenrock KA, Ganz R, Leunig M. Anterior femoroacetabular impingement: part I. Techniques of joint preserving surgery. Clin Orthop Relat Res. 2004;418:61–6.
33. Leopold S, Battista V, Oliverio JA. Safety and efficacy of intraarticular hip injection using anatomic landmarks. Clin Orthop Relat Res. 2001;391:192–7.
34. Loudon JK, Reiman MP. Conservative management of femoroacetabular impingement (FAI) in the long distance runner. Phys Ther Sport. 2014;15:82–90.
35. Maheshwari A, Malik A, Dorr L. Impingement of the native hip joint. J Bone Joint Surg Am. 2007;89(11):2508–18.
36. Maneiro E, de Andres MC, Fernández-Sueiro JL, Galdo F, Blanco FJ. The biological action of hyaluronan on human osteoartritic articular chondrocytes: the importance of molecular weight. Clin Exp Rheumatol. 2004;22:307–12.

37. McMahnon SE, Laroux JA, Smith TO, Hing CB. Total joint arthroplasty following intra-articular steroid injection; a literature review. Acta Orthop Belg. 2013;70:672–9.
38. Noyes FR, Grood ES, Nussbaum NS, Cooper SM. Effect of intra-articular corticosteroids on ligament properties: a biomechanical and histological study in rhesus knees. Clin Orthop Relat Res. 1977;123:197–209.
39. Ostergaard M, Halberg P. Intra-articular corticosteroids in arthritic disease: a guide to treatment. BioDrugs. 1998;9:95–103.
40. Park JS, Eun Jang YE, Nahm FS, Lee PB, Choi EJ. Efficacy of intra-articular steroid injection in patients with femoroacetabular impingement. Korean J Pain. 2013;26:154–9.
41. Pateder DB, Hungerford MW. Use of fluoroscopically guided intra-articular hip injection in differentiating the pain source in concomitant hip and lumbar spine arthritis. Am J Orthop. 2007;36:591–3.
42. Pollard TC. A perspective on femoroacetabular impingement. Skelet Radiol. 2011;40(7):815–8.
43. Pozo MA, Balazs EA, Belmonte C. Reduction of sensory responses to passive movements of inflamed knee joints by hylan, a hyaluronan derivative. Exp Brain Res. 1997;116:3–9 [PubMed].
44. Smith J, Hurdle MF. Office-based ultrasound-guided intra-articular hip injection: technique for physiatric practice. Arch Phys Med Rehabil. 2006;87:296–8.
45. Wall PD, Fernandez M, Griffin DR, Foster NE. Nonoperative treatment for femoroacetabular impingement: a systematic review of the literature. PM R. 2013;5(5):418–26.
46. Wobig M, Bach G, Beks P, Dickhut A, Runzheimer J, Schwieger G, Vetter G, Balazs E. The role of elastoviscosity in the efficacy of viscosupplementation for osteoarthritis of the knee: a comparison of hylan G-F 20 and a lower-molecular-weight hyaluronan. Clin Ther. 1999;21:1549–62.
47. Wright AA, Hegedus EJ. Augmented home exercise program for a 37-year-old female with a clinical presentation of femoroacetabular impingement. Man Ther. 2012;17:358–63.

Physiology of the Developing Hip and Pathogenesis of Femoroacetabular Impingement

7

Páll Sigurgeir Jónasson, Olufemi R. Ayeni, Jón Karlsson, Mikael Sansone, and Adad Baranto

Contents

P.S. Jónasson (✉) • J. Karlsson • M. Sansone
A. Baranto
Department of Orthopaedics,
Sahlgrenska Academy, University of Gothenburg,
Gothenburg, Sweden
e-mail: pallsj@gmail.com; jon.karlsson@telia.com; mikael.sansone@gmail.com; adad.baranto@vgregion.se

O.R. Ayeni
Division of Orthopaedic Surgery, Department of Surgery, McMaster University Medical Centre,
1200 Main Street West, 4E15,
Hamilton, ON L8N 3Z5, Canada
e-mail: ayenif@mcmaster.ca

7.1 Bone Growth

Bone development occurs through either intramembranous ossification (mesenchymal or connective tissue) or enchondral ossification, where bone is formed from hyaline cartilage. The flat bones of the skull and the mandible, maxilla and clavicles are formed by intramembranous ossification. The long bones and spine and most of the other bones of the axial skeleton are formed by enchondral ossification. In this chapter, the growth and development of the hip, particularly the proximal femur, is reviewed as well as the pathways for the development of adaptive bony changes leading to FAI.

7.1.1 Physiology of Bone Growth

All the long bones of a growing individual consist of an epiphysis, physis, metaphysis and diaphysis (Fig. 7.1).

The diaphysis is the primary centre of ossification. It grows circumferentially through appositional growth by the deposition of bone beneath the periosteum, but it does not grow longitudinally. The diaphysis is composed of lamellar bone with a strong cortical exterior.

The metaphysis is composed of spongious, trabecular bone with a thin layer of exterior cortical bone. It connects the diaphysis with the adjacent physis.

O.R. Ayeni et al. (eds.), *Diagnosis and Management of Femoroacetabular Impingement*,
DOI 10.1007/978-3-319-32000-7_7

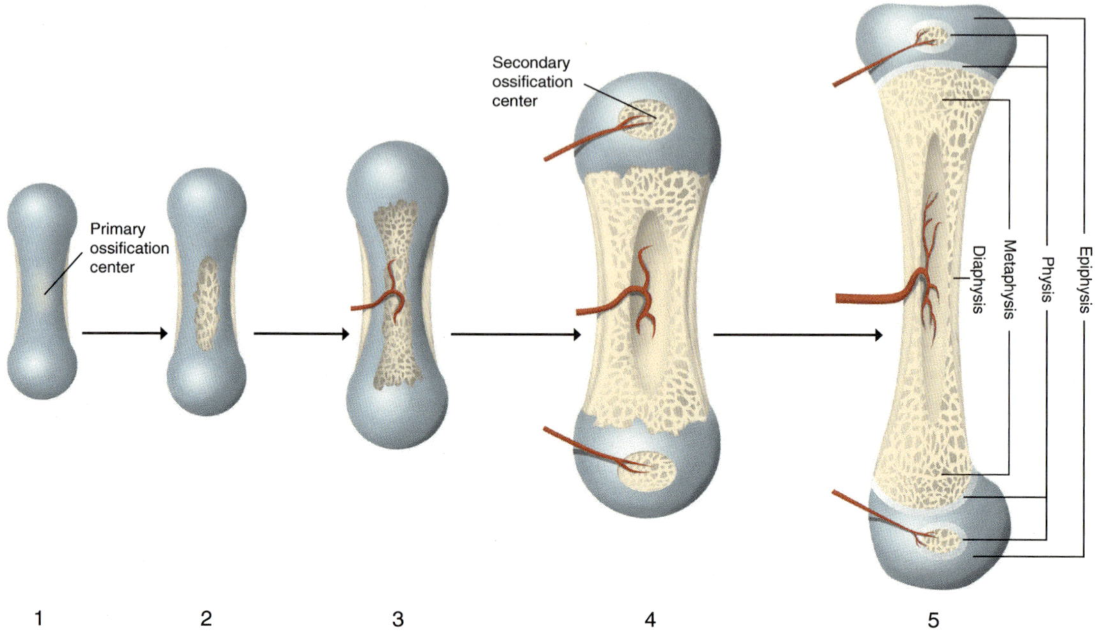

Fig. 7.1 All the long bones in the body are formed by enchondral ossification, where a bone collar is formed around a hyaline cartilage model and a primary ossification centre forms inside the model (*1*). The cartilage matrix deteriorates (*2*) and spongious bone in formed (*3*). The secondary ossification centre forms in the epiphysis and is invaded by an epiphyseal artery (*4*). After ossification of the epiphyses, hyaline cartilage only remains in the epiphyseal plates and the articular cartilage. The long bone now consists of an epiphysis, physis, metaphysis and diaphysis (*5*)

The epiphysis is located on top of the physis and forms an articulation with the adjacent bone. Almost all epiphyses contain one or more secondary ossification centres. These ossification centres grow spherically by enchondral ossification and are responsible for less than 5 % of the bone growth in length.

The physis forms a discoid structure between the metaphysis and epiphysis. It is often referred to as the epiphyseal plate/line or growth plate/line. More than 95 % of longitudinal growth of long bones occurs in the physis. When visualised under a microscope, it is a complex structure, with its cellular anatomy defined into different layers or zones (Fig. 7.2). In the *resting zone* (also called the germinal or reserve zone) on the epiphyseal side, the stem cells accumulate and the storage of nutrients occurs. In the adjacent *proliferative zone*, the stem cells divide and differentiate into chondrocytes, oriented in columns (sometimes called the columnar zone). The chondrocytes then enlarge in size to form the hypertrophic zone. In the *hypertrophic zone*, the chondrocytes show increased metabolic activity and go into apoptosis and die. The dead chondrocytes are invaded by vascular channels from the metaphysis and the mineralisation of the intercellular matrix occurs in the *calcification zone*.

The physis is avascular, receiving oxygen and nutrients at its periphery from epiphyseal and metaphyseal vessels. Small branches from the epiphyseal arteries pass through the resting zone and terminate at the top of the proliferative zone. On the metaphyseal side, the interosseous artery and metaphyseal arteries combine and form loops that penetrate into the zone of calcification and the hypertrophic zone, bringing nutrition to osteoprogenitor cells producing bone in the cartilage matrix scaffold [5–7, 18, 27, 37, 44, 48, 55].

At the periphery of the physis (the periphysis), the zone of Ranvier is responsible for the horizontal growth of the physis and the perichondrial ring (ring of La Croix) provides mechanical stability to the physis [45]. In the proximal femur, the perichondrial fibrocartilaginous complex replaces the zone of Ranvier and the ring of La

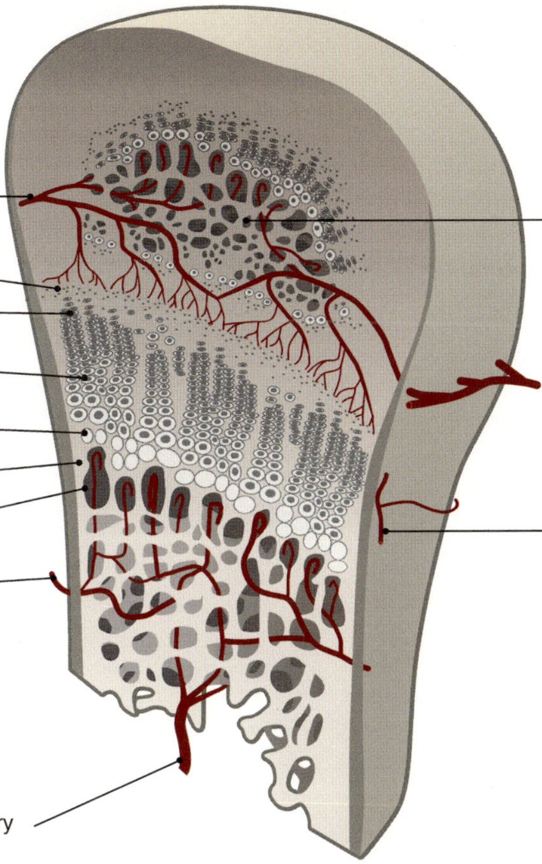

Fig. 7.2 The physis is avascular, but oxygen and nutrients arrive from the epiphyseal and metaphyseal arteries. At the periphery, the blood supply comes from periosteal arteries. Its cellular anatomy is defined into different layers or zones

Croix [11] (Fig. 7.3). Branches from a periosteal artery supply the zone of Ranvier.

7.2 Acetabular Development

During development the acetabulum is formed from the interposition of the os pubis, os ilium and the os ischium, forming a triradiate cartilage complex. Interstitial bone growth in the triradiate cartilage complex causes the acetabulum to expand during growth. The presence of a spherical femoral head leads to the concavity of the acetabulum. At puberty, three secondary centres of ossification form around the acetabular cavity, one from each epiphyses of the os pubis, os ilium and os ischium. The secondary ossification centre of the os pubis, sometimes referred to as the os acetabuli, forms the anterior wall of the acetabulum. The secondary ossification centre of the os ilium and os ischium form the superior and posterior wall of the acetabulum, respectively. They expand towards the periphery of the acetabulum and thus contribute to its depth. The physes of the triradiate cartilage complex close at around the age of 15–18 years [42, 43].

7.3 Proximal Femoral Bone Growth

The previously described fundamentals of bone growth and physeal anatomy apply to the proximal femur with certain modifications. At birth, the cartilaginous epiphysis forms the femoral head and greater trochanter that have the same shape as in an adult. The epiphysis is supported by a curved physis. With physeal growth, the

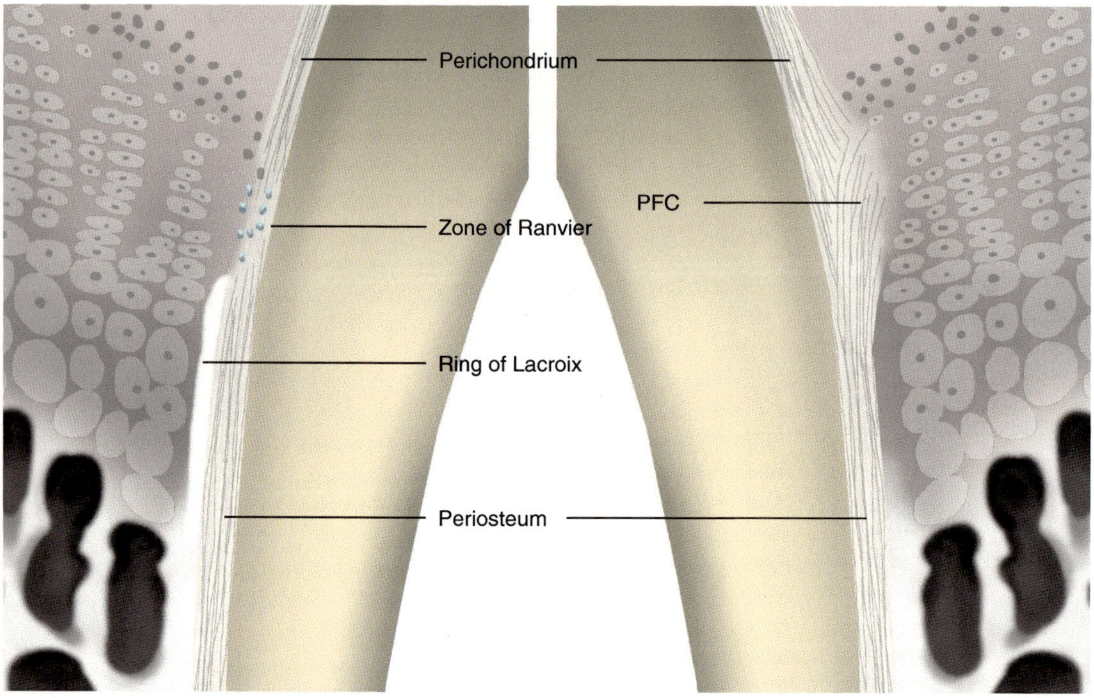

Fig. 7.3 In the proximal femur, the zone of Ranvier and ring of La Croix are replaced by the perichondrial fibrocartilaginous complex

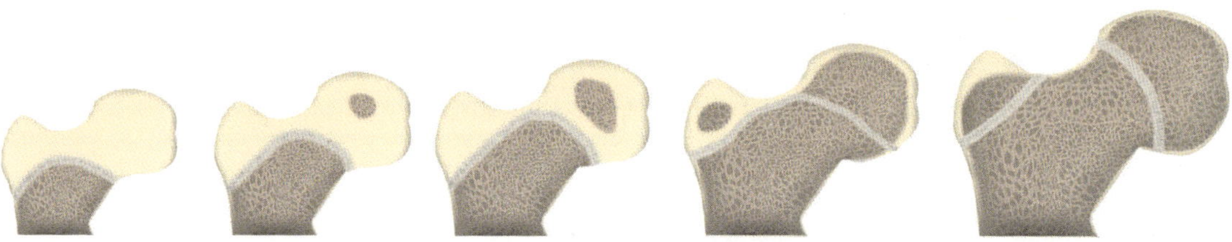

Fig. 7.4 At birth, the cartilaginous epiphysis forms the femoral head and greater trochanter. With physeal growth, the epiphysis divides into the femoral head epiphysis and the greater trochanter apophysis

epiphysis divides into the femoral head epiphysis and the greater trochanter apophysis (Fig. 7.4) [34, 38].

Blood supply to the proximal femoral physis changes during growth. Arteries in the ligamentum teres supplement the epiphyseal blood supply but only during the first 3–4 years. Between 4 and 7 years of age, the anterior half of the physis receives blood supply from the lateral circumflex artery and the posterior half from the medial circumflex artery. Eventually, after the age of 7 years, the blood supply to the femoral head is received mainly from branches of the medial circumflex artery. The posteroinferior artery supplies the inferior portion of the femoral head, while the posterosuperior artery travels in the intertrochanteric groove and supplies the superior portion of the femoral head. Both arteries traverse the physis superficially, leaving them vulnerable to damage if the femoral neck or physis is fractured (Fig. 7.5). Even though the proximal femoral physis is one of the least injured long-bone physes, the vulnerable blood supply leads to a high complication rate (such as avascular necrosis) when injuries occur [10, 13, 38, 55, 60, 61].

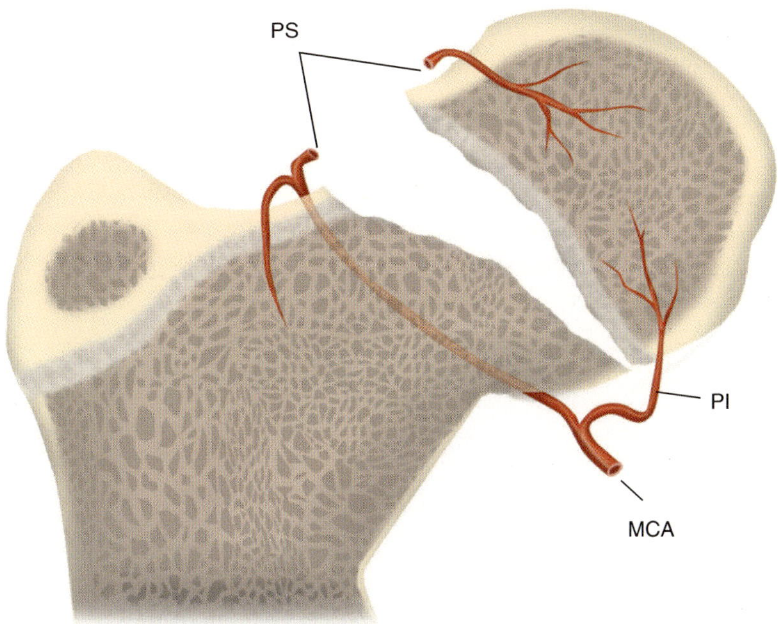

Fig. 7.5 Eventually, the blood supply to the femoral head is received from the posteroinferior (*PI*) and the posterosuperior (*PS*) branches of the medial circumflex artery (*MCA*). Both arteries traverse the physis superficially, leaving them vulnerable to damage if the femoral neck or physis is fractured

Closure of the proximal femoral physis begins superolaterally and continues inferomedially. Complete closure typically occurs in half of 14-year-old females and 17-year-old males [15, 17].

The microscopic anatomy of the proximal femoral physis differs slightly from what is seen in other physes, with the zone of Ranvier and ring of La Croix replaced by the perichondrial fibrocartilaginous complex [11]. The presence of a bony peg on the underside of the epiphysis projecting down into a socket on the metaphysis has also been described. In the literature, it is referred to as the 'epiphyseal tubercle' and it is believed to be an important stabiliser of the epiphysis [30, 53, 54] (Fig. 7.6).

7.4 Factors Affecting Bone Growth

The mechanisms controlling physeal growth are not well known. Factors known to influence physeal growth can be divided into general factors, which can affect many or all physes, and local factors, affecting only a single physis. Genetics, nutrition, hormones and general health are examples of general factors. Local factors include blood supply, mechanical forces, traumatic injuries and infection. In this section we will focus on how local factors affect bone growth.

7.4.1 Mechanical Forces

A certain physiological load is needed for normal bone growth [33]. The effect of load on bone growth can be summarised in two laws.

Heuter-Volkmann's Law establishes that physeal growth is retarded by increased load and accelerated by decreased load. This leads to the physis aligning itself perpendicularly to the force applied and usually at a right angle to the longitudinal axis of the bone [23].

Wolff's Law proposes that the bone in a healthy individual will adapt to the loads under which it is placed. Under increased load, the bone becomes stronger and thicker through appositional growth, while a reduced load leads to weakening of the bone. A fracture of a long bone that heals in an angulated manner therefore has a tendency to straighten when a

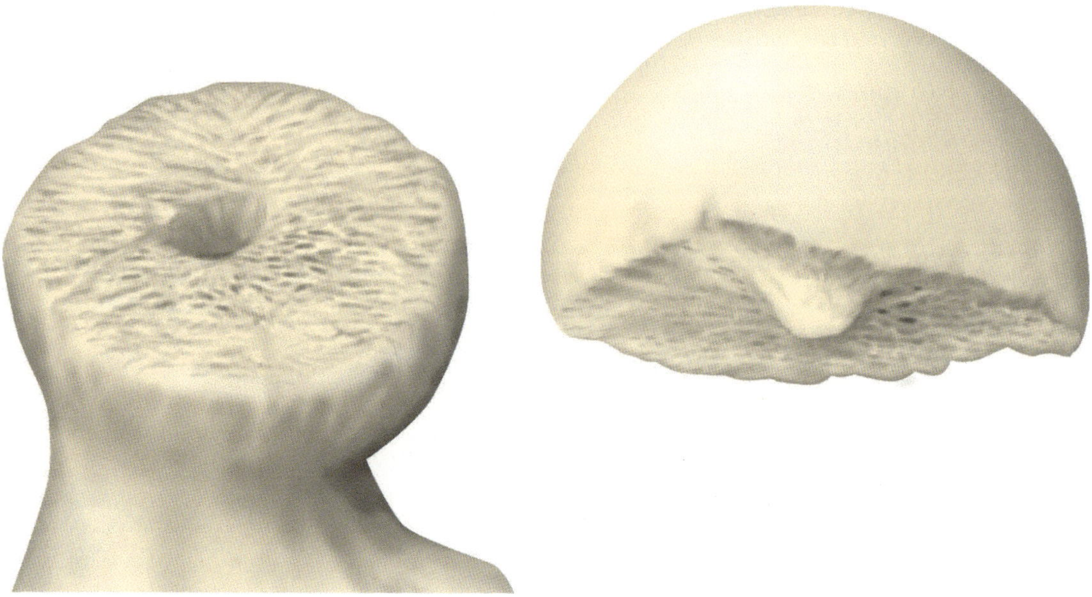

Fig. 7.6 The epiphyseal tubercle projects down into a socket on the metaphysis

load is applied because of increased appositional bone growth on the concave side of the fracture [62].

7.4.2 Blood Supply Disturbance

Compromised blood supply disturbs physeal growth, but the way this happens depends on the supply route that is affected.

If the blood supply from the metaphyseal side is compromised, the vascular loops stop invading the hypertrophic zone and the cells in the hypertrophic zone accumulate. The cells in the resting and proliferating zone receive blood supply from the epiphyseal vessels and continue to grow. Longitudinal growth therefore continues and the physis widens in the affected area.

In the event of a diminished blood supply through the epiphyseal vessels, cells in the resting and proliferating zones are deprived of oxygen and nutrients. Longitudinal growth ceases in the affected area, but the vascular loops continue invading the hypertrophic zone and the physis narrows. If only a portion of the physis is affected, the rest of the physis continues to grow and angular deformities occur [25, 56–59] (Fig. 7.7).

7.4.3 Trauma

Fractures in and around the physis also affect growth, most probably through disruption in blood flow. Hefti et al. [22] described four types of growth disturbance following fractures in children (Table 7.1).

The exact reason why overgrowth of the physis occurs following a fracture is unclear. One possible explanation is the increase in blood flow following healing of the fracture.

Physiolysis or fracture/physiolysis most often leads to diminished growth or, in the worst case, complete growth cessation. If the injury is confined to the cellular columns or hypertrophic zone of the physis and the epiphyseal blood supply is intact, normal growth usually resumes.

Table 7.1 The four types of growth disturbance seen following fractures in children according to Hefti et al. [22]

Type 1	Increased growth in the whole physis
Type 2	Decreased growth in the whole physis or complete growth arrest
Type 3	Increased growth in part of the physis, creating angular deformation
Type 4	Asymmetrical growth arrest, with the formation of a bone bridge

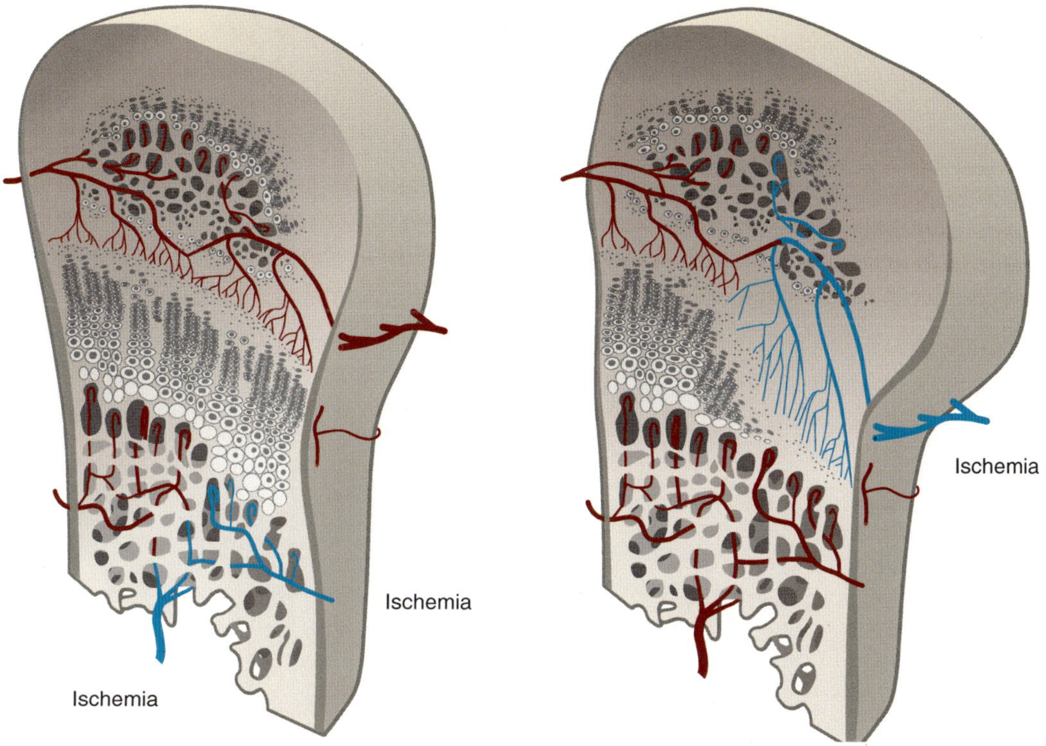

Fig. 7.7 A compromised blood supply on the metaphyseal side causes the continued growth and widening of the physis, but growth cessation and narrowing of the physis occurs if the blood supply is compromised on the epiphyseal side

7.4.4 Infection

Growth disturbances due to infections are due either to the direct destruction of the physis or, secondarily, to disturbed blood supply leading to decreased growth in the whole or part of the physis.

7.5 Bone Development and FAI

Knowledge of growth disturbances and chronic physeal damage to the upper and lower extremities and the spine of adolescent elite athletes is well established [4, 8, 16, 31, 32, 50].

The pincer deformity is a local or global overcoverage of the femoral head by the acetabulum leading to linear contact between the acetabular rim and the femoral head-neck junction. Pincer impingement seems to be more common in females [52].

The aetiology of the pincer deformity is unknown. Factors reported as affecting the development of the acetabulum are congenital instability of the hip and epiphyseal fractures of the triradiate cartilage complex. When acetabular development is affected in these cases, acetabular dysplasia usually occurs [12, 29, 40]. There is currently limited knowledge on factors that may predispose individuals to develop pincer-type deformities of the acetabulum.

The CAM deformity is a nonspherical shape of the femoral head at the femoral head-neck junction. It usually resides on the antero-superior surface and leads to a reduced offset of the femoral head and neck junction with resultant abutment of the head-neck junction against the acetabular rim, causing FAI (Fig. 7.8).

The aetiology of the CAM deformity is still not completely known. Theories, including evolutionary changes [24], genetic factors [41], abnormal ossification of the proximal femur

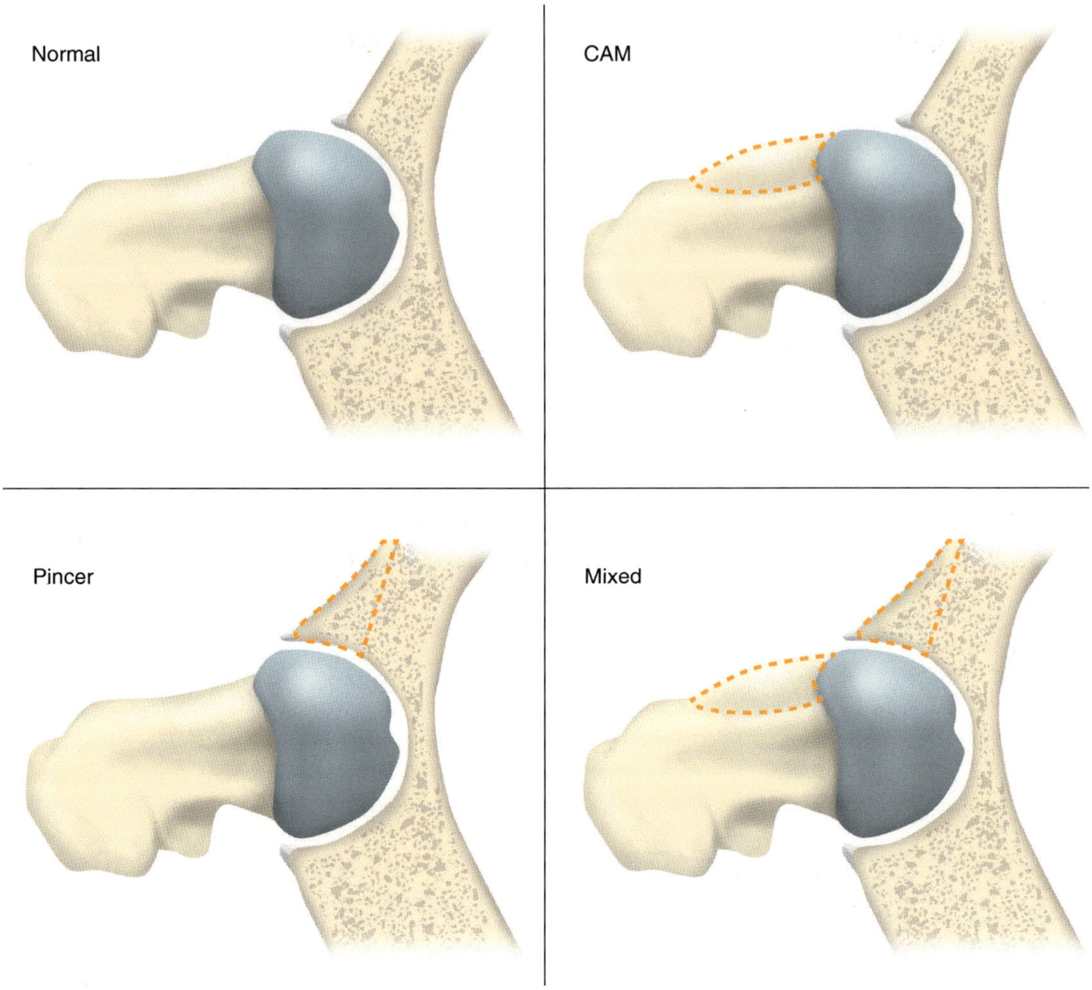

Fig. 7.8 Horizontal view of a left hip showing the different types of femoroacetabular impingement

[35] and growth disorder or childhood condition, like a silent or mild slipped capital epiphysis or Perthes disease [19, 21, 35, 49], have been proposed. The CAM deformity seems to be more common and larger in males compared to females [63].

In recent years, evidence has emerged supporting mechanical factors, affecting the proximal femoral physis, as a cause of CAM deformity [39]. As early as 1971, Murray showed that the tilt deformity was more prevalent in individuals who were more active in sports during adolescence as compared with their less active peers [36]. The CAM deformity has been shown to emerge from the physeal scar of the proximal femoral physis [47] and to develop during adolescence in response to vigorous sporting activity with the period immediately preceding and during physeal closure seeming to be of special susceptibility [1, 2, 9, 46, 51]. In a study on porcine hips, Jónasson et al. concluded that injuries in and around the porcine proximal femoral epiphyseal plate after repeated physiological loading could lead to growth disturbances and consequently to the development of the CAM deformity [26] (Fig. 7.9).

Although studies on asymptomatic individuals and nonathletes have shown that CAM mor-

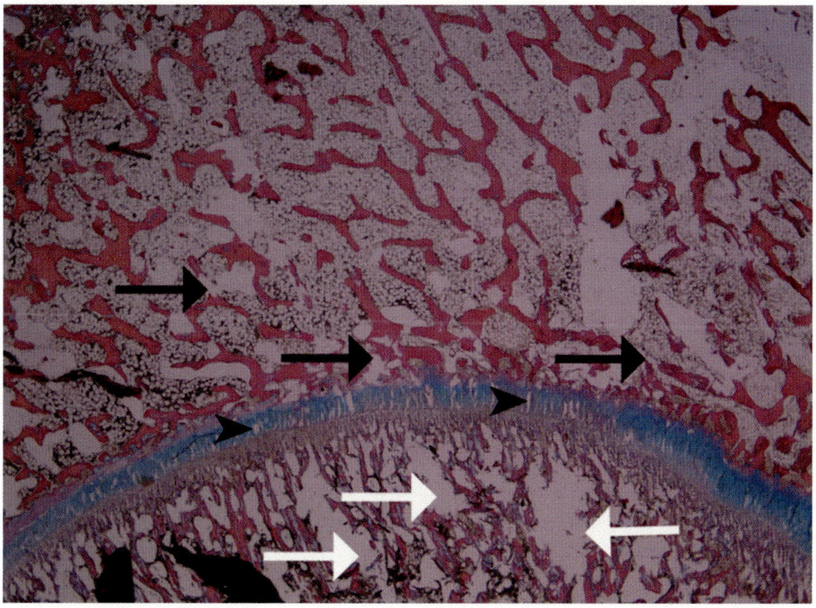

Fig. 7.9 A microscopic photograph of a specimen from a young porcine proximal femur after cyclical loading. Fractures of the epiphyseal bone (*above, black arrows*) and metaphyseal bone (*below, white arrows*) are seen and the injuries in the physeal line (*black arrowheads*) are aligned parallel to the cellular columns of the physeal line

phology exists in these populations, the prevalence amongst basketball players, ice-hockey players and soccer players is higher compared to nonathletes [1, 3, 20, 46]. This suggests that even though high loads during growth is an important factor in CAM development, other factors also play a role. Daily nonathletic activities vary between individuals, high body-mass index puts higher loads on the hips and ethnicity has been suggested as a factor in CAM development [14, 28].

Although injuries, osteonecrosis, infection and other occurrences later in life can lead to morphologic changes of the hip joint and subsequently lead to FAI, the changes connected to FAI are in the majority of cases caused by disturbances in skeletal growth and present from adolescence. Perthes disease and slipped capital femoral epiphysis often lead to considerable deformation of the hip joint and FAI. The aetiology of more subtle changes and their causality in symptom development is often more uncertain. In these cases diagnosis can be difficult but that is the subject of another chapter.

7.6 Future Perspectives

The development of the CAM and pincer deformity is likely multifactorial. In most cases the morphological changes are present when the individual is fully grown. Excessive loads on the hip during growth play a part but exact what type of loads (axial, rotational, shearing) and in what dosage that impacts development is unclear. Adjustment in activities of growing individuals might help in preventing CAM and pincer development, but further evidence is needed before recommendations can be made.

Take-Home Points

1. The growing skeleton is susceptible to mechanical loads.
2. High loads lead to disturbances in skeletal growth and skeletal deformities.
3. The CAM deformity of the femoral head-neck junction is common in athletes.
4. High loads on the adolescent athlete's hip can lead to the development of CAM.
5. The development of CAM and pincer deformities is likely multifactorial.

Key Evidence Related Sources

1. Agricola R, Heijboer MP, Ginai AZ, Roels P, Zadpoor AA, Verhaar JA, Weinans H, Waarsing JH. A cam deformity is gradually acquired during skeletal maturation in adolescent and young male soccer players: a prospective study with minimum 2-year follow-up. Am J Sports Med. 2014;42(4):798–806.
2. Carsen S, Moroz PJ, Rakhra K, Ward LM, Dunlap H, Hay JA, Willis RB, Beaule PE. The Otto Aufranc Award. On the etiology of the cam deformity: a cross-sectional pediatric MRI study. Clin Orthop Relat Res. 2014;472(2):430–6.
3. Jonasson P, Ekstrom L, Hansson H-A, Sansone M, Karlsson J, Sward L, Baranto A. Cyclical loading causes injury in and around the porcine proximal femoral physeal plate: proposed cause of the development of cam deformity in young athletes. J Exp Orthop. 2015;2:6.
4. Packer JD, Safran MR. The etiology of primary femoroacetabular impingement: genetics or acquired deformity? J Hip Preserv Surg. 2015. doi:10.1093/jhps/hnv046.

References

1. Agricola R, Bessems JH, Ginai AZ, Heijboer MP, van der Heijden RA, Verhaar JA, Weinans H, Waarsing JH. The development of Cam-type deformity in adolescent and young male soccer players. Am J Sports Med. 2012;40(5):1099–106.
2. Agricola R, Heijboer MP, Ginai AZ, Roels P, Zadpoor AA, Verhaar JA, Weinans H, Waarsing JH. A cam deformity is gradually acquired during skeletal maturation in adolescent and young male soccer players: a prospective study with minimum 2-year follow-up. Am J Sports Med. 2014;42(4):798–806.
3. Ayeni OR, Banga K, Bhandari M, Maizlin Z, de Sa D, Golev D, Harish S, Farrokhyar F. Femoroacetabular impingement in elite ice hockey players. Knee Surg Sports Traumatol Arthrosc. 2014;22(4):920–5.
4. Baranto A, Hellstrom M, Nyman R, Lundin O, Sward L. Back pain and degenerative abnormalities in the spine of young elite divers: a 5-year follow-up magnetic resonance imaging study. Knee Surg Sports Traumatol Arthrosc. 2006;14(9):907–14.
5. Bisgard JD. Longitudinal bone growth: the influence of sympathetic deinnervation. Ann Surg. 1933;97(3):374–80.
6. Brighton CT. Structure and function of the growth plate. Clin Orthop Relat Res. 1978;136:22–32.
7. Brighton CT. The growth plate. Orthop Clin North Am. 1984;15(4):571–95.
8. Caine D, DiFiori J, Maffulli N. Physeal injuries in children's and youth sports: reasons for concern? Br J Sports Med. 2006;40(9):749–60.
9. Carsen S, Moroz PJ, Rakhra K, Ward LM, Dunlap H, Hay JA, Willis RB, Beaule PE. The Otto Aufranc Award. On the etiology of the cam deformity: a cross-sectional pediatric MRI study. Clin Orthop Relat Res. 2014;472(2):430–6.
10. Chung SM. The arterial supply of the developing proximal end of the human femur. J Bone Joint Surg Am. 1976;58(7):961–70.
11. Chung SM, Batterman SC, Brighton CT. Shear strength of the human femoral capital epiphyseal plate. J Bone Joint Surg Am. 1976;58(1):94–103.
12. Delgado-Baeza E, Sanz-Laguna A, Miralles-Flores C. Experimental trauma of the triradiate epiphysis of the acetabulum and hip dysplasia. Int Orthop. 1991;15(4):335–9.
13. Dias JJ, Lamont AC. Ultrasonic imaging of the lateral artery of the capital femoral epiphysis: brief report. J Bone Joint Surg Br. 1989;71(2):322.
14. Dudda M, Kim Y-J, Zhang Y, Nevitt MC, Xu L, Niu J, Goggins J, Doherty M, Felson DT. Morphological differences between Chinese and Caucasian female hips: could they account for the ethnic difference in hip osteoarthritis? Arthritis Rheum. 2011;63(10):2992–9.
15. Dvonch VM, Bunch WH. Pattern of closure of the proximal femoral and tibial epiphyses in man. J Pediatr Orthop. 1983;3(4):498–501.
16. Epstein NE, Epstein JA. Limbus lumbar vertebral fractures in 27 adolescents and adults. Spine (Phila Pa 1976). 1991;16(8):962–6.
17. Flecker H. Time of appearance and fusion of ossification centers as observed by roentgenographic methods. Am J Roentgenol. 1942;47:97–159.
18. Fujii T, Takai S, Arai Y, Kim W, Amiel D, Hirasawa Y. Microstructural properties of the distal growth plate of the rabbit radius and ulna: biomechanical, biochemical, and morphological studies. J Orthop Res. 2000;18(1):87–93.
19. Goodman DA, Feighan JE, Smith AD, Latimer B, Buly RL, Cooperman DR. Subclinical slipped capital femoral epiphysis. Relationship to osteoarthrosis of the hip. J Bone Joint Surg Am. 1997;79(10):1489–97.
20. Hack K, Di Primio G, Rakhra K, Beaule PE. Prevalence of cam-type femoroacetabular impingement morphology in asymptomatic volunteers. J Bone Joint Surg Am. 2010;92(14):2436–44.

21. Harris WH. Etiology of osteoarthritis of the hip. Clin Orthop Relat Res. 1986;213:20–33.
22. Hefti F, von Laer L, Morscher E. Principles and pathogenesis of post-traumatic axial malalignment in the growth years. Orthopade. 1991;20(6):324–30.
23. Heuter C. Anatomische stidien an den extremitatengelenken neugeborener und erwachsener. Virchows Archiv Int J Pathol. 1862;25:572–99.
24. Hogervorst T, Bouma H, de Boer SF, de Vos J. Human hip impingement morphology: an evolutionary explanation. J Bone Joint Surg. 2011;93(6):769–76.
25. Jaramillo D, Laor T, Zaleske DJ. Indirect trauma to the growth plate: results of MR imaging after epiphyseal and metaphyseal injury in rabbits. Radiology. 1993;187(1):171–8.
26. Jonasson P, Ekstrom L, Hansson H-A, Sansone M, Karlsson J, Sward L, Baranto A. Cyclical loading causes injury in and around the porcine proximal femoral physeal plate: proposed cause of the development of cam deformity in young athletes. J Exp Orthop. 2015;2:6.
27. Kember NF. Cell division in endochondral ossification. A study of cell proliferation in rat bones by the method of tritiated thymidine autoradiography. J Bone Joint Surg Br. 1960;42B:824–39.
28. Kumar R, Aggarwal A. Femoroacetabular impingement and risk factors: a study of 50 cases. Orthop Surg. 2011;3(4):236–41.
29. Lindstrom JR, Ponseti IV, Wenger DR. Acetabular development after reduction in congenital dislocation of the hip. J Bone Joint Surg Am. 1979;61(1): 112–8.
30. Liu RW, Armstrong DG, Levine AD, Gilmore A, Thompson GH, Cooperman DR. An anatomic study of the epiphyseal tubercle and its importance in the pathogenesis of slipped capital femoral epiphysis. J Bone Joint Surg Am. 2013;95(6):e341–8.
31. Lundin O, Hellstrom M, Nilsson I, Sward L. Back pain and radiological changes in the thoraco-lumbar spine of athletes. A long-term follow-up. Scand J Med Sci Sports. 2001;11(2):103–9.
32. Maffulli N, Longo UG, Gougoulias N, Loppini M, Denaro V. Long-term health outcomes of youth sports injuries. Br J Sports Med. 2010;44(1):21–5.
33. Malina RM. Exercise as an influence upon growth. Review and critique of current concepts. Clin Pediatr. 1969;8(1):16–26.
34. Morgan JD, Somerville EW. Normal and abnormal growth at the upper end of the femur. J Bone Joint Surg Br. 1960;42-B:264–72.
35. Murray RO. The aetiology of primary osteoarthritis of the hip. Br J Radiol. 1965;38(455):810–24.
36. Murray RO, Duncan C. Athletic activity in adolescence as an etiological factor in degenerative hip disease. J Bone Joint Surg Br. 1971;53(3):406–19.
37. Nicholson JT, Nixon JE. Epiphyseal fractures. J Pediatr. 1961;59:939–50.
38. Ogden JA. Changing patterns of proximal femoral vascularity. J Bone Joint Surg Am. 1974;56(5): 941–50.
39. Packer JD, Safran MR. The etiology of primary femoroacetabular impingement: genetics or acquired deformity? J Hip Preserv Surg. 2015. doi:10.1093/jhps/hnv046.
40. Plaster RL, Schoenecker PL, Capelli AM. Premature closure of the triradiate cartilage: a potential complication of pericapsular acetabuloplasty. J Pediatr Orthop. 1991;11(5):676–8.
41. Pollard TC, Villar RN, Norton MR, Fern ED, Williams MR, Simpson DJ, Murray DW, Carr AJ. Femoroacetabular impingement and classification of the cam deformity: the reference interval in normal hips. Acta Orthop. 2010;81(1):134–41.
42. Ponseti IV. Growth and development of the acetabulum in the normal child. Anatomical, histological, and roentgenographic studies. J Bone Joint Surg Am. 1978;60(5):575–85.
43. Portinaro NM, Murray DW, Benson MK. Microanatomy of the acetabular cavity and its relation to growth. J Bone Joint Surg Br. 2001;83(3):377–83.
44. Robertson Jr WW. Newest knowledge of the growth plate. Clin Orthop Relat Res. 1990;253:270–8.
45. Shapiro F, Holtrop ME, Glimcher MJ. Organization and cellular biology of the perichondrial ossification groove of ranvier: a morphological study in rabbits. J Bone Joint Surg Am. 1977;59(6):703–23.
46. Siebenrock KA, Behning A, Mamisch TC, Schwab JM. Growth plate alteration precedes cam-type deformity in elite basketball players. Clin Orthop Relat Res. 2013;471(4):1084–91.
47. Siebenrock KA, Wahab KHA, Werlen S, Kalhor M, Leunig M, Ganz R. Abnormal extension of the femoral head epiphysis as a cause of cam impingement. Clin Orthop Relat Res. 2004;418:54–60.
48. Siffert RS. The growth plate and its affections. J Bone Joint Surg Am. 1966;48(3):546–63.
49. Stulberg SD, Cordell LD, Harris WH, Ramsey PL, MacEwen GD. Unrecognized childhood hip disease: a major cause of idiopathic osteoarthritis of the hip. In: The hip: proceedings of the third open scientific meeting of the hip society. St Louis: Mosby; 1975. p. 212–28.
50. Sward L, Hellstrom M, Jacobsson B, Peterson L. Back pain and radiologic changes in the thoraco-lumbar spine of athletes. Spine (Phila Pa 1976). 1990;15(2):124–9.
51. Tak I, Weir A, Langhout R, Waarsing JH, Stubbe J, Kerkhoffs G, Agricola R. The relationship between the frequency of football practice during skeletal growth and the presence of a cam deformity in adult elite football players. Br J Sports Med. 2015:49: 630–4.
52. Tannenbaum E, Kopydlowski N, Smith M, Bedi A, Sekiya JK. Gender and racial differences in focal and global acetabular version. J Arthroplasty. 2014;29(2): 373–6.
53. Tayton K. Does the upper femoral epiphysis slip or rotate? J Bone Joint Surg Br. 2007;89(10):1402–6.
54. Tayton K. The epiphyseal tubercle in adolescent hips. Acta Orthop. 2009;80(4):416–9.

55. Trueta J. The normal vascular anatomy of the human femoral head during growth. J Bone Joint Surg Br. 1957;39-B(2):358–94.
56. Trueta J, Amato VP. The vascular contribution to osteogenesis. III. Changes in the growth cartilage caused by experimentally induced ischaemia. J Bone Joint Surg Br. 1960;42-B:571–87.
57. Trueta J, Little K. The vascular contribution to osteogenesis. II. Studies with the electron microscope. J Bone Joint Surg Br. 1960;42-B:367–76.
58. Trueta J, Morgan JD. The vascular contribution to osteogenesis. I. Studies by the injection method. J Bone Joint Surg Br. 1960;42-B:97–109.
59. Trueta J, Trias A. The vascular contribution to osteogenesis. IV. The effect of pressure upon the epiphysial cartilage of the rabbit. J Bone Joint Surg Br. 1961;43-B:800–13.
60. Tucker FR. Arterial supply to the femoral head and its clinical importance. J Bone Joint Surg Br. 1949;31B(1):82–93.
61. Wertheimer LG, Lopes Sde L. Arterial supply of the femoral head. A combined angiographic and histological study. J Bone Joint Surg Am. 1971;53(3):545–56.
62. Wolff J. The law of bone remodeling. Berlin/Heidelberg: Springer; 1986.
63. Yanke AB, Khair MM, Stanley R, Walton D, Lee S, Bush-Joseph CA, Espinosa Orias AA, Inoue N, Nho SJ. Sex differences in patients with CAM deformities with femoroacetabular impingement: 3-dimensional computed tomographic quantification. Arthroscopy. 2015;31(12):2301–6.

Surgical Management of CAM-Type FAI: A Technique Guide

8

Darren de SA, Matti Seppänen,
Austin E. MacDonald, and Olufemi R. Ayeni

Contents

D. de SA, MD • O.R. Ayeni, MD, MSc, FRCSC (✉)
Division of Orthopaedic Surgery, Department of Surgery, McMaster University Medical Centre, 1200 Main Street West, 4E15, Hamilton, ON L8N 3Z5, Canada
e-mail: ayenif@mcmaster.ca

M. Seppänen, MD
Department of Orthopaedic Surgery, Turku University Hospital, Turku, Finland
e-mail: matti.seppanen@fimnet.fi

A.E. MacDonald, MD(Cand)
Department of Orthopaedic Surgery,Michael G. DeGroote School of Medicine, McMaster University, Hamilton, ON, Canada

8.1 Introduction

Conservative management of femoroacetabular impingement (FAI) remains a first-line treatment; however, the physical and structural abnormality often necessitates surgical intervention to restore impingement-free motion [1–3]. Surgical management, therefore, is often indicated in FAI, especially after a patient fails conservative management [3]. Although open, mini-open, and arthroscopic techniques have been described, both in the lateral decubitus and supine positions, the use of a particular technique is often dependent on surgeon preference [4]. This chapter will highlight the technique for arthroscopic management in the supine position for CAM-type FAI and will also briefly compare the supine position to the lateral decubitus position.

8.2 Surgical Technique

8.2.1 Patient Setup

Surgical management of CAM-type FAI involves the sequential progression of a diagnostic hip arthroscopy, followed by labral repair, acetabular rim trimming, and femoral neck osteochondroplasty. Intravenous antibiotics for infectious prophylaxis are administered. Anesthetic (e.g., spinal or general) is administered once the patient is supine on the fracture table (Fig. 8.1). Note that

O.R. Ayeni et al. (eds.), *Diagnosis and Management of Femoroacetabular Impingement*,
DOI 10.1007/978-3-319-32000-7_8

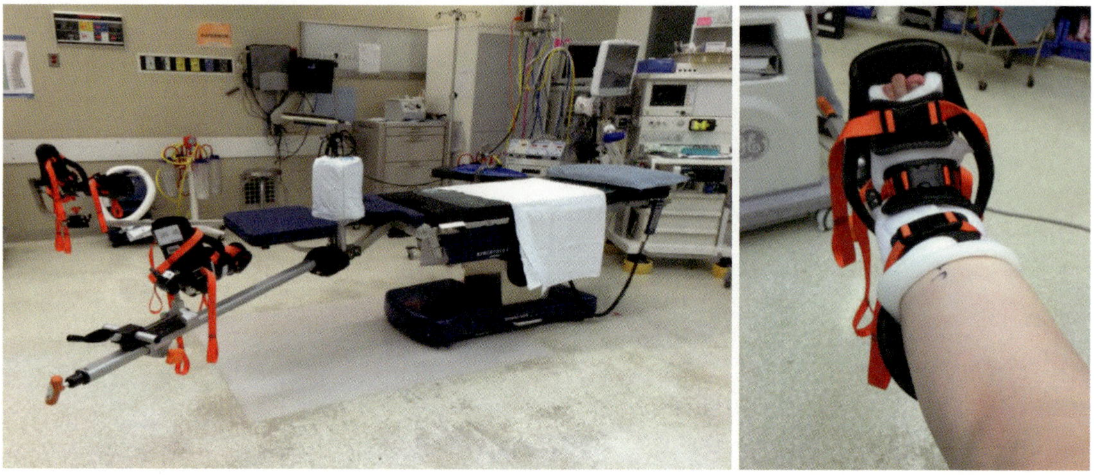

Fig. 8.1 Operating room setup. (*Left*) The operating table setup with a perineal foam post and traction setup. (*Right*) Patient's foot wrapped in protective foam pad and tightly secured to the traction boots

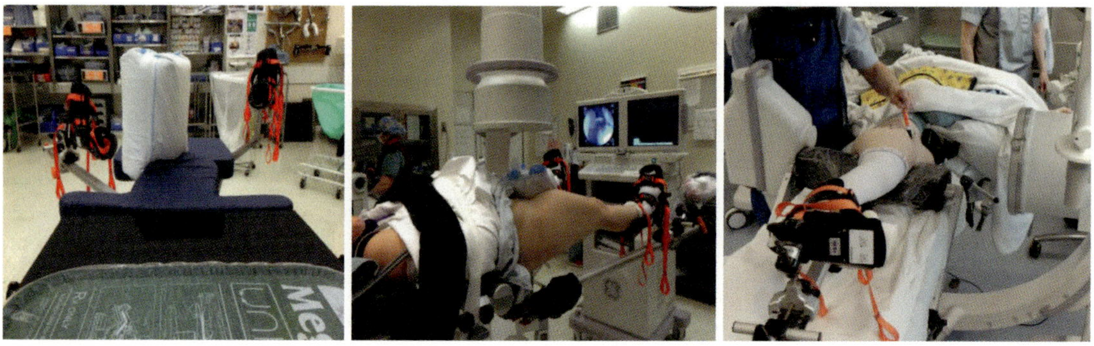

Fig. 8.2 Patient positioning. (*Left*) Perineal foam pad positioning to prevent pudendal nerve injury. (*Center*) Patient has been transported down the bed to allow the perineal foam pad to be an effective countertraction force. Note the fluoroscopic device positioned over the operative extremity from the opposite side of the surgeon. (*Left*) Patient and fluoroscopic device positioning if performing hip arthroscopy in the lateral decubitus position

this procedure can be done in the supine or lateral position, but this chapter will focus on the supine approach (and highlight aspects of the lateral approach). General anesthetic is advantageous for allowing muscle relaxation to aid with hip distraction.

The patient, now supine on the fracture table, has foam pads applied to their feet (Fig. 8.1). The patient is positioned on the operating table so that the large, well-padded perineal post (to prevent injury to the perineal soft tissue and pudendal nerve) is positioned to be an effective countertraction measure to a medially/adducted force (Fig. 8.2). The padded feet are securely fastened to the traction table using the appropriate straps and the operative leg positioned in full abduction. For lateral decubitus position, the fracture table is then rotated 90° so that the operative extremity is superior to the rest of the patient (Fig. 8.2, right). On occasion, an examination under anesthesia is performed to assess for hypermobility of the hip in all planes of motion in cases where clinically indicated (connective tissue disorders).

For the supine position, the fluoroscopic device is brought in from the opposite side of the operative extremity, at a 45° angle (Fig. 8.2, middle). In-line longitudinal traction (with the

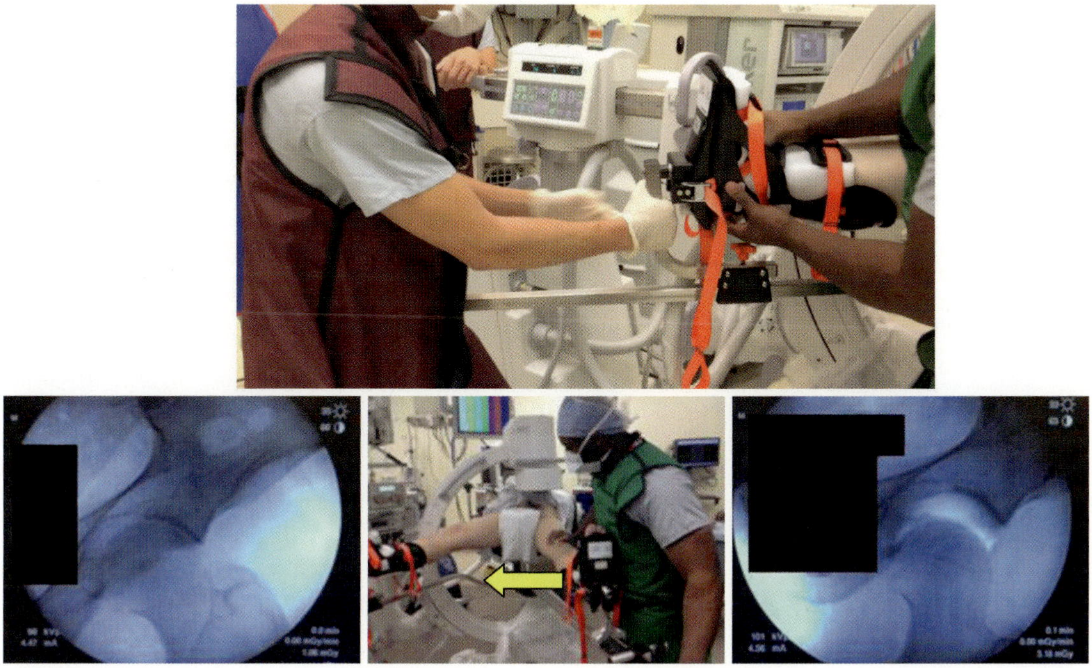

Fig. 8.3 Application of traction to distract the hip joint. (*Top*) Application of longitudinal traction in line with the femoral neck with the extremity in full abduction to provide distraction at the hip joint. (*Bottom, right*) Intraoperative fluoroscopic image prior to application of any hip traction. (*Bottom, center*) With longitudinal traction applied, the surgeon next sequentially adducts the operative extremity 5–10° at a time, with intermitted fluoroscopic images confirming appropriate distraction at the hip joint. (*Bottom, left*) Intraoperative fluoroscopic image with the extremity in the optimal operative position demonstrating distraction at the hip joint

femoral neck) is then applied (Fig. 8.3, top), and the operative extremity is adducted 5–10° at a time (Fig. 8.3, bottom center), with sequential fluoroscopic images confirming progressive joint distraction (Fig. 8.3, bottom right and left). Approximately 11–22 kg of traction is required to distract the operative joint 8–10 mm, looking for a "loss of seal" effect and often audible "pop." The final operative extremity should be in neutral abduction, slight internal rotation (i.e., approximately 5°), and a maximum 5–10° of flexion. The nonoperative extremity should be in 45–50° of abduction and slight external rotation (i.e., approximately 5°), serving as countertraction. This is usually completed prior to prepping and draping the hip.

When operating in the lateral decubitus position, traction is applied with 10° of flexion, 20° of abduction, and neutral rotation of the hip. Similar to above, adequate separation of the femoral head from the acetabulum is verified with fluoroscopy. Usually 40–50 kg of traction force is enough to create adequate 1–1.5 cm distraction.

Limiting traction time to 90–120 min maximum decreases the risk of traction-related complications.

8.2.2 Draping

Draping techniques vary, but it is standard practice to drape in sterile fashion and allow for complete exposure of the entire hemi-pelvis of the operative side. Adhesive clear dressing (such as Ioban) is applied to the hip region only to allow for preservation of landmarks drawn on the hip. This draping technique generally exposes the hip from above the inguinal ligament to the mid-thigh anteriorly. Care is also taken to expose the hip posteriorly to allow for a posterolateral portal placement (exposing

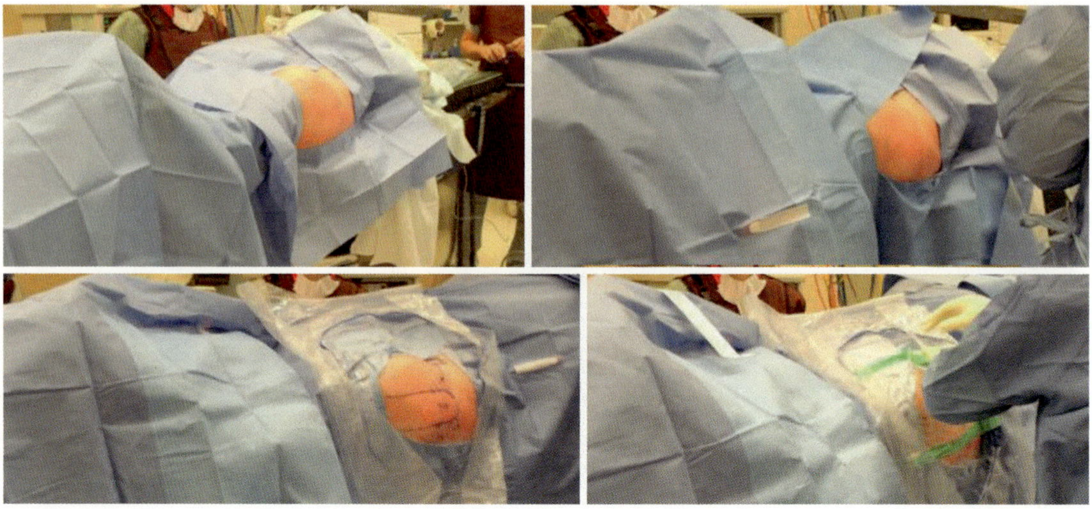

Fig. 8.4 Sterile draping of the operative site. (*Top*, *left*) Large approach sheets placed on the leg and torso and operative hip squared off. (*Top*, *right*) Extremity drape applied. (*Bottom*, *left*) Marking pen used to delineate anatomy and potential portal sites (see Fig. 8.5). (*Bottom*, *right*) Sterile skin adhesive dressing applied

approximately 5 cm posterior to the posterior border of the greater trochanter). Finally, the operative leg, below the knee, is free of draping to allow for a manual dynamic assessment of the hip when needed (Fig. 8.4).

8.2.3 Portal Placement for Supine Position

Upward of nine different central and peripheral arthroscopic portals have been described [5], and the ones that follow are those of the senior author's preference. Proper portal placement is essential for ease of execution of the surgical plan, and inadequate portal placement can predispose to complications such as damage to periarticular structure such as the sciatic nerve injury. Of note, there exists wide variability between patients of different weight, body mass index, and the locations of at-risk neurovascular structures to the arthroscopic portals used, and so great caution must be exercised [6]. Traditionally, four portals are used: anterolateral, anterior/mid-anterior portal, distal anterolateral portal, and posterolateral portal (Fig. 8.5). The majority of central compartment procedures however can be done through the anterolateral and anterior/mid-anterior portals, with the posterolateral portal serving mainly as an outflow portal. In general, do not hesitate to make additional portals if necessary or reposition already made ones for ease, remembering not to go medial of a line drawn vertically from the anterior superior iliac spine (ASIS), so as to avoid injury to the neurovascular bundle.

First, the standard anterolateral portal is created using a Seldinger technique. Using the anterior superior iliac spine (ASIS) and the most proximal tip of the greater trochanter (GT) as landmarks, the anterolateral portal (risk to superior gluteal nerve) is made using a skin entry that is 1 cm anterior and superior to the tip of the GT. The trajectory for the spinal needle is 15° cephalad and 15° posterior. Another method to obtain this portal is to insert the spinal needle at the level of the joint line approximately 1 cm anterior to the GT tip and direct the spinal needle 15–20° posterior. The muscle interval used is the tensor fasciae latae/gluteus maximus with rectus femoris/hip flexors. Once the spinal needle penetrates the joint, a loss of resistance is appreciated. The needle insert is withdrawn, and fluoroscopy is used to visualize an air arthrogram. Saline (approximately 10 cc) is then injected intra-articularly, and a flashback or

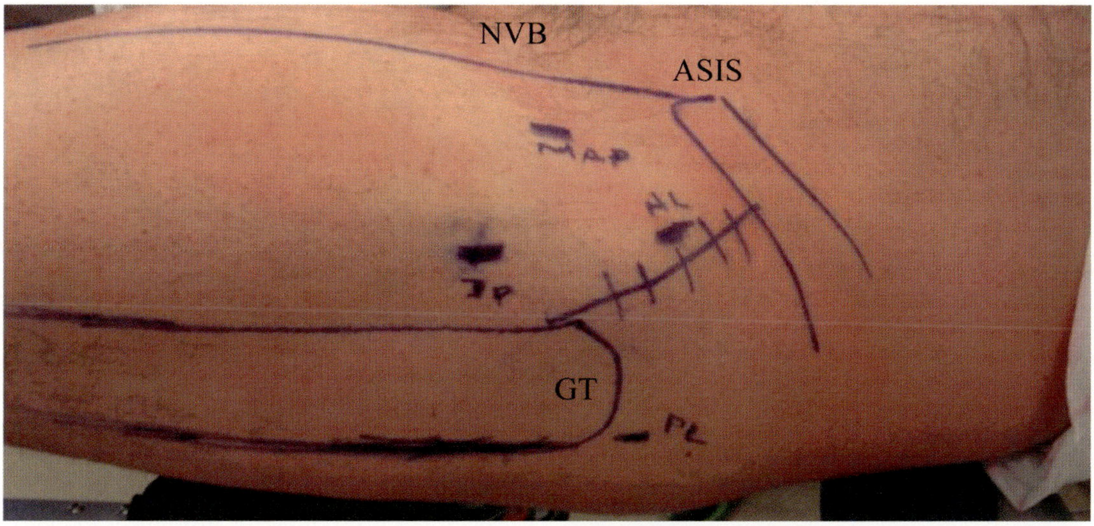

Fig. 8.5 Surgical landmarks of the operative extremity in supine position. Anatomy and possible portal sites marked on the operative site (left hip) with a sterile marking pen. *AL* anterolateral portal, *PL* posterolateral portal, *DP* accessory (distal) anterolateral portal, *MAP* mid-anterior portal, *GT* greater trochanter of femur, *ASIS* anterior superior iliac spine, *NVB* neurovascular bundle (lies medial to a vertical line originating at the ASIS)

backflow of fluid is visualized, confirming the correct location. Next, a long guidewire is passed through the cannulated spinal needle and advanced to the acetabular fossa. The spinal needle is withdrawn, and a scalpel is used to create a 1 cm skin incision for portal creation. The scope trochar is advanced over the guidewire and through the capsule, with caution taken to ensure the guidewire does not bend or break. Fluoroscopy is used to ensure the guidewire does not damage intra-articular structures. Once the trochar is placed correctly, the guidewire is withdrawn (Figs. 8.6 and 8.7).

The 70° arthroscope is inserted, and the anterior/mid-anterior portal (risks to lateral femoral cutaneous nerve (LFCN), femoral nerve, femoral artery, femoral vein, ascending branch of lateral circumflex artery) is made under direct visualization with fluoroscopic guidance as needed. The capsular triangle (Fig. 8.8), formed by the femoral head and acetabulum, is the target for spinal needle insertion to create this portal (approximate 3 o'clock position viewing from anterolateral portal). Again, a Seldinger technique is employed. We use a mid-anterior portal for the decreased risk of LFCN injury. The skin landmark is approximately 2–3 cm anterior and 2–3 cm distal to the anterolateral portal. The spinal needle trajectory is 45° cephalad and 10–15° medially. Once intra-articular confirmation is directly visualized, the inserter is withdrawn, a scalpel is used to make a 1 cm skin incision, care is taken to cut the skin only (and avoid branches of LFCN), the guidewire is passed through the

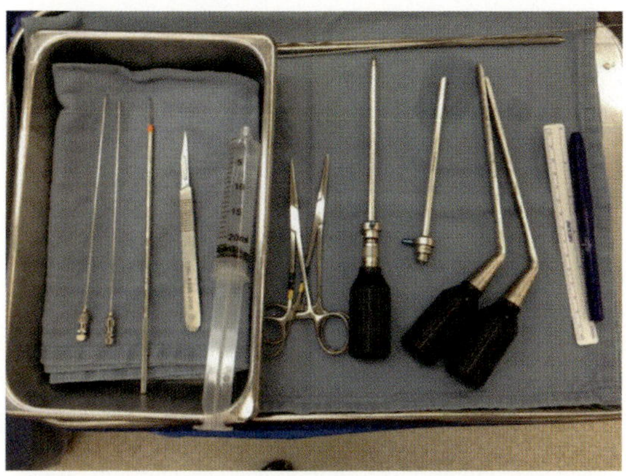

Fig. 8.6 Hip arthroscopy instruments. Instruments used to establish the portals (from *left to right*): spinal needles (×2), arthroscopic scalpel, scalpel, syringe with saline, snaps (×2), scope trochars (×2), half pipes, ruler, and marking pen. The guidewire and switching stick are located at the top of the sheet

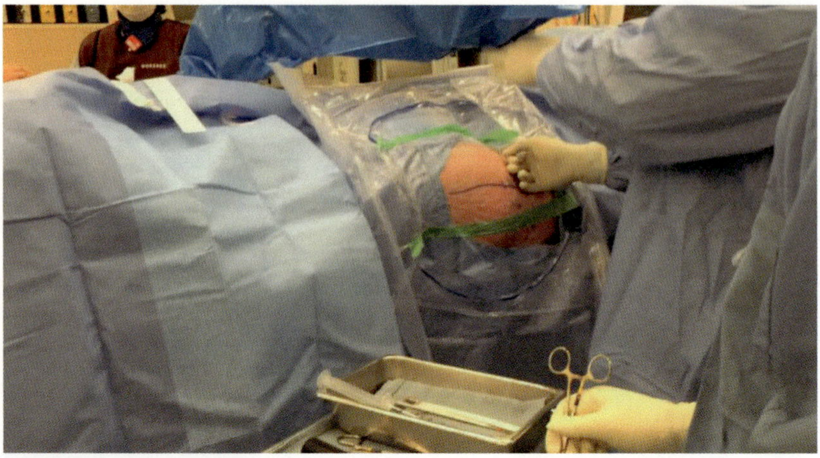

Fig. 8.7 Arthroscopic portal creation demonstrating surgical and fluoroscopic set up. The Seldinger technique is used to create the arthroscopic portals

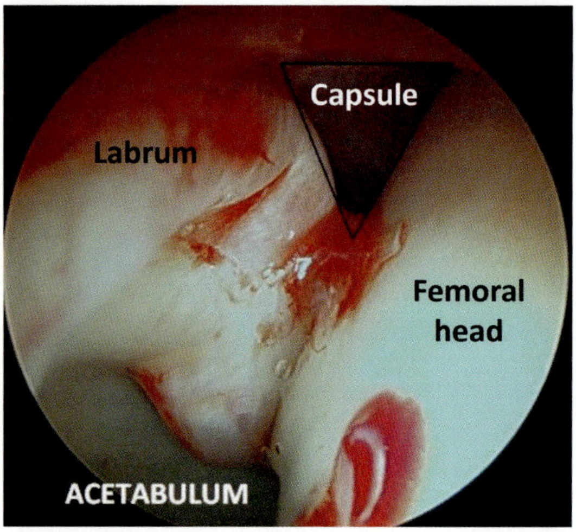

Fig. 8.8 Creation of the mid-anterior portal. Arthroscopic view of the hip joint for creation of the mid-anterior portal. The intraoperative landmark is an inverted triangle of hip capsule between the femoral head and labrum

cannulated spinal needle, the spinal needle is withdrawn, and the trochar is advanced over the guidewire – again, taking caution not to deform the wire.

Once anterolateral and mid-anterior portals are created, an interportal capsulotomy is created from 3 o'clock to 11 o'clock anterolaterally is made by connecting the two portals with an arthroscopic scalpel. The technique involves a coordinated use of the half pipe and switching stick to switch the arthroscope and arthroscopic scalpel between portals while protecting the surrounding soft tissue and maintaining portal placement. The limited capsulotomy is essential for instrument mobility, anchor placement, and arthroscopic knot tying and can be a "bailout" for a suboptimally positioned portal. The capsulotomy itself starts approximately 5–8 mm from the labrum and measures approximately 15–20 mm in total length [7]. This allows for repair of the capsule when indicated.

The distal anterolateral portal for the osteochondroplasty is made 3–5 cm distal to the anterolateral portal (Fig. 8.5, DP), using a similar trajectory and technique as that for creation of the anterolateral portal. The posterolateral portal (risk to sciatic nerve) is made 1–3 cm posterior to the greater trochanter, in line with the anterolateral portal (Fig. 8.5, PL).

8.2.4 Portal Placement for Lateral Decubitus Position

The portal placement in the lateral decubitus position is very similar to the supine portal placement as described above. One of the senior authors (MS), who operates in the lateral decubitus position, normally uses the same four described portals: an anterolateral or lateral (ALP), a modified mid-anterior (MMAP), a distal anterolateral or distal (DALP), and a posterolateral portal (PLP) (Fig. 8.9).

As in the supine technique, the GT and ASIS are landmarked and drawn onto the patient with a marking pen [8]. A vertical, medial line is drawn down from the ASIS that indicates where no inci-

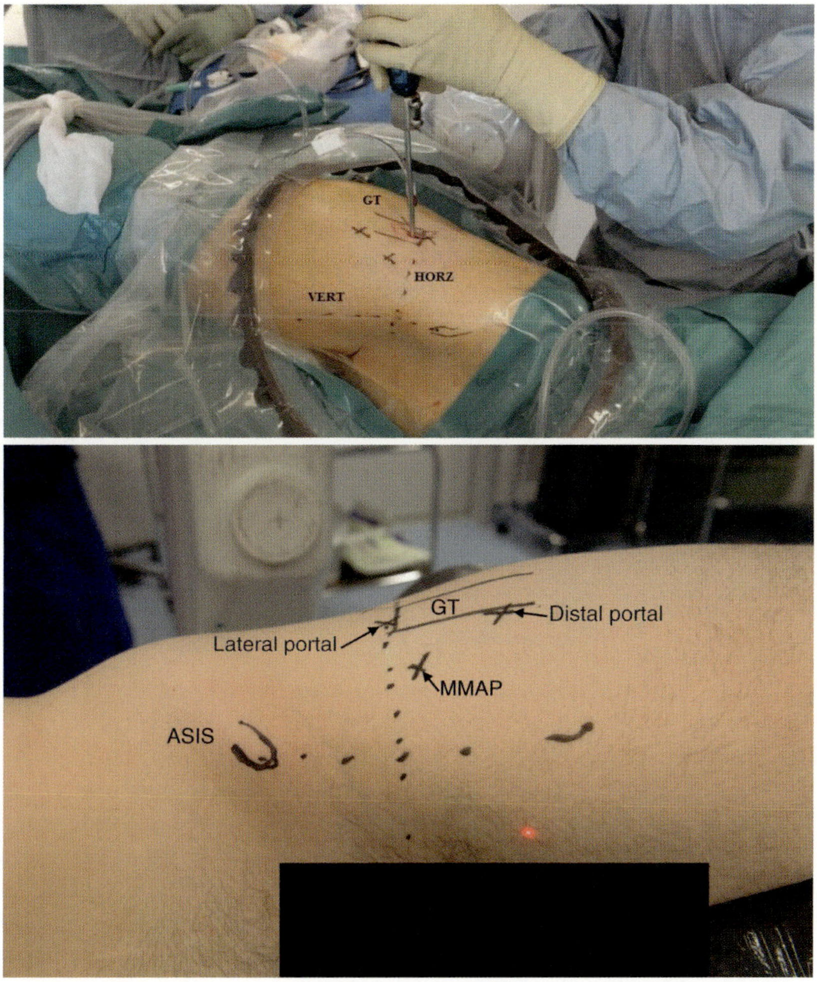

Fig. 8.9 Surgical landmarks of the operative extremity in lateral decubitus position. (*Top*) Anatomy and possible portal sites marked on the operative site (right hip) with a sterile marking pen. The GT has been outlined. *HORZ* horizontal line from the level of the superior border of the GT, *VERT* vertical line descending from the ASIS (anterior superior iliac spine). (*Bottom*) Anatomy and possible portal sites marked on the operative site (left hip) with a sterile marking pen. GT and ASIS have been outlined. The lateral portal (anterolateral), the distal portal (distal anterolateral), and the modified mid-anterior portal are marked

sions should be made in order to avoid the femoral artery and nerve [8]. The first portal that is made is the LP which is approximately halfway between the ALP and PLP (Fig. 8.9).

To distract the joint, a 17-gauge spinal needle (tip away from the femoral head and blunt wedge to the cartilage) is introduced to the central compartment from the site of the PLP. The spinal needle is introduced 35° medial and 20° cephalad. Space between the acetabulum and femoral head should be at least 10 mm, but not more than 15 mm, after the first needle is introduced into the joint capsule and the vacuum is released. Another 17-gauge spinal needle is introduced to the central compartment from the site of the LP in the same manner. A flexible metal guidewire is introduced through the spinal needle, and adequate position of the guidewire is verified with fluoroscopy. The switching stick and arthroscopy cannulas are introduced with help of the guidewire. The arthroscopy pump is connected to the arthroscopy cannula and a 70° arthroscope is inserted. The PLP can then be created. A posterior portal is necessary for posterior labral sutures and posterior rim trimming. The MMAP can then be created using direct visual control where the site of the skin incision is approximately 7 cm medial and 2 cm distal from the LP [9].

8.2.5 Diagnostic Arthroscopy

Diagnostic arthroscopy is first completed to examine the entirety of the labrum, looking for areas of injection and associated pathology. Any pathology is appropriately dealt with as outlined in previous chapters. The chondrolabral junction is also examined and areas of detachment and tearing identified. The femoral head is examined for evidence of foveal and/or articular cartilage damage. The ligamentum teres is next examined and the capsule diffusely examined as well.

8.2.6 Femoral Neck Osteochondroplasty Technique and Outcomes

The distal anterolateral portal is finally created using the aforementioned Seldinger technique, and a T-capsulotomy is completed to facilitate multiplanar deformity correction of the CAM lesion anterolaterally. The T-capsulotomy extends from the femoral head-neck junction to the intertrochanteric line, incising the iliofemoral ligament between the gluteus minimus and iliocapsularis muscle – a muscle overlying the anterior hip capsule with a role in stabilizing the femoral head within a deficient acetabulum [10, 11]. Care is taken not to extend the T capsulotomy beyond the zona orbicularis. Typically, 2 to 3 cm of exposure is required. While under traction, the lateral component of the CAM lesion is decompressed using the 5.5 mm arthroscopic burr. The starting point for bony resection is typically just distal to the physeal scar of the femoral head and neck and the starting point of an obvious bony prominence. Fluoroscopic guidance (Fig. 8.9) is used to observe decompression (Fig. 8.9, left and right), and bony debris is thoroughly evacuated using suction. The contour of the lateral head and neck junction of the femur is assessed and compared to the pre-operative image that was saved on an xray screen. At the completion of this lateral decompression with restoration of a normal lateral contour, the hip is released from traction and the hip is flexed (45°) and both fully internally and externally rotated to obtain a 180° view of the anterior portion of CAM lesion and to allow for completion of the CAM lesion decompression in the peripheral compartment [10]. The osteochondroplasty is then completed under dynamic conditions with hip rotation at 0°, 45° and also 90° of flexion to ensure that full decompression is achieved. The zona orbicularis marks the most distal extent of decompression and is a critical structure to avoid damaging when addressing the CAM lesion [12]. This landmark not only marks the terminal branch of the lateral femoral circumflex artery, but compromising the zona orbicularis may potentiate hip instability and loss of the "suction seal" of the hip capsuloligamentous complex [12]. Proximally, the resection line should be limited on the femoral head surface to 5 mm distal to the acetabular labrum from the 9 o'clock (anterior) to 12 o'clock (superior) positions [13]. Other proximal limits of proximal bony resection include the physeal scar. Fluoroscopic images are taken to confirm restoration of a normal head-neck offset and contour on multiple views (AP and Lateral) (Fig. 8.9). The arthroscope is then withdrawn, and the three portal sites are closed with nonabsorbable suture. Sterile dressings are applied, and the patient is awoken and transferred to the recovery room in stable condition. Intraoperative blood loss is minimal to nonexistent. Postoperative medications, activity and weight-bearing status, and rehabilitation are discussed in Chap. 16. We do not routinely prescribe any medication or radiation therapy for heterotopic ossification (HO) prophylaxis.

Generally, the alpha angle – defined as the angle created by a line between the anterior point, where the distance from the center of the head exceeds the radius of the subchondral surface of the femoral head, and a line from the center of the head through the narrowest part of the femoral neck [14] – is but one of many parameters used to assess adequate decompression. Of 20 radiographic parameters in the hip, Mast et al. [15] reported a high inter-rater and intra-rater reliability for the alpha angle, with respective intra-class correlation coefficients (ICCs) of 0.83 and 0.90, though depending on modality, studies would suggest that considerably inter- and intra-variability exists in alpha angle measurement – to

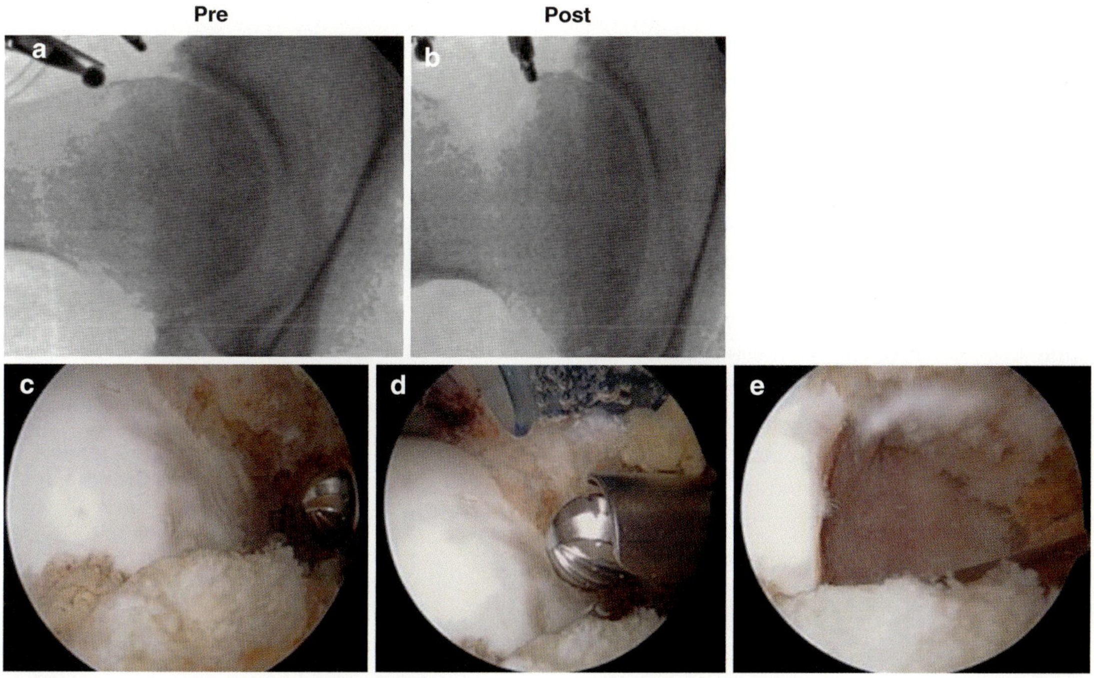

Fig. 8.10 (**a**, **b**) Pre-, post- fluoroscopic images confirming restoration of a normal head-neck offset and contour. (**c**–**e**) Arthroscopic also showing view and access with T capsulotomy and reshaping of the femoral head-neck junction. A 5.5 mm arthroscopic burr is used to resect the CAM lesion and restore offset

such a degree that it arguably may be of no statistical value for assessing CAM impingement [16]. The literature defines an abnormal alpha angle as greater than 50–55° [14, 17], and a systematic review by de SA et al. [18] showed improved patient outcomes and no complications when patients had a postoperative alpha angle restored to less than 55°. However, a cohort study examining 3D computed tomography navigation for FAI correction suggests that the alpha angle does not correlate with outcome, as Brunner et al. [19] noted no statistical differences in visual analog pain scores, non-arthritic hip scores, and range of motion in the 6/50 patients that did not achieve adequate CAM resection (i.e., alpha angle less than 50° or a mean difference of 20° from pre- and postoperative measurements). However, with small sample sizes (25 patients per cohort) it is questionable that the study was adequately powered to detect any meaningful statistical or clinical difference. Another intraoperative parameter used to assess the adequacy of resection includes restoration of head/neck offset and also direct visualization of impingement-free motion through all ranges of flexion/extension and internal/external rotation. Also, the current accepted parameter limits resection to a maximum area of 30 % of the femoral neck diameter, recognizing the potential for iatrogenic femoral neck fracture and compromised labral-sealing effect in hip flexion if more than 30 % is resected [20, 21]. We suggest using a combination of approaches to ensure adequate deformity correction, given that incomplete resection is the most frequent cause for revision surgery [22, 23] (Fig. 8.10). As a 5.5 mm burr is typically used, a useful guide is using 2 widths (or double) of the burr size ($5.5 \times 2 = 11$ mm) to obtain adequate resection depth.

Typically, the senior author does not routinely repair the capsulotomy except in cases with documented hyperlaxity subtle dysplasia or connective tissue disorders. Capsular repair is a controversial topic and there have recently been several studies that aim to demonstrate whether or not capsular repair is effective at improving hip arthroscopy outcomes. Proponents feel that it is a fast and easily reproducible technique to avoid postoperative instability and pain [24], especially in situations where the patient has a connective tissue disorder predisposing them to capsular laxity and/or dysplastic hip features [25]. Frank et al. [26] demonstrated that patients who underwent arthroscopy for FAI improved significantly at the 2.5-year mark after surgery regardless of whether they underwent capsular repair or not. They did find, however, that patients who had full closure of the capsule had (compared to partial closure) superior sport-specific outcomes and less revision surgery than those patients who did not [26]. Studies do exist [7, 27–29], suggesting that not repairing a capsulotomy may propagate microinstability; the consequences of which may include early degenerative changes, but further study is required to determine this. Domb et al. [30] on the other hand demonstrated that capsular repair was safe and did not negatively affect patients who had this procedure but that there was no difference in clinically significant outcomes between groups. Amar et al. [31] examined the incidence of heterotopic ossification (HO) post-hip arthroscopy in two groups of 50 patients with and without capsular closure, finding no significant difference in HO rate between the groups followed for a minimum of 9 weeks postoperatively. A case report by Austin et al. [32] suggests that failure to close the capsule post-hip arthroscopy could predispose to hip instability, though in a study examining over 4,000 hip arthroscopies where the capsule was not addressed, not one case of instability was reported [16, 33]. Interestingly, cadaveric studies by Bayne et al. [34] demonstrated that capsulotomy improved femoral translation with the hip in neutral position and femoral rotation with the hip in flexion – which may in fact be beneficial to those with FAI suffering from limited ROM. There likely exists a fine balance between insufficient capsulotomy to prevent adequate ease of procedure and sufficient improvements in range of motion and too much whereby hip instability ensues.

Take-Home Points

1. Arthroscopic restoration of impingement-free motion for FAI in the supine position using the anterolateral, mid-anterior, and distal anterolateral portals is safe.
2. Approximately 11–22 kg of traction is required to distract the operative joint 8–10 mm for intra-articular work, and traction-related complications are avoided by limiting traction time to a maximum of 120 min.
3. A T-capsulotomy provides adequate exposure to the hip joint, and repair postoperatively is controversial.
4. The limits of CAM resection proximally and distally on the femoral head are 5 mm distal to the acetabular labrum and the zona orbicularis, respectively. Resection should be limited to no more than 30 % of the femoral neck diameter to minimize risk of iatrogenic femoral neck fracture.
5. Adequate restoration of impingement-free motion can be assessed intraoperatively by restoration of an alpha angle less than 55°, a normal femoral head/neck offset (i.e., greater than 10 mm), and/or direct visualization of impingement-free motion.

Key Evidence Related Sources

1. Beaule PE, Le Duff MJ, Zaragoza E. Quality of life following femoral head-neck osteochondroplasty for femoroacetabular impingement. J Bone Joint Surg. 2007;89:773–9.
2. de SA D, Urquhart N, Philippon M, Ye JE, Simunovic N, Ayeni OR. Alpha angle correction in femoroacetabular impingement. Knee Surg Sports Traumatol Arthrosc. 2014;22(4):812–21. doi:10.1007/s00167-013-2678-6.

3. Domb BG, Philippon MJ, Giordano BD. Arthroscopic capsulotomy, capsular repair, and capsular plication of the hip: relation to atraumatic instability. Arthroscopy. 2013;29(1):162–73. doi:10.1016/j.arthro.2012.04.057.

Acknowledgments The authors wish to express their gratitude to Marie-Claude Leblanc, MD, FRCSC, for the intraoperative photographs taken for this chapter.

References

1. Bedi A, Kelly BT. Femoroacetabular impingement. J Bone Joint Surg Am. 2013;95(1):82–92. Retrieved Feb. 8, 2015 from http://dx.doi.org/10.2106/JBJS.K.01219.
2. Dolan MM, Heyworth BE, Bedi A, Duke G, Kelly BT. CT reveals a high incidence of osseous abnormalities in hips with labral tears. Clin Orthop Relat Res. 2011;469(3):831–8. doi:10.1007/s11999-010-1539-6.
3. Beaule PE, Le Duff MJ, Zaragoza E. Quality of life following femoral head-neck osteochondroplasty for femoroacetabular impingement. J Bone Joint Surg. 2007;89:773–9.
4. Wilson AS, Quanjun C. Current concepts in management of femoroacetabular impingement. World J Orthop. 2012;3(12):204–11. doi:10.5312/wjo.v3.i12.204.
5. Thorey F, Ezechieli M, Ettinger M, Albrecht UV, Budde S. Access to the hip joint from standard arthroscopic portals: a cadaveric study. Arthroscopy. 2013;29(8):1297–307. doi:10.1016/j.arthro.2013.05.017.
6. Watson JN, Bohnenkamp F, El-Bitar Y, Moretti V, Domb BG. Variability in locations of hip neurovascular structures and their proximity to hip arthroscopic portals. Arthroscopy. 2014;30(4):462–7. doi:10.1016/j.arthro.2013.12.012.
7. Harris JD, Slikker III, Gupta AK, McCormick FM, Nho SJ. Routine complete capsular closure during Hip arthroscopy. Arthrosc Tech. 2013;2(2):e89–94. doi:10.1016/j.eats.2012.11.007.
8. Glick JM, Sampson TG, Gordon RB, Behr JT, Schmidt E. Hip arthroscopy by the lateral approach. Arthroscopy. 1987;3(1):4–12.
9. Matsuda DK, Villamor A. The modified mid-anterior portal for hip arthroscopy. Arthrosc Tech. 2014;3: e469–74. doi:10.1016/j.eats.2014.05.005.
10. Suslak AG, Mather III RC, Kelly BT, Nho SJ. Improved arthroscopic visualization of peripheral compartment. Arthrosc Tech. 2012;1(1):e57–62. doi:10.1016/j.eats.2012.02.001.
11. Babst D, Steppacher SD, Ganz R, Siebenrock KA, Tannast M. The iliocapsularis muscle: an important stabilizer in the dysplastic hip. Clin Orthop Relat Res. 2011;469(6):1728–34. doi:10.1007/s11999-010-1705-x.
12. Ito H, Song Y, Lindsey DP, Safran MR, Giori NJ. The proximal hip joint capsule and the zona orbicularis contribute to hip joint stability in distraction. J Orthop Res. 2009;27:989–95.
13. Yamasaki S, Hashimoto Y, Terai S, Takigami J, Takahashi S, Nakamura H. Proposed referential index to resect femoroacetabular cam-type impingement during arthroscopy using a cadaveric hip model. Arthroscopy. 2015. doi:10.1016/j.arthro.2014.12.024 [Epub ahead of print].
14. Nötzli HP, Wyss TF, Stoecklin CH, Schmid MR, Treiber K, Holder J. The contour of the femoral head-neck junction as a predictor for the risk of anterior impingement. J Bone Joint Surg Br. 2002;84:556–60.
15. Mast NH, Impellizzeri F, Keller S, Leunig M. Reliability and agreement of measures used in radiographic evaluation of the adult hip. Clin Orthop Relat Res. 2011;469:188–99.
16. Lohan DG, Seeger LL, Motamedi K, Hame S, Sayre J. Cam-type femoral-acetabular impingement: is the alpha angle the best MR arthrography has to offer? Skeletal Radiol. 2009;38(9):855–62. doi:10.1007/s00256-009-0745-3.
17. Nouh MR, Schweitzer ME, Rybak L, Cohen J. Femoroacetabular impingement: can the alpha angle be estimated? Am J Roentgenol. 2008;190:1260–2. doi:10.2214/AJR.07.3258.
18. de SA D, Urquhart N, Philippon M, Ye JE, Simunovic N, Ayeni OR. Alpha angle correction in femoroacetabular impingement. Knee Surg Sports Traumatol Arthrosc. 2014;22(4):812–21. doi:10.1007/s00167-013-2678-6.
19. Brunner A, Horisberger M, Herzog RF. Evaluation of a computed tomography-based navigation system prototype for hip arthroscopy in the treatment of femoroacetabular cam impingement. Skeletal Radiol. 2009;38(9):855–62. doi:10.1007/s00256-009-0745-3.
20. Ilizaliturri V. Complications of arthroscopic femoroacetabular impingement treatment: a review. Clin Orthop Relat Res. 2009;467(3):760–8.
21. Papvasiliou AV, Bardakos NV. Complications of arthroscopic surgery of the hip. Bone Joint Res. 2012;1:131–44.
22. Philippon MJ, Stubbs AJ, Schenker ML, Maxwell RB, Ganz R, Leunig M. Arthroscopic management of femoroacetabular impingement: osteoplasty technique and literature review. Am J Sports Med. 2007;35(9):1571–80.
23. Heyworth BR, Shindle MK, Voos JE, Rudzki JR, Kelly BT. Radiologic and intraoperative findings in revision hip arthroscopy. Arthroscopy. 2007;23: 1295–302.
24. Mei-Dan O, Young DA. A novel technique for capsular repair and labrum refixation in hip arthroscopy using the SpeedStitch. Arthrosc Tech. 2012;1(1):e107–12. doi:10.1016/j.eats.2012.05.001.

25. Mei-Dan O, McConkey MO, Brick M. Catastrophic failure of hip arthroscopy due to iatrogenic instability: can partial division of the ligamentum teres and iliofemoral ligament cause subluxation? Arthroscopy. 2012;28:440–5. doi:10.1016/j.arthro.2011.12.005.
26. Frank RM, Lee S, Bush-Joseph CA, Kelly BT, Salata MJ, Nho SJ. Improved outcomes after hip arthroscopic surgery in patients undergoing T-capsulotomy with complete repair versus partial repair for femoroacetabular impingement: a comparative matched-pair analysis. Am J Sports Med. 2014;42(11):2634–42. doi:10.1177/0363546514548017.
27. Myers CA, Register BC, Lertwanich P, Ejnisman L, Pennington WW, Giphart JE, LaPrade RF, Philippon MJ. Role of the acetabular labrum and the iliofemoral ligament in hip stability: an in vitro biplane fluoroscopy study. Am J Sports Med. 2011;39(Suppl):85S–91. doi:10.1177/0363546511412161.
28. Martin HD, Savage A, Braly BA, Palmer IJ, Beall DP, Kelly B. The function of the hip capsular ligaments: a quantitative report. Arthroscopy. 2008;24:188–95. doi:10.1016/j.arthro.2007.08.024.
29. Hewitt JD, Glisson RR, Guilak F, Vail TP. The mechanical properties of the human hip capsule ligaments. J Arthroplasty. 2002;17:82–9.
30. Domb BG, Stake CE, Finley ZJ, Chen T, Giordano BD. Influence of capsular repair versus unrepaired capsulotomy on 2-year clinical outcomes after arthroscopic hip preservation surgery. Arthroscopy. 2014. doi:10.1016/j.arthro.2014.10.014.
31. Amar E, Warschawski Y, Sampson TG, Atoun E, Steinberg EL, Rath E. Capsular closure does not affect the development of heterotopic ossification after hip arthroscopy. Arthroscopy. 2015;31(2):225–30. doi:10.1016/j.arthro.2014.08.026.
32. Austin DC, Horneff JG, Kelly JD. Anterior hip dislocation 5 months after hip arthroscopy. Arthroscopy. 2014;30(10):1380–2. doi:10.1016/j.arthro.2014.04.099.
33. Domb BG, Philippon MJ, Giordano BD. Arthroscopic capsulotomy, capsular repair, and capsular plication of the hip: relation to atraumatic instability. Arthroscopy. 2013;29(1):162–73. doi:10.1016/j.arthro.2012.04.057.
34. Bayne CO, Stanley R, Simon P, Espinoza-Orias A, Salata MJ, Bush-Joseph CA, Inoue N, Nho SJ. Effect of capsulotomy on hip stability-a consideration during hip arthroscopy. Am J Orthop. 2014;43(4):160–5.

Arthroscopic Management of Pincer-Type Impingement

9

James B. Cowan, Christopher M. Larson, and Asheesh Bedi

Contents

J.B. Cowan, MD
Sports Medicine and Shoulder Service, Department of Orthopaedic Surgery, University of Michigan, MedSport, 24 Frank Lloyd Wright Dr. Lobby A, Ann Arbor, MI 48106, USA
e-mail: cowanj@med.umich.edu

C.M. Larson, MD
Minnesota Orthopedic Sports Medicine Institute, Twin Cities Orthopedics, Edina, MN 55435, USA
e-mail: chrislarson@tcomn.com

A. Bedi, MD (✉)
Sports Medicine and Shoulder Service, Department of Orthopaedic Surgery, University of Michigan, MedSport, 24 Frank Lloyd Wright Dr. Lobby A, Ann Arbor, MI 48106, USA

Department of Orthopaedic Surgery, University of Michigan, MedSport, 24 Frank Lloyd Wright Dr., Lobby A, Edina, MN 48106, USA
e-mail: abedi@med.umich.edu

9.1 Introduction

As mentioned in previous chapters, pincer-type femoroacetabular impingement (FAI) is due to repetitive and abnormal contact between the femoral head-neck junction and an area of either focal, relative, or global acetabular overcoverage [1]. Unlike CAM-type impingement, which causes a greater degree of intra-articular chondral damage, pincer-type impingement causes edge loading of the acetabular rim and labrum resulting in progressive tearing, degeneration, and ossification of the labrum and potential contrecoup chondral injury of the posteroinferior acetabulum or posteromedial femoral head (see Chap. 5 – Pathophysiology of Damage Associated with FAI) [2–4]. Cadaveric studies have shown that the labrum is important for maintaining hip stability, joint fluid seal, and intra-articular lubrication and fluid pressure to protect articular cartilage [5–9]. Subspine hip impingement is a distinct, though related, type of extra-articular pincer-type impingement between the anterior inferior iliac spine (AIIS) and the distal femoral neck [10, 11]. It is important to differentiate subspine impingement from acetabular retroversion as patients with these conditions may present with similar clinical and radiographic findings, but errant rim resection in this population can precipitate iatrogenic dysplasia [12, 13].

Previous chapters discuss the differential diagnosis, clinical diagnosis, and imaging of

O.R. Ayeni et al. (eds.), *Diagnosis and Management of Femoroacetabular Impingement*,
DOI 10.1007/978-3-319-32000-7_9

FAI. In general, when history, physical examination, and imaging studies are consistent with symptomatic pincer-type FAI, initial treatment should focus on symptomatic control, strengthening exercises, and activity modification. Formal physical therapy should avoid attempts to restore "normal" range of motion as this may aggravate symptoms due to repetitive impingement (see Chap. 7 – Nonoperative Management of FAI) [14]. However, improved core strength and control of pelvic tilt and obliquity may be important to improve functional range of motion. In patients with intermittent, activity-related pain that is refractory to at least 6 weeks of nonoperative management, arthroscopic surgical treatment may be considered in the absence of significant degenerative changes on plain radiographs (see Chap. 7 – Indications for FAI Surgery). The goal of FAI surgery is to eliminate areas of symptomatic focal impingement between the proximal femur and pelvis. The purpose of this chapter is to describe the contemporary techniques and outcomes of arthroscopic management of pincer-type FAI.

9.2 Intraoperative Setup

We prefer performing hip arthroscopy in the supine rather than lateral position, either on a standard fracture table or using a commercially available device/table for hip distraction (Fig. 9.1). Prior to positioning the patient, a thorough exam under anesthesia must be performed to determine the passive range of hip flexion, internal rotation, and external rotation. The patient's feet must be well padded and

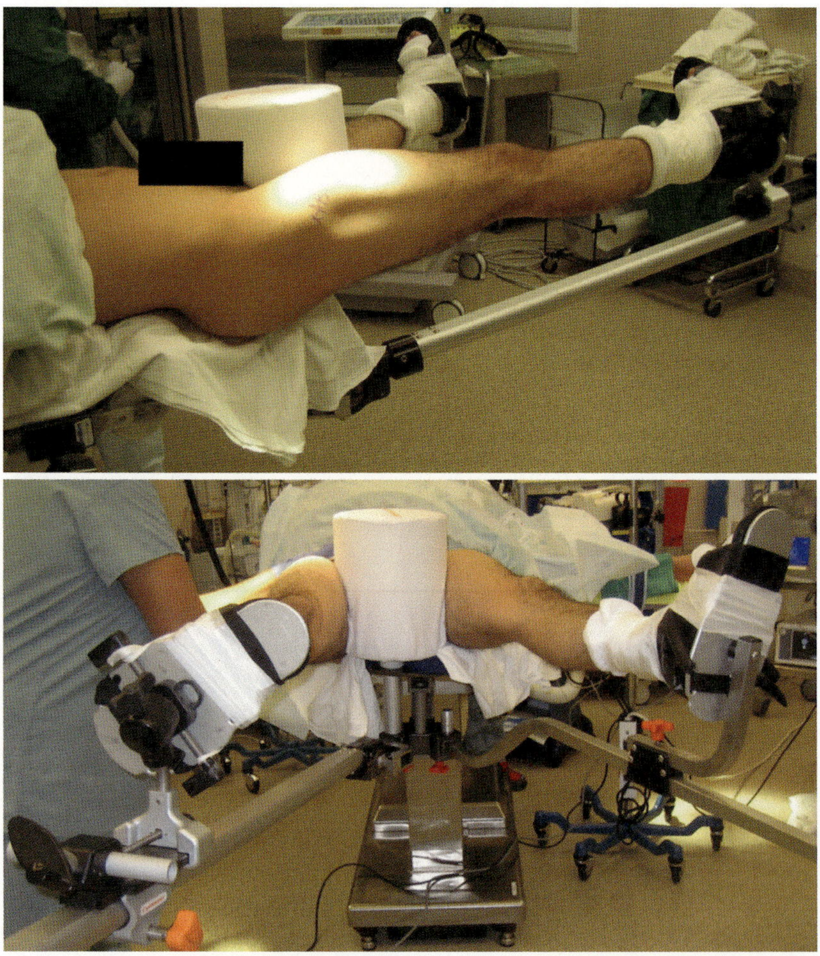

Fig. 9.1 Hip arthroscopy setup and patient positioning on operating table

adequately secured in the operative boots. A well-padded perineal post is positioned just lateral to midline toward the operative extremity to improve the vector of traction. The operative hip is positioned in 10° of flexion, 15° of internal rotation, and neutral abduction. Approximately 25–50 pounds of traction is applied to the operative extremity to ensure that approximately 6–8 mm of joint distraction may be achieved. Traction time should be ideally limited to less than 1 h and absolutely less than 2 h to reduce the risk of iatrogenic nerve injury [15]. The contralateral leg is positioned in slight abduction, external rotation, and with the minimal traction necessary to achieve adequate visualization, as the amount of traction may be a more important risk factor than the duration of traction for avoiding postoperative nerve dysfunction or injury [16].

Intraoperative fluoroscopy is arranged to match preoperative imaging. This is crucial for comparing the actual and planned procedures and avoiding over-resection, potentially leading to hip instability or dysplasia, or under-resection, particularly of posterosuperior pincer-type lesions [17, 18]. Such comparison may be useful as Philippon et al. [19] have shown than radiographic changes in lateral center-edge angle can be estimated by the amount of arthroscopic lateral rim resection. Neutral pelvic position is achieved by tilting the bed so that a line between each anterior superior iliac spine (ASIS) is parallel to the floor. Fluoroscopic assessment should include anteroposterior (AP), cross-table lateral, false profile, and 45° and 90° Dunn lateral images to ensure adequate intraoperative evaluation of all aspects of the proximal femur. Additionally, preoperative computer-assisted modeling using three-dimensional computed tomography (CT) may be useful for localizing areas of impingement and surgical planning [20, 21]. Certain consistent anatomic structures are also utilized (i.e., indirect head of the rectus femoris, psoas tendon, AIIS) to correlate zones of resection with the fluoroscopic anatomy.

9.3 Surgical Approach

The hip joint is first accessed via the anterolateral portal located approximately 1–2 cm anterior and 1–2 cm proximal to the anterosuperior aspect of the greater trochanter (Fig. 9.2). This is the viewing portal for the majority of the procedure. An 18-gauge spinal needle is inserted under fluoroscopic guidance to ensure adequate portal placement, taking care to avoid labral penetration or

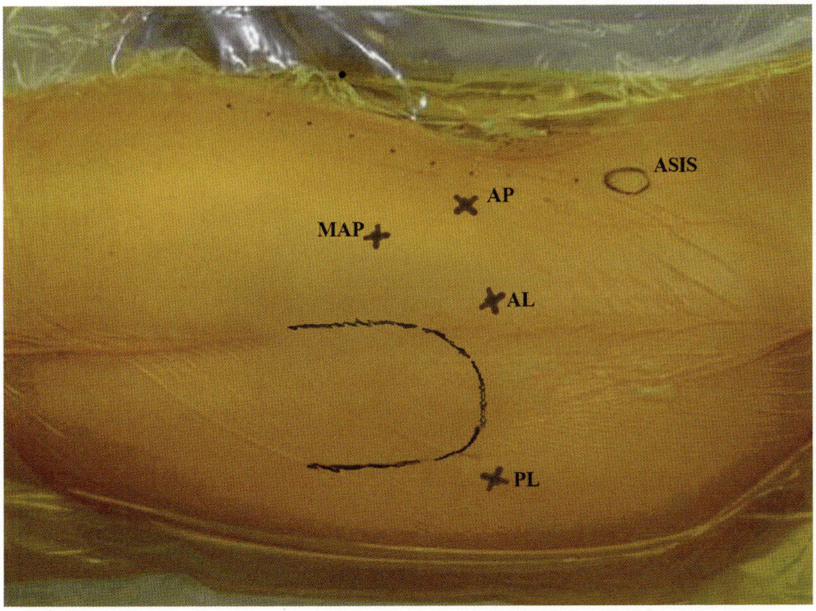

Fig. 9.2 Hip arthroscopy portals

iatrogenic femoral head chondral injury. Once intra-articular position is confirmed, the joint is distended with approximately 30 mL of normal saline. A guidewire is placed through the spinal needle, and a cannula is passed over the guidewire to enter the joint. After the arthroscope has been introduced, the anterior portal can be made using an 18-gauge spinal needle under direct visualization. Traditionally the anterior portal is made at the intersection between a line from the ASIS down the shaft of the femur and a horizontal line at the level of the superior aspect of the greater trochanter. However, we favor a modified anterior portal that is placed more laterally and distally to the standard anterior portal to increase margin of safety from the lateral femoral cutaneous nerve and improve trajectory for instrumentation of the labrum and acetabular rim.

A transverse interportal capsulotomy is made sharply to ensure adequate exposure (Fig. 9.3) [17]. Care is taken to remain between the labrum and femoral head to avoid iatrogenic labral or chondral injury. A blade is used rather than radiofrequency ablation to preserve full-thickness capsular margins for later repair [22]. A radio-frequency ablation wand is used to clear the extracapsular rim and expose the pincer lesion. The labral attachment and transitional zone cartilage are preserved whenever possible, but formal detachment and refixation may be required in certain cases of significant overcoverage (i.e., profunda) in which an extensive resection is required. A beaver blade is placed through the modified anterior portal, and the junction between the labrum and acetabular rim is identified. The labrum is detached from inferior to superior while taking care to avoid damage to the adjacent articular cartilage or labral amputation (Fig. 9.4). A thorough examination of the central compartment and pincer lesion is useful to define the type and extent of the pathology [4, 23]. The indirect head of the rectus femoris originating from the lateral acetabular rim uses a useful landmark for guiding rim resection (Fig. 9.5). Intraoperative findings consistent with pincer-type FAI include labral ecchymosis, ossification, and cystic degeneration; anterosuperior acetabular wave sign; posterior linear acetabular wear; extension of the acetabular rim at least 3–5 mm beyond the labrochondral junction; and anterior or superior acetabular rim fractures or os acetabuli [14]. The interportal capsulotomy can be extended posteriorly to the piriformis tendon or anteromedially to the psoas tendon depending on the extent of the pathology encountered [22]. Delaminated cartilage should be debrided to a stable edge. Microfracture may be selectively employed for focal full-thickness defects with well-shouldered margins. When small os acetabuli or rim fractures are encountered, typically

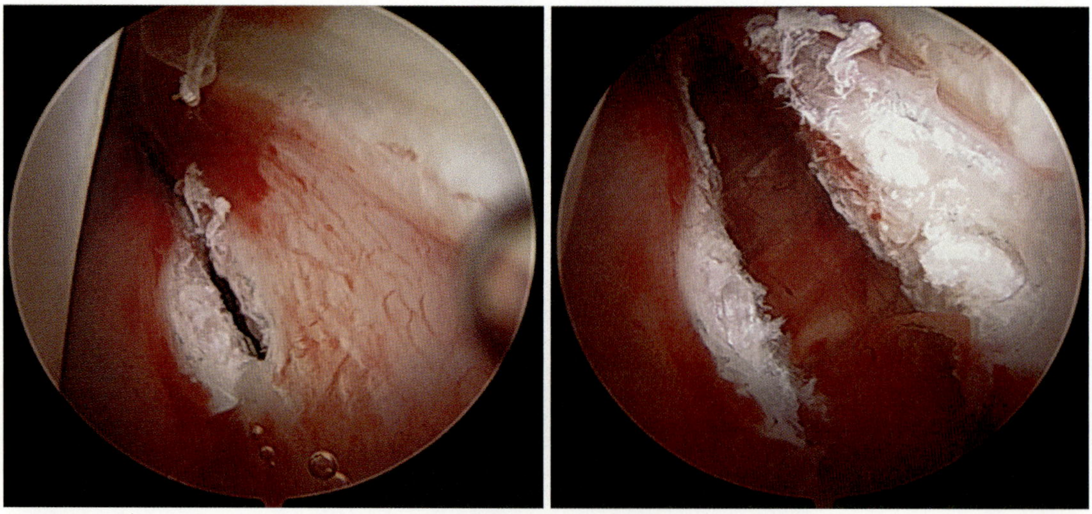

Fig. 9.3 Arthroscopic images demonstrating the interportal capsulotomy in a right hip

they may be excised to help resolve the pincer-type impingement (Fig. 9.6). However, larger fragments or those involving weight-bearing portions of the acetabulum may be treated with arthroscopic reduction and cannulated screw fixation to avoid iatrogenic dysplasia [24, 25].

A thorough assessment of the labrum is crucial to determine the need for labral preservation, debridement, or excision. Preservation is preferred, but debridement may be necessary in the presence of significant intrasubstance cystic degeneration or ossification. If the labrum appears relatively normal with an intact labrochondral junction, smaller areas of bony prominence of the acetabular rim may be resected via extracapsular exposure without formal detachment of the labrum. When a greater area of pathology is present, labral takedown is recommended prior to rim resection. Rim resection is performed with a burr placed via the modified anterior or lateral portal based on preoperative imaging and arthroscopic findings, with the goal being to contour the rim to correct the focal coverage or extra-articular subspine deformity extending to or caudal to the

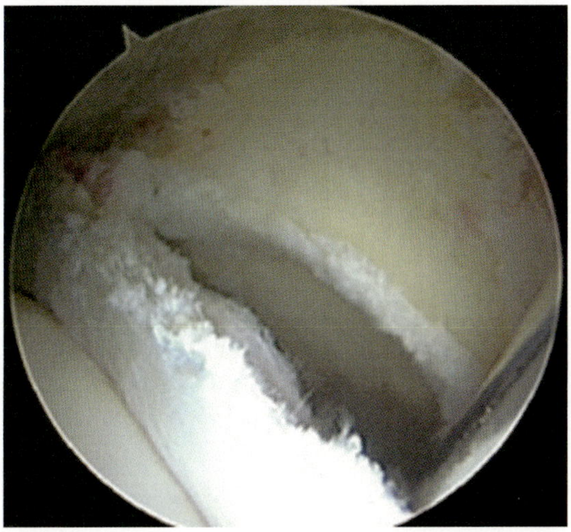

Fig. 9.4 Arthroscopic image demonstrating labral detachment to facilitate access to a pincer-type lesion

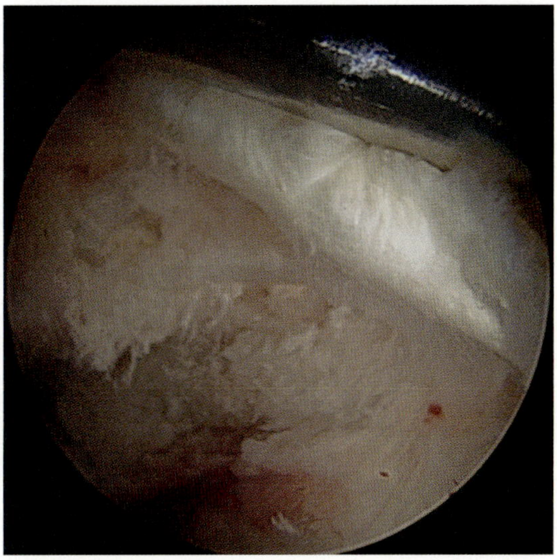

Fig. 9.5 Arthroscopic image demonstrating the origin of the indirect head of the rectus femoris from the acetabular rim

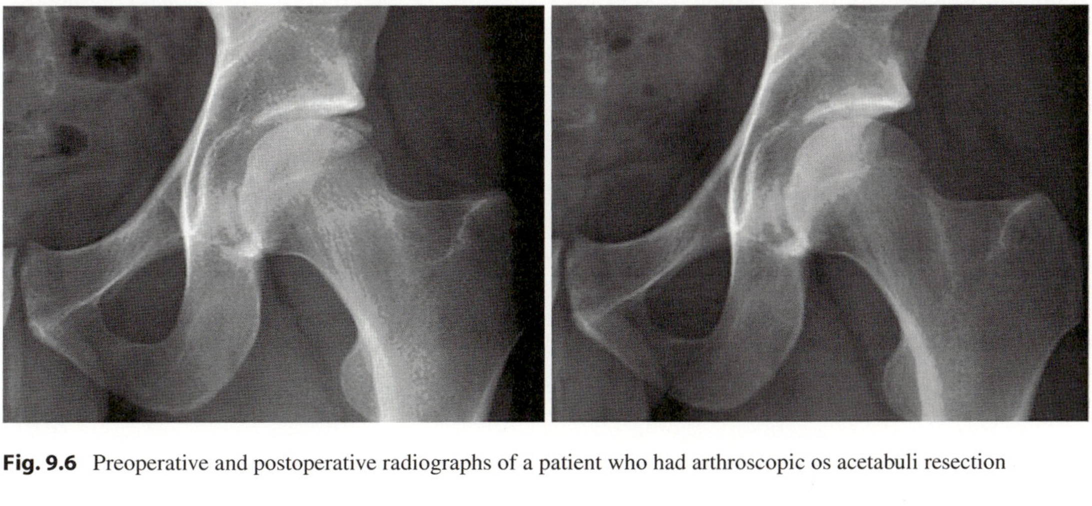

Fig. 9.6 Preoperative and postoperative radiographs of a patient who had arthroscopic os acetabuli resection

acetabular margin (Fig. 9.7). Fluoroscopy is used to identify the starting point for resection, which is typically just inferior to the location of the crossover sign. For focal anterior overcoverage, rim resection is performed to correct the area of focal retroversion as templated on preoperative imaging; the width of the burr can help to estimate the magnitude of resection. The amount of the bony resection should be sufficient to eliminate rim extension beyond the labrochondral junction and to eliminate the crossover sign and restore a lateral center-edge angle of 25–40° on fluoroscopic imaging. The deepest area of resection should occur at the midpoint of the pincer lesion with more gradual resection occurring peripherally. Resection of the harder, yellowish, pincer lesion should reveal the underlying softer, pinkish cancellous bone [17]. Some surgeons recommend microfracture of the subchondral bone until punctate bleeding occurs [4]. The amount of rim resection is confirmed and/or adjusted by comparing intraoperative fluoroscopy with preoperative imaging. Intermittent release of traction, fluoroscopic evaluation of acetabular coverage, and intraoperative assessment of range of motion may be useful to assess the extent of the correction.

The presence of subspine impingement should also be recognized and addressed as needed. This is best appreciated on false-profile plain radiographs and three-dimensional CT imaging [11]. Adequate visualization may require reflection of the joint capsule proximally up to the AIIS or creation of a window through the direct head of the rectus tendon. Decompression should be considered when there is AIIS extension to the level of, or caudal to, the anterior acetabular rim (Fig. 9.8). Other intraoperative findings suggestive of AIIS impingement include calcific deposits within the proximal rectus femoris and synovitis or peripheral labral ecchymosis anteriorly at the level of the AIIS [12]. An adequate resection may require making a small longitudinal split in the rectus femoris; however, detachment of the tendon should be avoided to prevent postoperative hip flexion weakness. Studies have shown that the broad footprint of the rectus tendon is protective, and a large series of arthroscopic resections performed for symptomatic deformity with this technique yielded excellent clinical outcomes with no cases of postoperative avulsion [26].

Once labral takedown and adequate rim resection is complete, labral refixation is indicated to reestablish femoral stability and physiologic joint seal (Fig. 9.9) [6, 27]. Preparation of the labrum and acetabulum may be completed with a motorized shaver and burr, respectively, to promote labral healing. Anchors should be placed with a distal-to-proximal trajectory to prevent intra-articular penetration. Fluoroscopy may be used to confirm that the drill is superior to the acetabular sourcil. We frequently utilize an accessory distal anterolateral portal to improve trajectory and safety. To avoid iatrogenic cartilage damage, the anchor should be placed 2 mm off the articular margin on the acetabular rim. During drilling and suture anchor placement, direct visualization of the articular surface is recommended

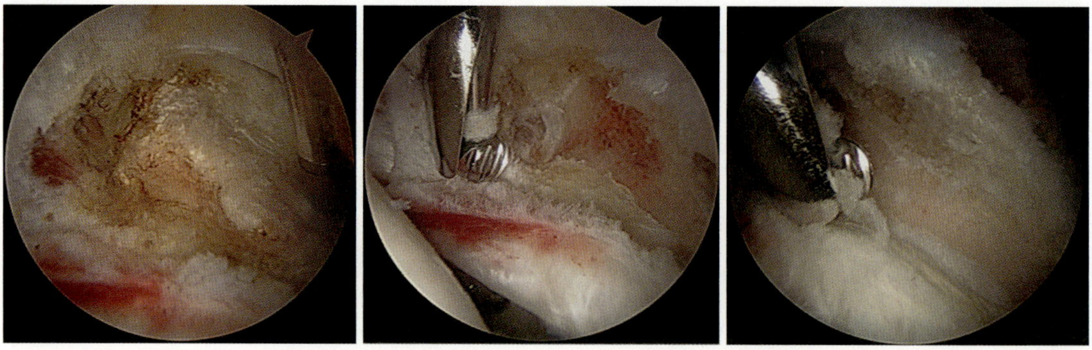

Fig. 9.7 Arthroscopic images demonstrating a pincer-type lesion prior to (far left) and during arthroscopic resection

to ensure that the articular surface is not penetrated. Labral base fixation stitches are utilized when possible to minimize eversion and preserve the suction seal, but formal detachment of the labrum or marginal tissue quality may necessitate simple "loop around" stitch configuration [14]. The suture is tied using standard arthroscopic knot-tying technique. The arthroscope is then moved to the anterolateral portal, and an anterior suture anchor is placed using the same technique. In total, at least one and as many as eight anchors may be required depending on the extent of the labral takedown.

To address superior and superoposterior pathology, the arthroscope is placed through the anterior portal. The beaver blade and burr are placed through the anterolateral portal as needed for additional labral takedown and rim resection.

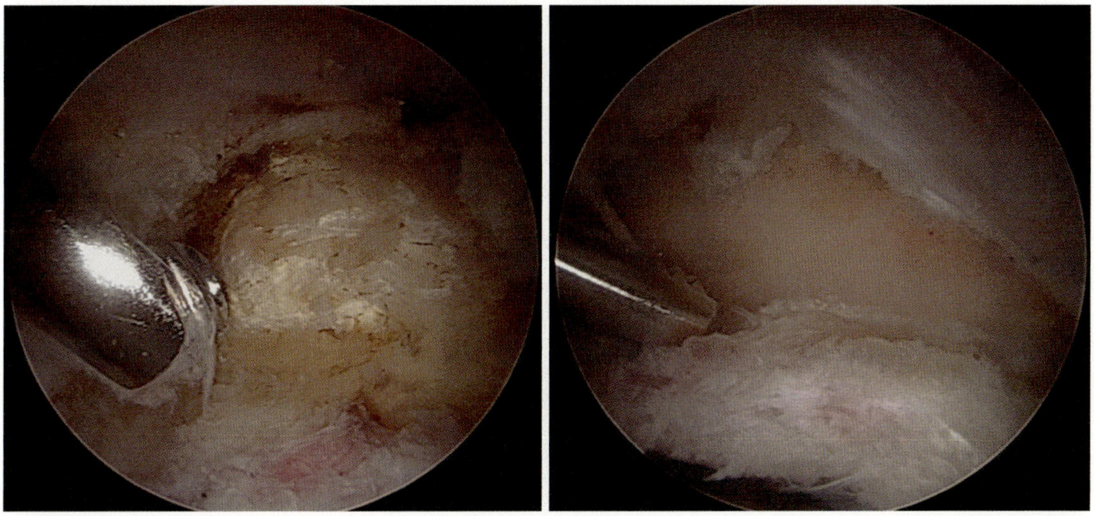

Fig. 9.8 Arthroscopic images demonstrating an anterior inferior iliac spine impingement lesion prior to (*left*) and during arthroscopic resection

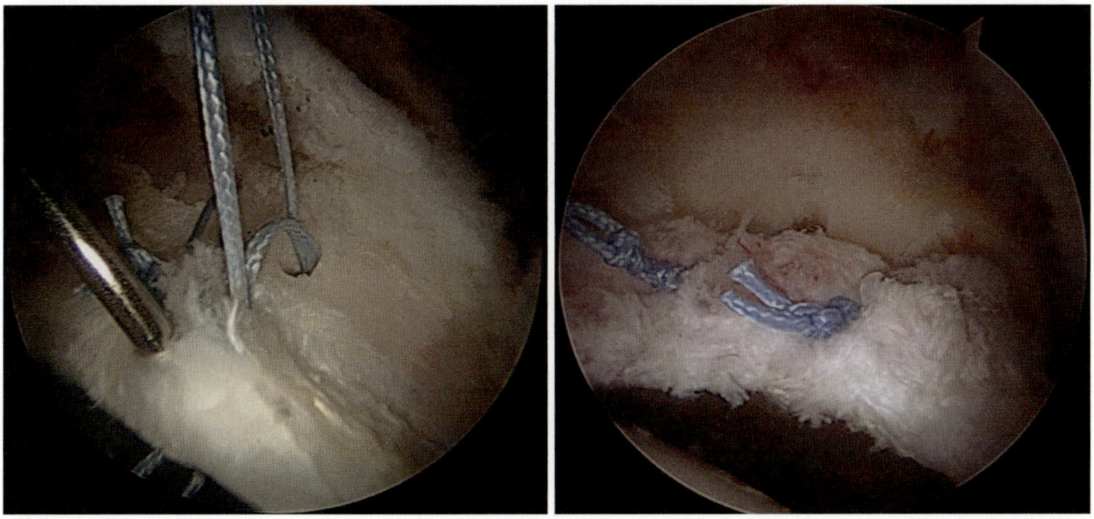

Fig. 9.9 Arthroscopic images demonstrating labral repair following labral detachment from the acetabular rim to facilitate pincer lesion resection

Again, fluoroscopy should be used to correlate intraoperative rim resection with preoperative imaging. When pincer-type FAI extends more posteriorly than is accessible through the anterior or anterolateral portals, a posterolateral portal may be established approximately 2 cm proximal to the greater trochanter at its posterosuperior margin. During placement of the posterolateral portal, the leg should be internally rotated to further protect the sciatic nerve.

At this point, thorough fluoroscopic and dynamic evaluation of the hip is crucial to assess for areas of residual impingement (Fig. 9.10). Fluoroscopic evaluation should include AP, cross-table lateral, and 45° and 90° Dunn lateral views to confirm improved acetabular morphology. While the presence or absence of CAM-type pathology should be confirmed during preoperative evaluation and imaging, "around the world" fluoroscopic views should confirm normal head-neck junction and femoral head sphericity. Ross et al. [28] described the six critical fluoroscopic images to assess the most common zones of proximal femoral deformity and assure a thorough correction in all of these planes. Dynamic evaluation should assess for residual impingement in extension, abduction, internal rotation, external rotation, FABER (maximum flexion, abduction, external rotation), and FADIR (maximum flexion, adduction, internal rotation). Once it is confirmed that no additional bony work is required, the motorized shaver should be reintroduced into the joint to remove bony debris to decrease the risk of postoperative heterotopic bone formation. Portal incisions are closed using simple interrupted nylon suture, and a soft dressing is applied.

9.4 Postoperative Management

Postoperative management and rehabilitation involve protecting any repaired or reconstructed structures while progressing with range-of-motion and strengthening exercises to minimize joint stiffness and muscle weakness, respectively (see Chap. 16 – Rehabilitation after FAI Surgery). In the early postoperative period, we restrict weight bearing and range of motion, particularly hip flexion and rotation. Passive range of motion begins immediately after surgery, followed by formal physical therapy guided by a therapist familiar with managing patients after hip arthroscopy.

9.5 Outcomes

To our knowledge, no studies report exclusively the results of arthroscopic treatment of isolated pincer-type FAI. This is not surprising as most patients presenting with FAI have mixed-type morphology involving both CAM and pincer lesions. Level III and IV studies of arthroscopic treatment of FAI report good to excellent results among outcome measures, including modified

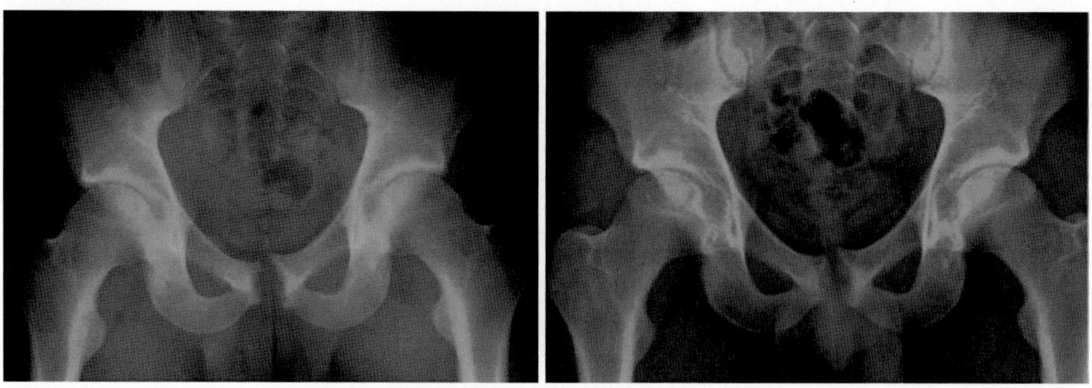

Fig. 9.10 Preoperative and postoperative anteroposterior pelvis radiographs of a patient with bilateral pincer-type impingement treated with arthroscopic rim resection. The crossover is present bilaterally on the preoperative radiograph (*left*)

Harris Hip Score (HHS), Hip Outcome Score (HOS), visual analog pain score, hip morphology, patient satisfaction, quality of life, and return to activity [29–34]. A study by Bedi et al. [20] confirmed that arthroscopic CAM and/or rim osteoplasty results in significant improvement in hip kinematics and range of motion in symptomatic patients. Although it has not been shown that arthroscopic treatment of FAI changes natural history or progression to osteoarthritis, elimination of impingement lesions hopefully decreases associated chondral injuries and preserves labral function to improve load transmission and joint-loading mechanics. Studies have also reported good clinical outcomes with labral preservation or repair, as compared with debridement or excision, during arthroscopic treatment of combined- and pincer-type FAI [35–40]. Hetsroni et al. [10] found significantly improved hip flexion and HHS in ten patients with AIIS impingement at an average follow-up of 14.7 months. In nine patients with an ipsilateral anterior CAM lesion, a preoperative intra-articular anesthetic injection did not relieve anterior hip pain. The authors interpreted this finding as being indicative of an extra-articular etiology of their symptoms. These studies support our preferred technique of arthroscopic acetabular rim osteoplasty, labral preservation or repair, and AIIS decompression in the setting of focal pincer-type FAI.

For all types of FAI, there is limited high-level evidence to support a given surgical technique. Systematic reviews have found comparable clinical outcomes among open, mini-open, and arthroscopic techniques [38, 41–44]. Arthroscopic techniques may have fewer major complications and allow for faster rehabilitation and sooner return to activity as compared with open surgery. Among various studies, negative predictors of clinical outcome include preoperative radiographic joint-space narrowing, higher grade of articular cartilage damage seen intraoperatively or on magnetic resonance imaging, and longer duration of preoperative symptoms [38, 39, 41, 45].

Hip arthroscopy may have a more limited application in certain types of pincer impingement such as global acetabular overcoverage (coxa profunda, protrusio acetabuli) and relative acetabular retroversion with decreased posterior coverage. Arthroscopic techniques to address these conditions have been described; however, concerns remain regarding the technical expertise required and the ability to adequately access and correct the deformity [46–48]. Furthermore, studies have suggested that protrusio deformity is far more complex than simply global overcoverage and that associated medial acetabular dysplasia and relative neck shortening are contributory to the pathology and not addressed with isolated rim recession [49, 50]. In the setting of acetabular retroversion with posterior undercoverage, arthroscopic resection of the anterior acetabulum may result in global undercoverage and hip instability. In such cases of complex deformity, techniques such as open surgical dislocation or anteverting periacetabular osteotomy may be more appropriate [51]. Additional clinical studies are needed to determine how to best address these complex morphologic problems.

Conclusions

Arthroscopic treatment of pincer-type FAI is a relatively safe treatment option that results in improved outcomes when nonoperative management has been ineffective. Thorough clinical evaluation and preoperative imaging are crucial for confirming the absence of ipsilateral pathology such as CAM-type FAI, coxa profunda, protrusio acetabuli, and hip dysplasia. Most studies report level III or IV evidence, such that future prospective studies with long-term follow-up and validated outcome measures will improve the quality of the literature regarding the treatment and outcomes of FAI.

Take-Home Points

1. Pincer Type FAI includes a variety of anatomical variants that range from focal to global acetabular overcoverage.
2. Pre operative planning using imaging is essential in determining location and extent of lesion resection.
3. Concurrent subpsine impingement should be addressed when present.

4. Labral and cartilage damage should be addressed comprehensively after the resection of the Pincer Lesion.
5. Dynamic clinical and intra operative radiographic assessment should confirm adequacy of resection at the completion of procedure.

Key Evidence Related Sources

1. Beck M, Kalhor M, Leunig M, Ganz R. Hip morphology influences the pattern of damage to the acetabular cartilage: femoroacetabular impingement as a cause of early osteoarthritis of the hip. J Bone Joint Surg Br. 2005;87(7):1012–8.
2. Larson CM, Kelly BT, Stone RM. Making a case for anterior inferior iliac spine/subspine hip impingement: three representative case reports and proposed concept. Arthroscopy. 2011;27(12):1732–7.
3. Zaltz I, Kelly BT, Hetsroni I, Bedi A. The crossover sign overestimates acetabular retroversion. Clin Orthop Relat Res. 2013;471(8):2463–70.
4. Chow RM, Krych AJ, Levy BA. Arthroscopic acetabular rim resection in the treatment of femoroacetabular impingement. Arthrosc Tech. 2013;2(4):e327–31.
5. Philippon MJ, Wolff AB, Briggs KK, Zehms CT, Kuppersmith DA. Acetabular rim reduction for the treatment of femoroacetabular impingement correlates with preoperative and postoperative center-edge angle. Arthroscopy. 2010;26(6):757–61.

References

1. Ganz R, Parvizi J, Beck M, Leunig M, Notzli H, Siebenrock KA. Femoroacetabular impingement: a cause for osteoarthritis of the hip. Clin Orthop Relat Res. 2003;417:112–20.
2. Beck M, Kalhor M, Leunig M, Ganz R. Hip morphology influences the pattern of damage to the acetabular cartilage: femoroacetabular impingement as a cause of early osteoarthritis of the hip. J Bone Joint Surg Br. 2005;87(7):1012–8.
3. Beck M, Leunig M, Parvizi J, Boutier V, Wyss D, Ganz R. Anterior femoroacetabular impingement: part II. Midterm results of surgical treatment. Clin Orthop Relat Res. 2004;418:67–73.
4. Philippon MJ, Schenker ML. Arthroscopy for the treatment of femoroacetabular impingement in the athlete. Clin Sports Med. 2006;25:299–308.
5. Cadet ER, Chan AK, Vorys GC, Gardner T, Yin B. Investigation of the preservation of the fluid seal effect in the repaired, partially resected, and reconstructed acetabular labrum in a cadaveric hip model. Am J Sports Med. 2012;40(10):2218–23.
6. Crawford MJ, Dy CJ, Alexander JW, et al. The biomechanics of the hip labrum and the stability of the hip. Clin Orthop Relat Res. 2007;465:16–22.
7. Ferguson SJ, Bryant JT, Ganz R, Ito K. Acetabular labrum seal: a poroelastic finite element model. Clin Biomech. 2000;15:463–8.
8. Ferguson SJ, Bryant JT, Ganz R, Ito K. An in vitro investigation of the acetabular labral seal in hip joint mechanics. J Biomech. 2003;36:171–8.
9. Smith MV, Panchal HB, Ruberte Thiele RA, Sekiya JK. Effect of acetabular labrum tears on hip stability and labral strain in a joint compression model. Am J Sports Med. 2011;39:103S–10.
10. Hetsroni I, Larson CM, Dela Torre K, Zbeda RM, Magennis E, Kelly BT. Anterior inferior iliac spine deformity as an extra-articular source for hip impingement: a series of 10 patients treated with arthroscopic decompression. Arthroscopy. 2012;28(11):1644–53.
11. Hetsroni I, Poultsides L, Bedi A, Larson CM, Kelly BT. Anterior inferior iliac spine morphology correlates with hip range of motion: a classification system and dynamic model. Clin Orthop Relat Res. 2013;471(8):2497–503.
12. Larson CM, Kelly BT, Stone RM. Making a case for anterior inferior iliac spine/subspine hip impingement: three representative case reports and proposed concept. Arthroscopy. 2011;27(12):1732–7.
13. Zaltz I, Kelly BT, Hetsroni I, Bedi A. The crossover sign overestimates acetabular retroversion. Clin Orthop Relat Res. 2013;471(8):2463–70.
14. Larson CM. Arthroscopic management of pincer-type impingement. Sports Med Arthrosc Rev. 2010;18(2):100–7.
15. Philippon MJ, Stubbs AJ, Schenker ML, Maxwell RB, Ganz R, Leunig M. Arthroscopic management of femoroacetabular impingement: osteoplasty technique and literature review. Am J Sports Med. 2007;35(9):1571–80.
16. Telleria JJ, Safran MR, Harris AH, Gardi JN, Glick JM. Risk of sciatic nerve traction injury during hip arthroscopy-is it the amount or duration? an intraoperative nerve monitoring study. J Bone Joint Surg Am. 2012;94(22):2025–32.

17. Chow RM, Krych AJ, Levy BA. Arthroscopic acetabular rim resection in the treatment of femoroacetabular impingement. Arthrosc Tech. 2013;2(4): e327–31.
18. Zumstein M, Hahn F, Sukthankar A, Sussmann PS, Dora C. How accurately can the acetabular rim be trimmed in hip arthroscopy for pincer-type femoral acetabular impingement: a cadaveric investigation. Arthroscopy. 2009;25(2):164–8.
19. Philippon MJ, Wolff AB, Briggs KK, Zehms CT, Kuppersmith DA. Acetabular rim reduction for the treatment of femoroacetabular impingement correlates with preoperative and postoperative center-edge angle. Arthroscopy. 2010;26(6):757–61.
20. Bedi A, Dolan M, Hetsroni I, et al. Surgical treatment of femoroacetabular impingement improves hip kinematics: a computer-assisted model. Am J Sports Med. 2011;29(1):43S–9.
21. Bedi A, Dolan M, Magennis E, Lipman J, Buly R, Kelly BT. Computer-assisted modeling of osseous impingement and resection in femoroacetabular impingement. Arthroscopy. 2012;28(2): 204–10.
22. Bedi A, Galano G, Walsh C, Kelly BT. Capsular management during hip arthroscopy: from femoracetabular impingement to instability. Arthroscopy. 2011;27(12):1720–31.
23. Guanche CA, Bare AA. Arthroscopic treatment of femoroacetabular impingement. Arthroscopy. 2006; 22(1):95–106.
24. Epstein NP, Safran MR. Stress fracture of the acetabular rim: arthroscopic reduction and internal fixation. J Bone Joint Surg Am. 2009;91(6):1480–6.
25. Larson CM, Stone RM. The rarely encountered rim fracture that contributes to both femoroacetabular impingement and hip stability: a report of 2 cases of arthroscopic partial excision and internal fixation. Arthroscopy. 2011;27(7):1018–22.
26. Hapa OH, Bedi A, Gursan O, et al. Anatomic footprint of the direct head of the rectus femoris origin: cadaveric study and clinical series of hips after arthroscopic anterior inferior iliac spine/subspine decompression. Arthroscopy. 2013;29(12):1932–40.
27. Philippon MJ, Schenker ML. A new method for acetabular rim trimming and labral repair. Clin Sports Med. 2006;25:293–7.
28. Ross JR, Bedi A, Stone RM, et al. Intraoperative fluoroscopic imaging to treat cam deformities: correlation with 3-dimensional computed tomography. Am J Sports Med. 2014;42(6):1370–6.
29. Fabricant PD, Heyworth BE, Kelly BT. Hip arthroscopy improves symptoms associated with FAI in selected adolescent athletes. Clin Orthop Relat Res. 2012;470(1):261–9.
30. Larson CM, Giveans MR. Arthroscopic management of femoroacetabular impingement: early outcomes measures. Arthroscopy. 2008;24(5):540–6.
31. Malviya A, Stafford GH, Villar RN. Impact of arthroscopy of the hip for femoroacetabular impingement on quality of life at a mean follow-up of 3.2 years. J Bone Joint Surg Br. 2012;94(4):466–70.
32. Nho SJ, Magennis EM, Singh CK, Kelly BT. Outcomes after the arthroscopic treatment of femoroacetabular impingement in a mixed group of high-level athletes. Am J Sports Med. 2011;39(1): 14S–9.
33. Philippon M, Schenker M, Briggs K, Kuppersmith D. Femoroacetabular impingement in 45 professional athletes: associated pathologies and return to sport following arthroscopic decompression. Knee Surg Sports Traumatol Arthrosc. 2007;15:908–14.
34. Philippon MJ, Weiss DR, Kuppersmith DA, Briggs KK, Hay CJ. Arthroscopic labral repair and treatment of femoroacetabular impingement in professional hockey players. Am J Sports Med. 2010;38(1):99–104.
35. Krych AJ, Thompson M, Knutson Z, Scoon J, Coleman SH. Arthroscopic labral repair versus selective labral debridement in female patients with femoroacetabular impingement: a prospective randomized study. Arthroscopy. 2013;29(1):46–53.
36. Larson CM, Giveans MR. Arthroscopic debridement versus refixation of the acetabular labrum associated with femoroacetabular impingement. Arthroscopy. 2009;25(4):369–76.
37. Larson CM, Giveans MR, Stone RM. Arthroscopic debridement versus refixation of the acetabular labrum associated with femoroacetabular impingement: mean 3.5-year follow-up. Am J Sports Med. 2012;40(5):1015–21.
38. Ng VY, Arora N, Best TM, Pan X, Ellis TJ. Efficacy of surgery for femoroacetabular impingement: a systematic review. Am J Sports Med. 2010;38(11): 2337–45.
39. Philippon MJ, Briggs KK, Yen YM, Kuppersmith DA. Outcomes following hip arthroscopy for femoroacetabular impingement with associated chondrolabral dysfunction: minimum two-year follow-up. J Bone Joint Surg Br. 2009;91(1):16–23.
40. Redmond JM, El Bitar YF, Gupta A, Stake CE, Domb BG. Arthroscopic acetabuloplasty and labral refixation without labral detachment. Am J Sports Med. 2014;43:105–12.
41. Bedi A, Chen N, Robertson W, Kelly BT. Management of labral tears and femoroacetabular impingement of the hip in the young, active patient. Arthroscopy. 2008;24(10):1135–45.
42. Botser IB, Smith TW, Nasser R, Domb BG. Open surgical dislocation versus arthroscopy for femoroacetabular impingement: a comparison of clinical outcomes. Arthroscopy. 2011;27(2):270–8.
43. Matsuda DK, Carlisle JC, Arthurs SC, Wierks CH, Philippon MJ. Comparative systematic review of the open dislocation, mini-open, and arthroscopic surgeries for femoroacetabular impingement. Arthroscopy. 2011;27(2):252–69.
44. Papalia R, Del Buono A, Franceschi F, Marinozzi A, Maffulli N, Denaro V. Femoroacetabular impingement syndrome management: arthroscopy or open surgery? Int Orthop. 2012;36:903–14.

45. Larson CM, Giveans MR, Taylor M. Does arthroscopic FAI correction improve function with radiographic arthritis? Clin Orthop Relat Res. 2011;469:1667–76.
46. Matsuda DK. Protrusio acetabuli: contraindication or indication for hip arthroscopy? and the case for arthroscopic treatment of global pincer impingement. Arthroscopy. 2012;28(6):882–8.
47. Matsuda DK, Gupta N, Hanami D. Hip arthroscopy for challenging deformities: global pincer femoroacetabular impingement. Arthrosc Tech. 2014;3(2):e197–204.
48. Safran MR, Epstein NP. Arthroscopic management of protrusio acetabuli. Arthroscopy. 2013;29(11):1777–82.
49. Leunig M, Nho SJ, Turchetto L, Ganz R. Protrusio acetabuli: new insights and experience with joint preservation. Clin Orthop Relat Res. 2009;467(9):2241–50.
50. Liechti EF, Ferguson SJ, Tannast M. Protrusio acetabuli: joint loading with severe pincer impingement and its theoretical implications for surgical therapy. J Orthop Res. 2014;33:106–13.
51. Zaltz I, Kelly BT, Larson CM, Leunig M, Bedi A. Surgical treatment of femoroacetabular impingement: what are the limits of hip arthroscopy? Arthroscopy. 2014;30(1):99–110.

Open Management of CAM Deformities in FAI

10

Colleen A. Weeks and Douglas D.R. Naudie

Contents

C.A. Weeks, MD, FRCSC
Division of Orthopaedic Surgery, Department of Surgery, University of Alberta, 400 – Community Service Center, Royal Alexandra Hospital, 10240 Kingsway Avenue, Edmonton, AB T5H 3V9, Canada
e-mail: cweeks1@ualberta.ca

D.D.R. Naudie, MD, FRCSC (✉)
Division of Orthopaedics, Department of Surgery, Western University, Schulich School of Medicine, A9-028, 339 Windermere Road, London, ON N6A 5A5, Canada

Division of Orthopaedic Surgery, Department of Surgery, London Health Sciences Center, University Hospital, London, ON, Canada

Joint Replacement Institute, London, ON, Canada
e-mail: Douglas.Naudie@lhsc.on.ca

10.1 Introduction and Background

Femoroacetabular impingement (FAI) is defined as an anatomic abnormality causing impingement of the femoral head-neck region against the acetabular rim. The abnormal contact forces cause damage to the labrum and shearing of the chondrolabral junction. Impingement occurs at both supraphysiologic extremes of motion in a normal joint and secondary to morphological abnormalities of the hip joint. A CAM lesion is a result of an asphericity of the femoral head-neck junction. The deformity causes jamming of the femoral head into a non-compliant acetabulum. Morphological abnormalities can result as a consequence of pathologic conditions, including slipped capital femoral epiphysis and previous periacetabular or proximal femoral osteotomy, but can also arise idiopathically. These lesions occur most commonly in young males. Presentation is most commonly a complaint of deep groin pain, worsened with prolonged sitting or activity requiring flexion of the hip.

O.R. Ayeni et al. (eds.), *Diagnosis and Management of Femoroacetabular Impingement*,
DOI 10.1007/978-3-319-32000-7_10

The increased contact force caused by the CAM lesion and consequent damage to the labrum and chondrolabral junction is a proposed cause of early-onset arthritis in the non-dysplastic hip [13]. Hip joint preservation surgery is aimed at both the alleviation of symptoms by restoring a normal range of hip motion and elimination of the abutment of the femoral head on the acetabulum and prevention of damage leading to arthritic changes in the young patient.

10.2 Indications and Decision-Making in Surgical Treatment of FAI

Decision-making in the young patient with hip impingement is complex in both timing and technique, with multiple options available. Hip joint preservation surgery is indicated in the young, symptomatic patient who has failed conservative treatment for their symptoms. Evidence does not provide any solid recommendations for optimal timing of surgery; however, earlier treatment may prevent the irreversible chondral damage that leads to early arthritic changes in young adults. Beaule et al. [3] have proposed that indications for surgery include patient age less than 45 years, moderate to severe symptoms, greater than 2 mm of joint space, and presence of a correctible radiographic deformity. Mardones et al. [16] also recommend surgical treatment in young patients with a correctible structural problem in the joint; this includes deformities resulting from a slipped capital femoral epiphysis, posttraumatic deformity, decreased femoral head-neck offset, and a nonspherical femoral head. Significant degenerative changes in the hip joint and deformities that cannot be surgically corrected are contraindications to hip joint preservation surgery. Hip joint preservation surgery is also relatively contraindicated in patients with advanced age and with inflammatory arthritis.

Hip joint preservation surgery in patients with CAM lesions consists of surgical osteochondroplasty of the femoral head-neck junction. This can be achieved through multiple techniques, which include open surgical dislocation of the hip as described by Ganz et al. [12], hip arthroscopy, or a minimally invasive open approach that can be combined with arthroscopy. Decision-making regarding approach depends on multiple patient and radiographic factors. Beaule et al. [3] recommend open surgical dislocation for CAM-type lesions with or without proximal femoral deformity and lesions on the posterosuperior aspect of the neck that are difficult to access from an arthroscopic or mini-open approach.

The minimally invasive open approach to CAM deformity utilizes a small anterior or anterolateral approach for osteochondroplasty. It does not allow for circumferential exposure of the head-neck junction and thus is not indicated for posterior lesions, circumferential CAM deformity, or those associated with significant femoral or acetabular deformity that may be better corrected with an open surgical dislocation. Furthermore, loss of the femoral offset that extends superiorly or posterosuperiorly requires elevation of the retinacular vessels for corrections and may be better addressed by open surgical dislocation.

In order to better guide decision-making in terms of approach to CAM resection, Diaz-Ledezma and Parvizi [11] created an analytic hierarchical analysis to compare the three main treatment options in FAI. Decision-making was guided by a combination of cost analysis, expert opinion, evidence, and the understanding of the pathophysiology causing impingement. Cost was based on monetary value at a single US center, and complications specific to the procedures were used. Software analysis recommended the mini-open approach as the superior procedure, but cost was the most influential criteria, and with this removed, arthroscopy was recommended but showed minimal benefit over the other treatment options. Their analysis did not factor in the significant learning curve associated with hip arthroscopy and mini-open procedures.

Zingg et al. [22] prospectively examined the outcomes of surgical hip dislocation in direct comparison to hip arthroscopy. Patients with a positive impingement test and the presence of a CAM lesion on MRI were included. Patients with previous surgery and arthritis of Tönnis grade greater than 1 were excluded. A total of 38 patients, 23 in the hip arthroscopy and 15 in the surgical dislocation group, were included and followed by means of the Western Ontario and McMaster Universities Arthritis Index (WOMAC) and a visual pain analogue score. Patients were also followed radiographically by MRI, and the alpha angle, the anterior head-neck offset, the anterior acetabular coverage angle, and the resection depth and width were recorded. The groups had similar preoperative characteristics. The surgical dislocation group required a longer hospital stay and had higher subjective pain scores and lower Harris hip scores at 6 weeks and 3 months, but there were no significant clinical differences in outcome scores at 1 year. The arthroscopy group had a larger alpha angle correction and a higher rate of labral resection rather than repair. The arthroscopy group also had a significantly lower visual analogue scale evaluating pain experienced during activities of daily living at 12 months compared to the group who had open surgery. Those patients in the open surgical hip dislocation group required a longer absence from work. With respect to numbers of patients able to return to high-level sport, there were no significant differences reported between the two groups; however, at 12 months, 10 of 23 patients in the arthroscopic group were able to return to high-level sport, compared to 5 of 15 in the open group.

The results of FAI treatment by arthroscopic and open surgical hip dislocation have been compared by radiographic and clinical results. While arthroscopy is increasing in popularity, open surgical hip dislocation still provides the benefit of access to posterosuperior lesions and allows for treatment of more significant proximal femoral deformity. Bedi et al. [6] reported on a series of 60 patients undergoing correction of CAM lesions by means of arthroscopy or open surgical dislocation. The groups were compared radiographically with anteroposterior pelvis and (Dunn) lateral radiographs by assessment of anterior femoral head-neck offset, anteroposterior and lateral α angle, and β angle on preoperative and postoperative radiographs. Patients in the open group were found to have a significantly better improvement in the alpha angle correction and anterior head-neck offset than the patients in the arthroscopic group. However, the authors reported that arthroscopic osteochondroplasty did restore head-neck offset and achieve comparable efficacy to open surgical dislocation for anterior and anterosuperior CAM and focal rim impingement deformities. The authors concluded that the open technique may allow greater correction of posterosuperior loss of femoral offset and may be favorable for FAI patterns that demonstrate considerable proximal femoral deformity on AP radiographs. It is important to note that other studies have shown that alpha angle measurements have been shown to have a high rate of intraobserver and interobserver variability [7].

10.3 Technique of Open Surgical Dislocation

The technique of surgical dislocation has been well described by Ganz et al. [5, 12]. A summary of the technique is as follows. The patient is positioned in the lateral decubitus position, and the approach can be initiated through either a Kocher-Langenbeck or Gibson approach (Fig. 10.1). The posterior border of the gluteus medius is identified, and an incision is made along the posterior edge of the muscle to the vastus ridge. An osteotomy of the greater trochanter, approximately 1.5 cm in thickness, is made in line with the incision and should exit anterior to the most posterior aspect of the gluteus medius, in order to protect the profundus branch of the MFCA (Fig. 10.2). It is important to keep the fibers of the vastus lateralis attached to the trochanter distally to resist proximal escape of the fragment. A modification of the traditional osteotomy to a stepped cut has also been described and popularized for more stable fixation [2]. The osteotomized fragment is mobilized anteriorly, and with the leg flexed and externally rotated, the vastus lateralis and intermedius are elevated from the proximal femur.

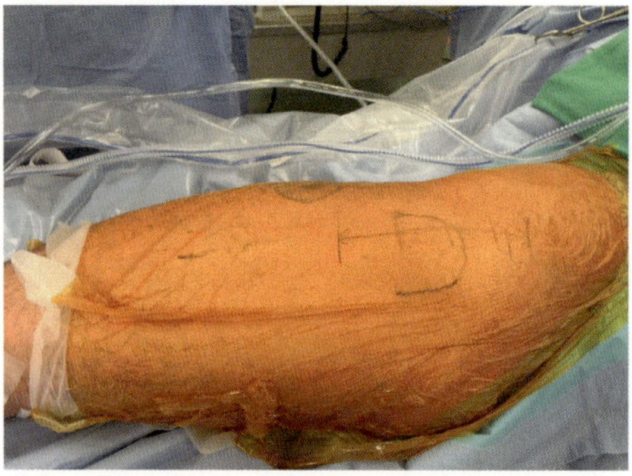

Fig. 10.1 Intraoperative view of the traditional positioning and incision for open surgical dislocation of the hip

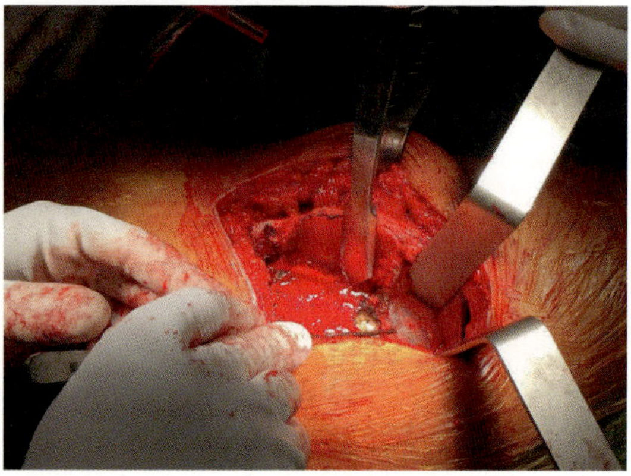

Fig. 10.2 Intraoperative view of the same patient (in Fig. 10.1) illustrating the osteotomy of the greater trochanter, approximately 1.5 cm in thickness, reflected from anterior to posterior

The tendon of piriformis is identified, and the inferior border of the gluteus minimus is separated from the tendon and underlying capsule. The muscle of gluteus minimus is retracted anteriorly and superiorly to expose the hip joint capsule. A capsulotomy is made along the neck of the femur and extended anteroinferiorly, avoiding injury to the MFCA. Elevation of the flap allows for visualization of the labrum (Fig. 10.3). At this point, a "Z" capsulotomy is completed with the third incision turning posteriorly along the superior margin of the acetabulum running parallel the cartilage. It is very important not to damage the labrum performing this limb of the capsulotomy. The hip can then be dynamically ranged into flexion and internal rotation to assess and identify any areas of anterior femoral acetabular impingement. The hip can also be extended and externally rotated to identify any areas of posterior impingement.

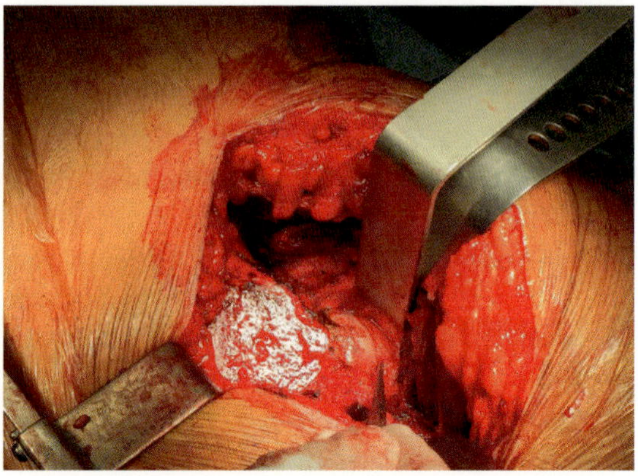

Fig. 10.3 Intraoperative view of the same patient illustrating reflection of the anterior sleeve of capsule and excellent visualization of the deformity at the femoral head-neck junction and the intact labrum

The hip is then formally dislocated anteriorly through flexion and external rotation. It is often necessary to cut the ligamentum teres with curved capsular scissors to enable complete dislocation. It is also necessary to bring the leg over the front of the OR table to maximize exposure. This technique allows complete visualization of the acetabulum and femoral head through manipulation of the leg. Resection of the CAM lesion is completed under direct visualization with a combination of osteotomes and a high-speed burr. Correction of the sphericity of the femoral head can be assessed with the use of commercially available plastic templates (Figs. 10.4 and 10.5). Any remnants of the ligamentum teres, thickening of the pulvinar, acetabular rim lesions, and chondrolabral pathology are visualized addressed (Fig. 10.6). The posterior and posterosuperior portions of the acetabulum can be visualized with further flexion and external rotation of the leg. The hip is then relocated, and dynamic reassessment of the impinging region is performed. It is necessary to confirm complete resection of any residual impingement. Bone wax can be applied to the resected area to prevent intra-articular bleeding and capsular adhesions. The hip is then

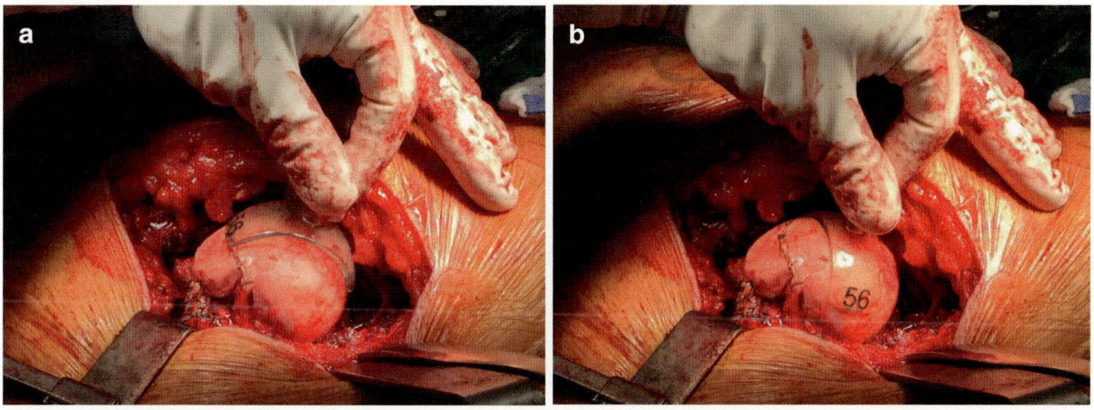

Fig. 10.4 (**a**, **b**) Intraoperative views of the same patient illustrating the use of commercially available templates in a severe CAM deformity of the femoral neck junction

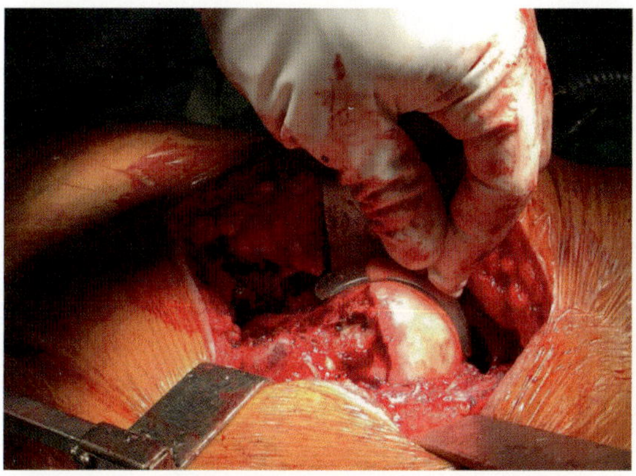

Fig. 10.5 Intraoperative view of the same patient illustrating the use of commercially available templates to confirm adequate offset restoration following open osteochondroplasty

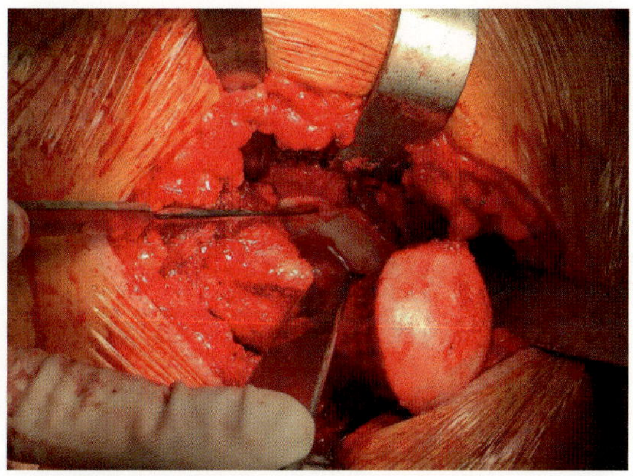

Fig. 10.6 Intraoperative view of the same patient following osteochondroplasty of the femoral head-neck junction and illustrating chondral damage to the anterior portion of the acetabulum

reduced and the capsule is repaired side to side with a running suture. The trochanteric osteotomy is fixed with 2 or 3 3.5 mm or 4.5 mm screws (Fig. 10.7).

Postoperatively, patients are mobilized the day after surgery touch weight bearing to their operated extremity. Range of motion is sometimes restricted to 90° if a labral repair is performed. Patients received routine antibiotic and deep vein thrombosis prophylaxis. Patients are typically discharged home on day two and are initiated with immediate physical therapy. They return to the clinic at 6 weeks, at which time radiographs are performed to confirm union of the trochanteric osteotomy. Patients are then gradually advanced to protected (typically 50%) weight bearing after 6 weeks' duration. The patient returns for a 10-week visit, and repeat radiographs are performed. If the patients remain well clinically and radiographically, then they are advanced to full weight bearing without restrictions at 10 weeks postoperatively.

10.4 Evidence for Open Surgical Dislocation in CAM Lesions

Significant improvement in quality-of-life parameters has been shown in the treatment of isolated CAM deformity by open surgical dislocation and

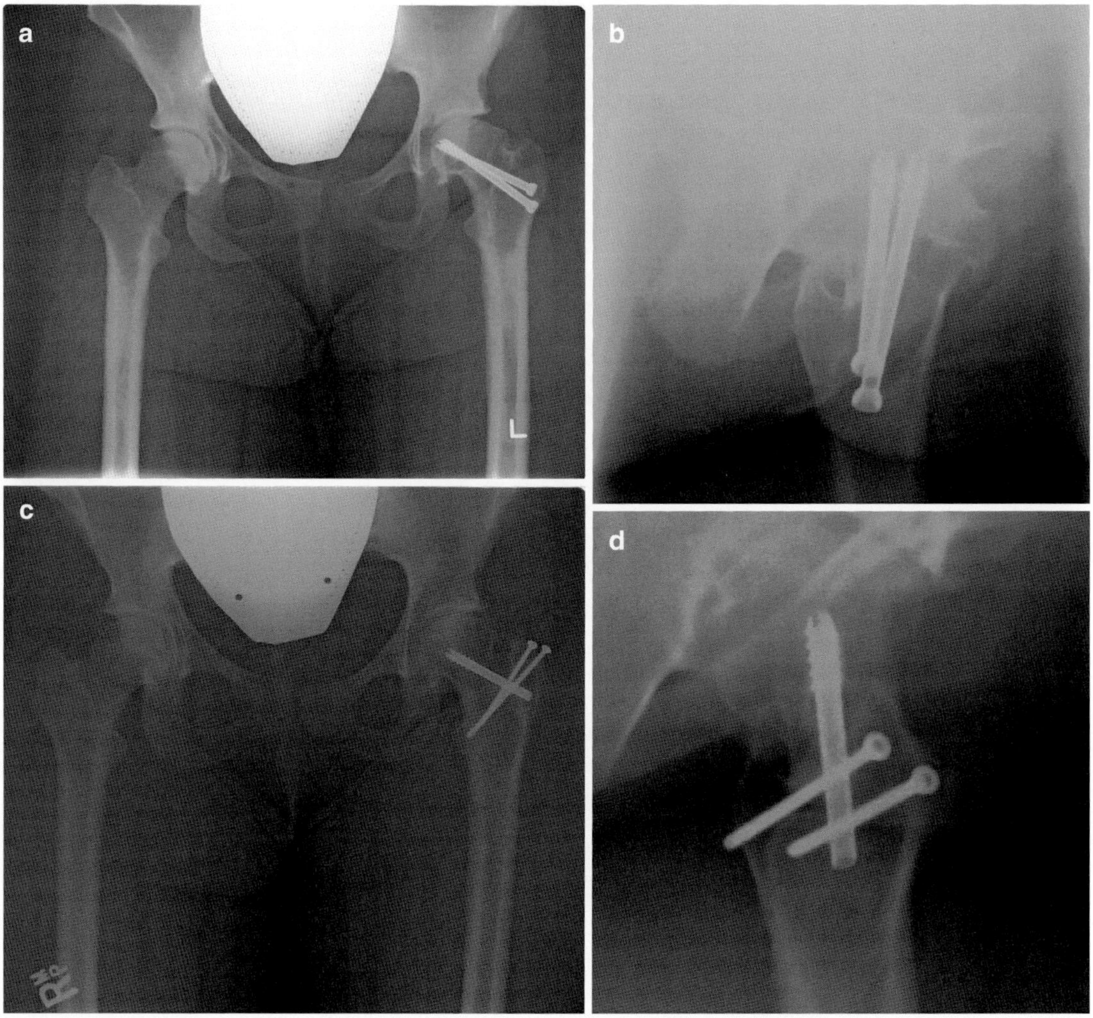

Fig. 10.7 Radiographic (**a**) anteroposterior and (**b**) lateral views of a 22-year-old female with a healed slipped capital femoral epiphysis and clinical symptoms and signs of left hip FAI. Radiographic (**c**) anteroposterior and (**d**) lateral views of the same patient 5 years after open surgical dislocation and removal of hardware to left hip

osteochondroplasty. Beaule et al. [4] followed a cohort of 37 hips in 34 patients with a WOMAC, UCLA, and SF-12 score at a mean of 3.1 years. Preoperative markers confirmed that FAI has a significant negative impact on quality of life, even with the absence of radiographic arthritis. In this group, 28 of 34 patients showed improvement in all clinical outcome scores and were either satisfied or very satisfied with the surgical outcome. Of the patients who had poor results, the Tönnis grade and the amount of chondral damage at the time of surgery was increased, further supporting the recommendation to avoid hip preservation surgery in arthritic hips. Despite the encouraging early clinical results, there were a significant number of reoperations for hardware removal and trochanteric complications.

Graves and Mast [14] followed a cohort of 48 hips in 46 patients with postsurgical hip dislocation, studying the Merle D'Aubigne-Postel score, rate of trochanteric nonunions, and incidence of femoral neck fracture. Surgical hip dislocation was performed through the Gibson approach, and an osteochondroplasty was performed at the femoral head-neck junction. In some patients, additional procedures were indicated, including relative neck lengthening, intertrochanteric osteotomy, lateralization of the GT, osteochondral allografting, osteophyte resection, sciatic neurolysis, and loose body removal. A total of 96 % of patients showed improvement at the final follow-up of an average of 38 months, by means of clinical outcomes scores and radiographic restoration of head-neck offset. Nine of the 48 patients had at least grade one heterotopic ossification (ossification islands around the hip) formation, but no nonunions occurred, and two patients required screw removal. Peters and Erickson [19] had similar results in a review of 30 hips in 29 patients who underwent a debridement by means of surgical hip dislocation. These patients were followed for a mean of 2 years and showed an improvement in HHS from 70 to 87 points. Eight hips showed radiographic progression of arthritis, with 4 patients progressing to hip arthroplasty. As with the previous series, those patients requiring a secondary procedure to convert to total hip arthroplasty had more severe cartilage damage on initial presentation.

Mardones et al. [16] investigated the structural effect of surgical resection of the head-neck junction on the risk of postoperative femoral neck fractures. The amount of femoral neck that could be safely resected was studied using cadaveric specimens. Osteochondroplasty was performed using a surgical dislocation as per Ganz with a saw and burr using an appropriately sized plastic template to confirm sphericity. The peak load to fracture was significantly reduced in specimens with greater than 50 % of the neck resected, while the 10 % and 30 % resections were equal.

The treatment of high-level athletes with FAI is a challenge given the need to return to professional level of sporting activity and the unique motivations of these patients. Naal et al. [17] looked specifically at the outcomes of professional athletes undergoing debridement of CAM and mixed lesions treated with open surgical hip dislocation. A series of 30 hips in 22 athletes were followed at an average of 45.2 months postoperatively with return to professional-level sporting activity being the primary outcome. In this patient group, 96 % were able to return to prior level of sporting activity, with 18 of 22 patients being satisfied or very satisfied with the outcome. Improvements were seen also in the SF-12, UCLA, HOS, HHS, and Tegner scale and a unique sports activity score. Patients had an average improvement of the alpha angle from 69.3 to 43.4 and the internal rotation of 6–14.5°. As with prior series, a significant rate of trochanteric complications was seen, with 20 % of patients requiring removal of the screws. No cases of AVN were recorded, and only one patient showed progression of their Tönnis grade. Results were comparable to hip arthroscopy and hip dislocation in a nonprofessional athlete population. These authors suggest that surgical hip dislocation may be preferable to other techniques as it allows for access to lesions that may be difficult to treat arthroscopically and may justify the increased recovery time and complication rate.

Unique complications of open surgical hip dislocation include the incidence of nonunion of the greater trochanteric osteotomy and symptomatic hardware from the trochanteric fixation. The rate of secondary procedures is higher than other techniques, mostly due to the need for screw removal in a significant number of patients, which is required in up to 20 % of patients ([17], Yun et al. [21]). This procedure also carries the risk of avascular necrosis of the femoral head. However, no cases of AVN were reported in the original series of patients reported by Ganz et al. [12]. Clinically significant heterotopic ossification, sciatic nerve injury, and progression of arthritis have also been reported.

10.5 Techniques for Minimally Invasive Open Approach

Multiple minimally invasive approaches to the hip joint for the treatment of CAM deformities have also been well described in the literature [1, 8, 10]. The proposed benefits of this procedure include direct visualization of CAM lesions without the morbidity associated with a surgical dislocation and the avoidance of complications associated with traction and the steep learning curve and expertise required for adequate resection by means of hip arthroscopy. The most commonly utilized techniques include the mini-open anterior approach described by Cohen et al. [10] and the Hueter technique described by Barton et al. [1] or Chiron et al. [8].

A minimally invasive anterior approach for the treatment of FAI has been described by Cohen et al. [10]. A 2–3 cm incision is made 2 cm distal and posterior to the anterior superior iliac spine (ASIS), in line with the medial border of the TFL muscle belly. Dissection is carried down to expose the medial fatty stripe of the Smith-Peterson interval. The fascia of the TFL is incised along the medial edge, and dissection is continued bluntly to palpate the femoral neck, around which blunt retractors are placed to expose the capsule. Pericapsular fat is excised, and the interval between the rectus and capsule is developed with a Cobb elevator. A final sharp Hohmann retractor is placed over the anterior acetabular rim to expose the entire capsule. A T-shaped capsule incision is made oriented proximally to expose the acetabulum and head-neck junction. The retractors are then repositioned within the capsule to expose the acetabular margin and the anterior femoral head. The exposure may be improved by having an assistant apply longitudinal traction and rotation to the limb. Bone is resected at the area of impingement using osteotomes and a 5 mm burr. Resection is completed when impingement is no longer observed during dynamic assessment with the hip brought through a full range of motion.

A second minimally invasive approach using the Hueter technique has also been published [1]. This approach utilizes a vertical incision starting 2 cm distal to the ASIS and extending 3–4 cm distally along the medial aspect of the TFL muscle. The fascia of the TFL is incised along the medial fibers and it is retracted laterally. Dissection is continued bluntly within the sheath of the TFL to avoid damage to the LFCN. Once the deep fascia of the TFL is exposed, the fascia in the interval between the gluteus medius and rectus femoris is exposed. The reflected head of the rectus can be retracted laterally to expose the underlying capsule without further muscle dissection. A proximally based T- or L-shaped capsular incision is then used to expose the acetabular rim and is reflected laterally to visualize the labrum and the femoral head-neck junction. Blunt retractors are placed around the femoral neck to enhance the exposure of the head-neck junction. At this point, the hip is brought into a position of impingement and the area of abutment is confirmed at the acetabular rim. Osteochondroplasty is completed as previously described with a combination of osteotomes and a high-speed burr. The extent of resection is determined by recreation of a smooth head-neck contour and an impingement-free range of motion.

Another anterolateral approach has been described by Chiron et al. [8]. This approach utilizes the interval between the TFL and rectus femoris, with the theoretical advantage of preventing damage to the LFCN. The incision is made from the anteroinferior edge of the greater trochanter to the ASIS. The iliotibial band is incised posterior to the TFL, and the intermuscular space is developed to expose the capsule from the intertrochanteric line to the reflected tendon of the rectus muscle. A crossbow-type incision is made into the capsule, and a spiked Hohmann retractor is used to expose the anterior wall of the acetabulum. Rotation of the limb by an assistant improves the visualization of the head-neck junction. The pathologic area of the CAM lesion is then treated with the hip in flexion and neutral rotation. The greatest limitation of all these approaches remains to be the inability to fully visualize the central portion of the joint and therefore address intra-articular pathology and the difficulty in visualizing the posterosuperior femoral neck.

10.6 Evidence for Minimally Invasive Open Approach for CAM Lesions in FAI

The minimally invasive approach to CAM resection provides a midpoint between open surgical dislocation and hip arthroscopy. Used alone or in combination with hip arthroscopy, it has been shown to be safe and effective in the treatment of isolated CAM lesions in FAI. The use of the mini-open approach in isolation for the treatment of FAI has been supported in the literature. In a series of 156 hips in 149 patients followed for a minimum of 2 years postoperatively after a direct anterior mini-open approach, clinical results have been promising in the short term [18]. Patients showed significant improvement in most areas of clinical outcomes assessment, including SF-36, WOMAC, UCLA, modified HHS, and super simple hip scores. Complications of the procedure, however, included the requirement of a number of secondary procedures for the treatment of neuroma, trochanteric bursitis, repeat labral tear, or subtrochanteric fracture. Twelve patients in the series by Parvizi et al. [18] also went on to require an arthroplasty procedure.

Only a few prospective trials have been designed to study the outcomes of the minimally invasive procedures for the treatment of CAM lesions. Using an anterolateral approach as previously described, Chiron et al. [8] examined a series of 120 FAI cases, including 69 isolated CAM-type lesions, which were done in succession and followed for a minimum of 1 year with multiple clinical outcome scores. The authors' choice of approach was based on a desire to minimize the risks associated with the other treatments of FAI, including trochanteric complications with surgical hip dislocation, nerve injuries (including to the lateral femoral cutaneous nerve to the thigh), radiation, incomplete resection, and the steep learning curve with hip arthroscopy. The authors report 77.3 % of patients being satisfied or very satisfied with the results of the procedure. The majority or patients were able to return to the desired level of sport or work. Despite radiographic progression of arthritis on imaging in 18 patients, only 4 required conversion to an arthroplasty procedure at the conclusion of the study. The alpha angle improved significantly to below 46° in all patients, showing that the exposure provides adequate visualization for complete resection of the CAM deformity. The authors of this series did not advocate debridement and reattachment of the labrum, and the central compartment was not visualized during the procedure. Complications included repeat procedures for drainage of hematoma, incomplete CAM resection, release of capsular adhesions, and a heterotopic ossification rate of 36 % on radiographs. The benefits included a shorter procedure time and minimization of serious complications.

In a study by Cohen et al. [10] specifically looking at athletes treated using a minimally invasive direct anterior approach, results were also promising. In the series of 234 patients, 59 of whom were competitive athletes, the percentage of patients able to return to the previous level of sporting activity was 55 %, consistent with series reporting on open surgical hip dislocation. Additionally, 18 patients were able to increase their level of activity postoperatively, but were not able to attain the activity level they had prior to symptoms onset. The majority had isolated CAM lesions. All but two patients experienced improvement in clinical symptoms, WOMAC and HHS scores, and none required conversion to an arthroplasty procedure. Complications of the procedure included a 20 % rate of mild neuralgia parasthetica and one transient femoral nerve palsy. The authors conclude that the mini-anterior approach allows for visualization of the CAM lesion while being less traumatic than the surgical dislocation. The disadvantages in this study include lack of visualization of the inferoposterior labrum and chondral lesions in the central compartment and a significant risk of complications related to the LFCN.

Ribas et al. [20] examined the effect of preexisting degenerative changes in patients treated for FAI with the mini-open approach. These authors studied a series of 117 hips in 105 patients divided into three groups based on severity of arthritis (2010). A DEXEUS-combined outcome score showed significant improvement in clinical outcomes and impingement test in patients with no or low-grade arthritic changes. Patients with higher Tönnis grade (>2) had poor outcomes despite correction of the anatomic deformities. Complications of the procedure included an 18 % rate of symptoms related to the lateral femoral cutaneous nerve of the thigh. Due to the position of the scar, patients were also at a higher risk for hypertrophic scar formation and had a 27 % rate of scar complications. The results of this study show that the mini-open procedure is a viable option, providing a middle ground between arthroscopy and surgical hip dislocation, but the identification of the deformity before the development of significant arthritis is critical to achievement of successful outcomes.

All approaches to the treatment of FAI have unique benefits and complications. Benefits of the mini-open approach include shorter operative time, decreased blood loss, elimination of radiation exposure, and decreased surgeon learning curve, lack of damage to ligamentum teres, pudendal nerve injury, and elimination of trochanteric complications. However, with the use of the anterior mini-open approach, the risk to the lateral femoral cutaneous nerve is significant, with up to 20 % complication rate reported [10, 20]. Postoperative hematomas requiring surgical drainage are also reported by the same authors, and meticulous care to eliminate bleeding from the femoral circumflex vessels must be taken. Higher levels of heterotopic bone formation have been reported with the mini-open approach than with either dislocation or arthroscopy, but this did not appear to be clinically significant. Due to the position of the scar, hypertrophic scar formation appears to be more common than in the other surgical approaches [8, 20].

10.7 Combined Arthroscopic and Open Treatment

A combination of the mini-open approach with hip arthroscopy has also been proposed for treatment of CAM lesions in FAI. Arthroscopic management of labral tears and CAM and pincer deformities is addressed in other chapters. The technique of central compartment arthroscopy to address labral and chondral pathology in combination with a mini-open approach for management of the CAM lesions has been popularized. Proposed benefits of the procedure include improved visualization of intra-articular and cartilage lesions, with increased accuracy of CAM resection with the open approach (Fig. 10.8).

Lincoln et al. [15] described a series of 14 patients with 16 hips treated using a combined hip arthroscopy and modified Hueter approach. At a 2-year follow-up, clinical improvement in range of motion was seen in all patients, specifically in internal rotation and flexion. Radiographs showed significant improvement in both alpha angle and head-neck offset. The study concluded that a combined approach is a safe and effective technique for treatment of CAM lesions and is a reasonable alternative to surgical dislocation or arthroscopy alone.

Clohisy et al. [9] also examined the results of a combined approach. These authors investigated the clinical and radiographic results of combined hip arthroscopy and a limited open osteochondroplasty in 35 patients at a 2-year follow-up [9]. Patients were treated with a standard hip arthroscopy to address labral and chondral pathology followed by an open procedure to complete the CAM resection. Patients showed a significant improvement in modified HHS scores and radiographic alpha angle and only two had progression of Tönnis grade at the final radiographic follow-up. Complications included heterotopic bone formation, wound infection, and deep vein thrombosis. No patients required conversion to total hip arthroplasty. These results confirm the efficacy and accuracy of this treatment method in the setting of an isolated CAM lesion.

Take-Home Points

1. Multiple open treatment options are available for debridement of CAM lesions and have been shown to be effective in relieving symptoms and correcting radiographic deformity in FAI.
2. Decision-making should be based on the location of the patient characteristics, CAM lesion, associated pathology, deformity of the proximal femur, and the surgeon's technical preferences.
3. Open surgical dislocation may be advantageous for CAM-type lesions on the posterosuperior aspect of the femoral neck that are difficult to access from an arthroscopic or mini-open approach.
4. Patients with significant joint degeneration (Tönnis grade > 2) are better served with an arthroplasty procedure, as outcomes with joint preservation surgery in this group are inferior.

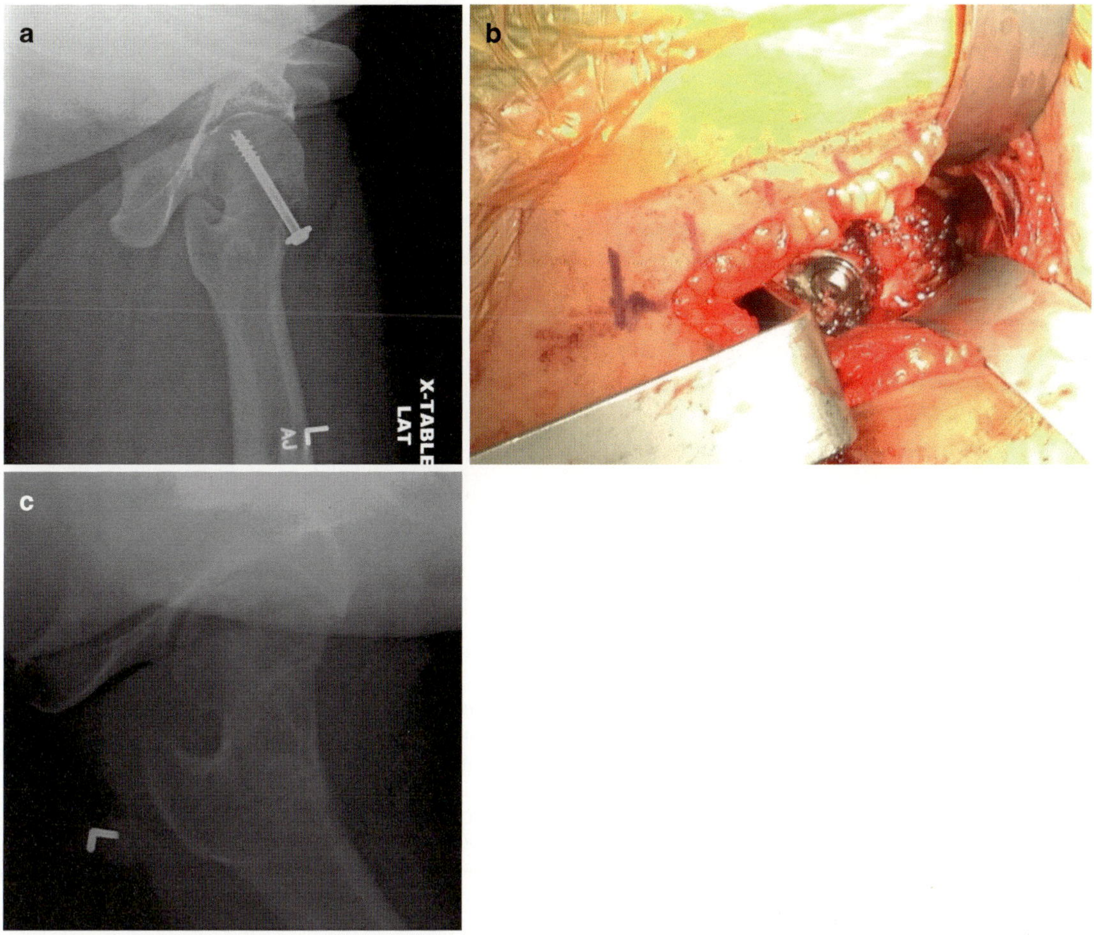

Fig. 10.8 Radiographic (**a**) lateral views of a 24-year-old female with a healed slipped capital femoral epiphysis and clinical symptoms and signs of left hip femoroacetabular impingement. Intraoperative (**b**) view of the same patient during mini-open screw removal and osteochondroplasty. Radiographic (**c**) lateral view of the same patient 5 years after arthroscopic removal of loose bodies and mini-open femoral osteochondroplasty and removal of hardware to left hip

5. Complications are specific to treatment type, with trochanteric nonunions and symptomatic hardware most commonly associated with surgical hip dislocation and injury to the lateral femoral cutaneous nerve of the thigh with mini-open approaches.
6. While short-term and mid-term results are promising, long-term follow-up is required to investigate the success of prevention of degenerative changes with hip preservation surgeries.

Key Evidence Related Sources

1. Beaule PE, Le Duff MJ, Zaragoza E. Quality of life following femoral head-neck osteochondroplasty for femoroacetabular impingement. J Bone Joint Surg. 2007;89(4):773–9.
2. Bedi A, Zaltz I, De La Torre K, Kelly BT. Radiographic comparison of surgical hip dislocation for the treatment of cam deformity in femoroacetabular impingement. Am J Sports Med. 2011;39(Suppl):20S–8.

3. Cohen SB, Huang R, Ciccotti MG, Dodson CC, Parvizi J. Treatment of femoroacetabular impingement in athletes using a mini-direct anterior approach. J Sports Med. 2012;40(7):1620–7.
4. Ganz R, Gill TJ, Gautier E, Ganz K, Krugel N, Berlemann U. Surgical dislocation of the adult hip: a technique with full access to the femoral head and acetabulum without risk of avascular necrosis. J Bone Joint Surg (Br). 2001;83(B-8):1119–24.
5. Lincoln M, Johnston K, Muldoon M, Santore R. Combined arthroscopic and modified open approach for CAM femoroacetabular impingement: a preliminary experience. Arthroscopy. 2009;25(4): 392–9.

References

1. Barton C, Banga K, Beaule PE. Anterior Hueter approach in the treatment of femoro-acetabular impingement: rationale and technique. Orthop Clin of North Am. 2009;40:389–95.
2. Bastian JD, Wolf AT, Wyss TF, Notzli HP. Stepped osteotomy of the trochanter for stable anatomic refixation. Clin Orthop Relat Res. 2009;467:732–8.
3. Beaule PE, Allen DJ, Beck M, Clohisy JC, Schoenecker P, Leunig M. The young adult with hip impingement: deciding on the optimal intervention. J Bone Joint Surg. 2009;91(1):210–21.
4. Beaule PE, Le Duff MJ, Zaragoza E. Quality of life following femoral head-neck osteochondroplasty for femoroacetabular impingement. J Bone Joint Surg. 2007;89(4):773–9.
5. Beck M, Leunig M, Parvizi J, Boutier V, Wyss D, Ganz R. Anterior femoroacetabular impingement. Part II. Midterm results of surgical treatment. Clin Orthop Relat Res. 2004;418:67–73.
6. Bedi A, Zaltz I, De La Torre K, Kelly BT. Radiographic comparison of surgical hip dislocation for the treatment of cam deformity in femoroacetabular impingement. Am J Sports Med. 2011;39(Suppl):20S–8.
7. Carlisle JC, Zebala LP, Shia DS, Hunt D, Morgan PM, Prather H, Wright RW, Steger-May K, Clohisy JC. Reliability of various observers in determining common radiographic parameters of adult hip structural anatomy. Iowa Orthop J. 2011;31:52–8.
8. Chiron P, Espie A, Reina N, Cavaignac E, Molinier F, Laffosse J-M. Surgery for femoroacetabular impingement using a minimally invasive anterolateral approach: analysis of 118 cases at 2.2 years follow up. Orthop Traumatol. 2012;98(1):30–8.
9. Clohisy JC, Zebala LP, Nepple JJ, Pashos G. Combined hip arthroscopy and limited open osteochondroplasty for anterior femoroacetabular impingement. J Bone Joint Surg Am. 2010;92(8):1697–706.
10. Cohen SB, Huang R, Ciccotti MG, Dodson CC, Parvizi J. Treatment of femoroacetabular impingement in athletes using a mini-direct anterior approach. J Sports Med. 2012;40(7):1620–7.
11. Diaz-Ledezma C, Parvizi J. Surgical approaches for CAM femoroacetabular impingement: the use of a multicriteria decision analysis. Clin Orthop Relat Res. 2013;471(8):2509–16.
12. Ganz R, Gill TJ, Gautier E, Ganz K, Krugel N, Berlemann U. Surgical dislocation of the adult hip: a technique with full access to the femoral head and acetabulum without risk of avascular necrosis. J Bone Joint Surg (Br). 2001;83(B-8):1119–24.
13. Ganz R, Parvizi J, Beck M, Leunig M, Notzli H, Siebenrock KA. Femoroacetabular impingement: a cause for osteoarthritis of the hip. Clin Orthop Relat Res. 2003;417:112–20.
14. Graves ML, Mast JW. Femoroacetabular impingement: Do outcomes predictably improve with surgical dislocations. Clin Orthop Relat Res. 2009;467(3):717–23.
15. Lincoln M, Johnston K, Muldoon M, Santore R. Combined arthroscopic and modified open approach for CAM femoroacetabular impingement: a preliminary experience. Arthroscopy . 2009;25(4):392–9.
16. Mardones RM, Gonzalez C, Chen Q, Zobitz M, Kaufman KR, Trousdale RT. Surgical treatment of femoroacetabular impingement: evaluation of the effect of the size of the resection. J Bone Joint Surg. 2005;87(2):273–9.
17. Naal FP, Miozarri HH, Wyss TF, Notzli HP. Surgical Hip dislocation for the treatment of femoroacetabular impingement in athletes. Am J Sports Med. 2011; 39(3):544–50.
18. Parvizi J, Huang R, Diaz-Ledezma C, Og B. Mini-open femoroacetabular osteoplasty: how do these patients do? J Arthroplasty. 2012;27(8):122–5.
19. Peters CL, Erickson JA. Treatment of femoroacetabular impingement with surgical dislocation and debridement in young adults. J Bone Joint Surg. 2006;88(8):1735–41.
20. Ribas M, Ledesma R, Cardenas C, Marin-Pena O, Toro J, Caceres E. Clinical results after anterior mini-open approach for femoroacetabular impingement in early degenerative stage. Hip Int. 2010;20 Suppl 7:S36–42.
21. Yun HH, Shon WY, Yun JY. Treatment of femoroacetabular impingement with surgical dislocation. Clin Orthop Surg. 2009;1(3):146–54.
22. Zingg PO, Ulbrich EJ, Buehler TC, Kalberer F, Poutawera VR, Dora C. Surgical hip dislocation versus hip arthroscopy for femoroacetabular impingement: clinical and morphological short-term results. Arch Orthop Trauma Surg. 2013;133(1):60–79.

Open Surgical Management of Pincer Lesions in FAI

11

Etienne L. Belzile

Contents

E.L. Belzile, MD, FRCS (C)
Division of Orthopaedic Surgery, Faculty of Medicine, Université Laval, Quebec City, QC, Canada

Department of Orthopaedic Surgery, CHU de Québec-Université Laval, 11 Côte du Palais, Quebec City, QC, Canada
e-mail: etienne.belzile@mail.chuq.qc.ca

11.1 Introduction

Hip pain caused by femoroacetabular impingement was first described by Ganz and the Bern group in a landmark article in 2003 [1]. The simplest definition of a *pincer-type* femoroacetabular impingement is the impaction-type injury [1–3] sustained over an area of the anterior/lateral acetabular labrum during hip motion caused by the repetitive abutment at the end of flexion between the femoral head–neck and the acetabular rim [4]. This lesion can result from different primary morphological variants, including lack of femoral head–neck offset, acetabular retroversion, focal anterosuperior (focal) overcoverage, or global overcoverage. And this can also result from early closure of the triradiate cartilage secondary to trauma of the acetabulum [5] as the injury may cause a premature growth arrest leading to the underdevelopment of the posterior wall, in certain childhood conditions [6, 7] or following corrective pelvic redirection osteotomy due to malposition of the acetabular fragment [8–10].

A complete picture of the prevalence and clinical impact of *pincer-type* hip impingement in one's practice is difficult to paint. First, as the expansion in knowledge on the subject of femoroacetabular impingement (FAI) grew in later years, it is of concern that very few, if any, authors have elected to study cohorts affected by *pincer-type* hip morphology in isolation. Thus, we

O.R. Ayeni et al. (eds.), *Diagnosis and Management of Femoroacetabular Impingement*,
DOI 10.1007/978-3-319-32000-7_11

extracted and present the most important information published to date on global and focal overcoverage. Most early studies on FAI included patients presenting with all morphologies of FAI including *CAM type*, *pincer type*, and *mixed type*. This last category is, however, very confusing since it is dependent on the subjectivity of the respective researchers as inclusion criterion varies greatly across studies. To have a better understanding of the prevalence of *pincer-type* hip morphology, one shall look at asymptomatic cohort or population studies. Secondly, FAI nomenclature has evolved in the last 10 years, rendering direct comparison across time potentially flawed. As an example of this, authors now propose that the radiological findings associated with coxa profunda may no longer be appropriate for determining global coverage [11–13]. These authors have shown that this classical radiological definition (when the floor of the acetabular fossa on an AP pelvic radiograph touches or is medial to the ilioischial line [14]) can be identified in dysplasia as much as in normal hips [11, 13, 15, 16]. More quantitative radiological parameters should now be used to define the depth of the acetabulum [12, 16]. Moreover, insufficient standardization of the radiographic techniques, in particular for pelvic rotation and tilt [17], is known to affect the evaluation of the acetabular rim position in space and thus may have influenced diagnostic criteria of acetabular retroversion over time in the literature.

11.2 Clinical Presentation

The clinical investigation of the patient should be focusing on family history of hip disease, personal history of childhood hip disease, as well as past history of hip surgery. A careful history of the character, location, onset, duration, and severity of the pain is also mandatory. Furthermore, the patient should be questioned about aggravating and alleviating factors as well as any past hip treatment modalities including activity modification, physical therapy regiment, nonsteroidal anti-inflammatories, pain medication use, and intra-articular hip injections. An appreciation of the patient's expectations from the surgical opinion should also be an integral part of the initial medical encounter.

Patients with *pincer-type* hip morphology usually present with an insidious onset of a dull and aching anterior hip pain or groin pain [18]. At times, the pain can be present in the gluteal, the greater trochanteric, or the lower back areas [18, 19]. This pain may radiate down the thigh when aggravated by certain physical activities or deep seating positions [19]. Recent onset of pain may have been provoked by the recent increase in the patient's physical activity or sporting activity [18]. Specific activities like getting out of the car, seating with legs crossed, or upon positioning in internal rotation with the affected leg in the weight-bearing position or deep flexion will worsen the discomfort [20]. Moreover, activities that do not reproduce impingement mechanism like walking, jogging, and even running will be well tolerated [21]. Sports prone to stimulate hip pain will usually involve rapid acceleration and deceleration, twisting, or pivoting, and monopodal weight-bearing on the affected hip such as ballet dancing [22], martial arts, yoga [23], ice hockey [24], golf, and European football.

Typically, patients present either in their second decade in life [18] or, later in their late thirties, early forties [23]. Pincer lesions are more common in the middle-aged, active women [1, 25], while CAM FAI has a male predominance [26]. In a study of 3620 subjects in the Copenhagen Osteoarthritis cohort, male and female prevalence of a deep acetabular socket (LCEA >45°) was 15.2 and 19.4 % respectively [27]. While authors in a recent population-based study of 2081 young asymptomatic adults, 34 % of the males and 17 % of the females demonstrated pincer morphology on radiographs [28]. This prevalence may vary with genetic backgrounds as in a population study comparing asymptomatic non-arthritic hips, white US women had a higher prevalence of overcoverage (LCEA >40°) than their Chinese counterparts [29]; 9 % versus 4 %. A recent study of female collegiate athletes identified 1 % of all 126 hips with radiographic pincer deformity (LCEA >40°) [30]. It is crucial for the reader to understand that the majority of the information pertaining to the clinical expression of pincer lesions is blended in and indissociable from CAM-type FAI in most clinical trials. Since the majority of FAI patients will present with a *mixed type* of FAI, the dissociation of the *pincer-type* FAI data is almost impossible. Of 302 hips treated in the first FAI cohort, only 26 had an isolated CAM and 16 an isolated pincer impingement [4]. More recently, Allen et al. [31] showed that 42 % of 201 hips in 113 patients presenting with a symptomatic cam-type lesion also had a pincer-type deformity on AP pelvic radiographs. Again, of note, the diagnostic criteria for pincer-type morphology have evolved over recent time, rendering direct comparison across studies spanning the latest 15 years difficult.

11.3 Pathophysiology of Pincer

Pincer-type impingement causes a distinct pattern of articular cartilage damage. As the abnormal contact occurs repetitively onto the acetabular rim due to direct impact of the femoral head or neck upon hip flexion and internal rotation, the labrum is crushed and will show eventual bruising and circumferential degeneration. Early in the process, the cartilage damage is mainly localized along a narrow circumferential strip along the acetabular rim [1, 4]. With time, the impact area on the femoral neck abutting onto the anterior osseous acetabular prominence will show callus formation and cortical thickening [4, 23], while the adjacent acetabular cartilage will show linear wear patterns [4, 32]. The labrum will develop intra-substance fissuring and ganglion formation [23]. Since the prominent acetabular rim is the instigator of cartilage damage, a more global injury pattern [33] is observed in *pincer-type* morphology as the femoral contact point changes with hip motion and position. Moreover, acetabular cartilage will demonstrate characteristic focal, well-circumscribed and localized area of severe damage [32]. With damage progression, microfractures at the acetabular rim lead to subperiosteal bony apposition onto labral tissue [34, 35], leaving it encased or simply pushed forward by the bony apposition. In early stages, the labrum is not histologically ossified and may not be associated with clinically important acetabular cartilage degeneration [34]. In later stages, the accumulated tissue damage may provoke labral ossification [36], further increasing impingement. At the position of maximal hip flexion/internal rotation, the femoral neck will lever on the overhanging acetabular rim and will apply a sheering force onto the posterior acetabular facet, leading to a typical "contrecoup" acetabular cartilaginous lesion [1, 4, 37]. In cases of protrusion, medial cartilage thinning is observed [38] (see Fig. 11.1). The negatively oriented weight-bearing zone of severe pincer hips leads to medial osteoarthritis [38].

11.4 Classification of Pincer Impingement

The classification of *pincer-type* hip morphology rests on acetabular radiological reference values defining acetabular depth including the lateral center-edge angle (LCEA) [39], the acetabular index known as the Tönnis angle [40], the femoral head extrusion index (FHEI) [41], the retroversion index [42–44] also known as the crossover overlap ratio [45], the crossover sign (COS) [15,

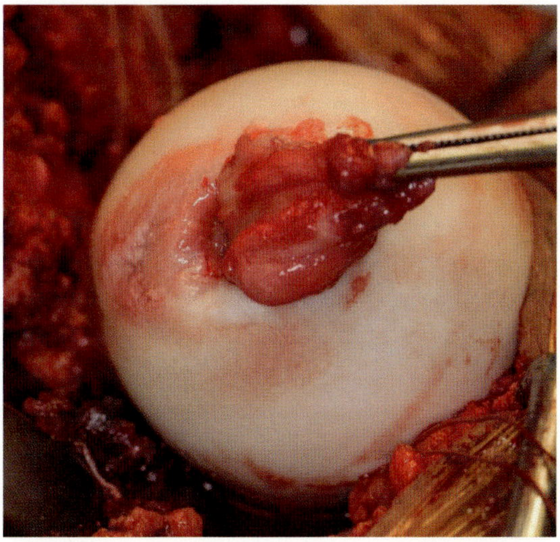

Fig. 11.1 Medial cartilage damage can be seen in early protrusion of the hip of a 19-year-old basketball player during hip dislocation surgery to correct a pincer-type FAI

18], and the posterior wall sign (PWS) [18, 22, 43]. The retroversion index, the crossover sign, and the posterior wall sign will be affected by pelvic position and tilt during the radiographic evaluation [46]. It is unclear how these radiological signs relate to each other in the presence of a deformed acetabulum and how sensitive they are to pelvic position. As an example, the PWS can exist in hip dysplasia and in the absence of any acetabular malrotation. First, an adequate radiological investigation must be conducted respecting current best clinical practices [14, 17] (Fig. 11.2). Second, one must recognize that the acetabular retroversion is a condition on a continuum of acetabular deformity. Werner et al. [47] have shown that as the COS appears alone, the retroversion index has a mean value of 20.5 %. With the combination of the COS and the PWS, the mean retroversion index value raises to 25.1 %, while the presence of a COS, a PWS, and a prominent ischial spine [48] leads to a mean retroversion index of 32.3 %. In fact, the retroversion index may represent a better radiological reference to quantify acetabular retroversion given that the AP pelvis radiograph measured is without rotation.

Subdividing *pincer-type* bony anatomy into subgroups can help the surgeon better understand the acetabular morphology leading to the development of a possible impinging anatomy [50]:

- Global overcoverage
- Focal overcoverage
  - Focal cranial (superolateral) retroversion
  - Acetabular retroversion
  - Total acetabular retroversion

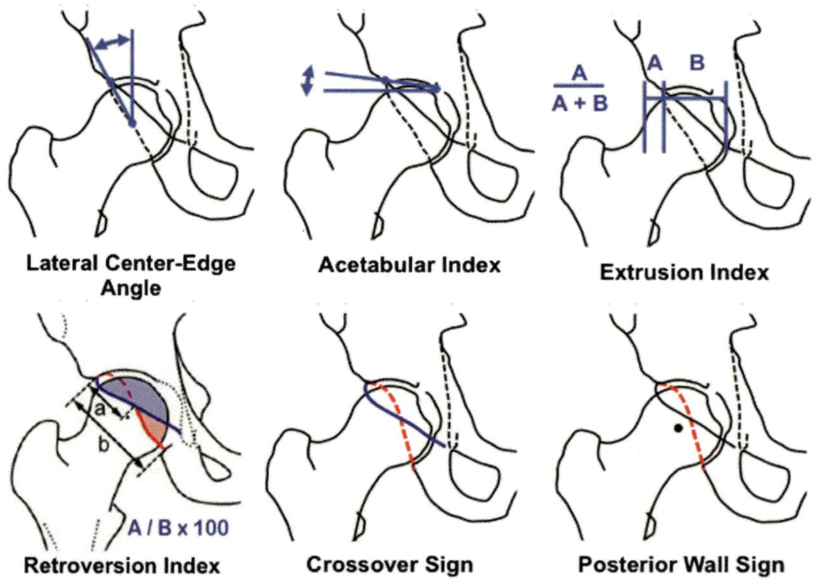

Fig. 11.2 Acetabular depth and wall position relative to the femoral head center of rotation can be defined by the following parameters (*from left to right*): lateral center-edge angle, angle between a vertical line drawn from the center of the femoral head and a line going to the most lateral point of sclerosis of the acetabular sourcil; acetabular index, plane of inclination of the acetabular sourcil represented by the angle between a line drawn from the most medial point of sclerosis to the most lateral point of sclerosis of the acetabular sourcil and the horizontal plane; extrusion index, proportion of the femoral head uncovered by the acetabulum as referenced by the measured segment of the femoral head lateral to the most lateral point of sclerosis of the acetabular sourcil (*A*) divided by the sum of the uncovered (*A*) and covered portion of the femoral head (*B*); retroversion index, degree of severity of the retroversion as defined by the measured distance from the most lateral point of sclerosis of the acetabular sourcil to the point of crossover between the anterior and posterior wall projections (*a*) as a proportion of the overall size of the acetabular opening (*b*); crossover sign, condition encountered when the projection of the anterior and posterior edges of the acetabular walls meet over the femoral head instead of at the most lateral point of sclerosis of the acetabular sourcil; and posterior wall sign, condition encountered when the projection of the posterior acetabular wall lies medial to the femoral head center (Figure adapted and reprinted with permission Tannast et al. [49])

Global overcoverage is the classically described deep acetabula. It can be better defined as a hip with a LCEA >40°, an acetabular index >0°, and the absence of a posterior wall sign. Such deformity can reach the protrusio position when the acetabular line crosses the ilioischial line by >3 mm (male) or >6 mm (female) on the AP pelvic radiograph [51] (Fig. 11.3c). The anterior wall and the posterior wall extend equally farther lateral to their normal position medial and at the center of the femoral head, respectively (Fig. 11.3b, c).

Focal overcoverage is, by contrast, defined as a hip with less than global overcoverage. This category can then be further subdivided into *focal cranial retroversion* when the overcoverage is concentrated in the proximal one-third of the acetabulum. According to its radiographic definition, the crossover sign is visible [15, 18], the posterior wall is within normal limits, but the retroversion index is less than 30 % while the LCEA is above 25° and less than 40°[52]. Focal cranial retroversion is more common in men [53] and has been shown to increase with age [54]. The observation of the crossover sign on the AP pelvic radiograph must be performed with care since the downward projection of the anterior inferior iliac spine may misleadingly interfere with its interpretation [55]. A CT measurement may provide supplemental information on the degree of cranial versus central versus caudal acetabular version [18] to properly guide the clinician at the cost of more radiation to the patient and without significant advantage over plain radiographs [52, 56, 57].

Acetabular retroversion results in a crossover sign along with a posterior wall sign with a retroversion index that can be variable but greater than 10 %. True retroversion of the acetabulum thus involves the central portion of the socket and is the representation of a developmental maltorsion of the distal hemipelvis. Acetabular retroversion occurs in 5–7 % of the population [7, 58, 59] and coexists in 12–37 % of hip dysplasia [7, 60–64], proximal femoral focal deficiency [65], and in 42 % of Legg–Calvé–Perthes disease [7]. Some authors have suggested that a deficiency in the posterior wall of the acetabulum [58] is required to produce such entity but recent work tends to counter such theory [15, 48, 64, 66, 67]. Moreover,

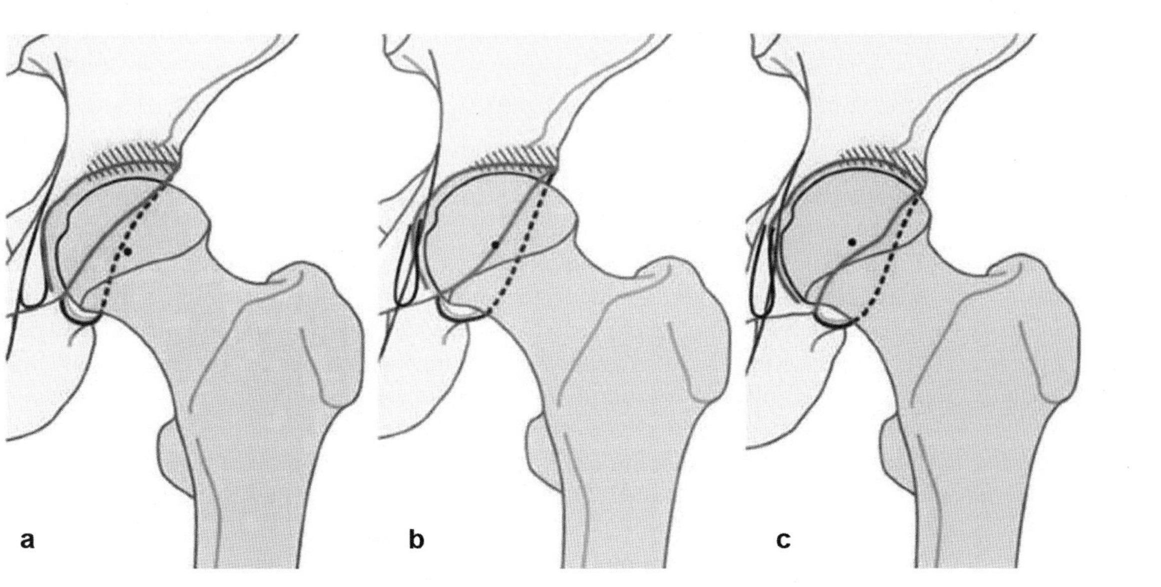

Fig. 11.3 Hip morphology is qualified via specific radiological reference values pertaining to acetabular depth: (**a**) normal hip, (**b**) moderate global overcoverage with LCEA >35° to <40° and acetabular index of 0°, and (**c**) severe global overcoverage with LCEA >40° and acetabular index of <0° (Figure reprinted with permission Leunig et al. [38])

this morphology can be the result of previous pelvic osteotomy [8, 9, 68].

Total acetabular retroversion is finally the ultimate *pincer-type* hip morphology. This rare condition will result in the combination of a posterior wall sign, a retroversion index of 100 %, and a misleadingly absent crossover sign. The anterior and posterior rims of the acetabulum typically converge at the most cranial part of the acetabular opening to form an obtuse angle [10]. It occurs when the entire acetabular opening is oriented posteriorly [10, 65]. All patients described in the literature had previous pelvic surgery and presented with less than 90° of hip flexion and weak abductors.

11.5 Exacerbating Factors

The different types of hip morphology discussed at this point in this chapter are mostly bony conditions affecting the pelvis and acetabulum. Certain associated conditions may affect how the hip morphology will express its pathology. Previous chapters have described the pathophysiology of FAI and impact that a lack of anterior femoral head–neck offset or *CAM-type* morphology has on hip biomechanics.

11.5.1 Soft Tissue Laxity

The soft tissue envelope surrounding the hip is complex and includes tendons, ligaments, and joint capsule. As the ability for these structures to respond to repetitive stresses and loads depends mostly on their composition, ligamentous laxity has been shown to influence hip biomechanics [69]. Focal laxity in the anterior capsule as a result of repetitive external rotation and/or extension has been suggested to create an instability and thus potentially subject the acetabular labrum to abnormal stresses [70, 71]. Poor abdominal muscle control may fail to stabilize the pelvis during hip range of motion during activity and may also worsen anterior impingement symptoms by affecting dynamic pelvic tilt.

11.5.2 Femoral Version

Proximal femoral version will dictate the position of the anterior aspect of the femoral neck in space relative to the femoral shaft. Hence, depending on hip flexion, the greater the femoral anteversion, the later the acetabular rim collision with the anterior femoral head–neck will occur. Femoral retroversion is considered relative when <15° and absolute when <0°, in the axial plane, to the posterior femoral condyles [72, 73]. The recognition of femoral retroversion is capital in understanding the dynamic interaction between the femoral neck and the anterior acetabular rim during flexion–internal rotation activities. For example, in the setting of a large CAM-type morphology associated with a focal overcoverage and relative femoral retroversion, it may be more appropriate to consider addressing only the CAM lesion [74]. On the other hand, in cases with the same amount of focal overcoverage and femoral retroversion <0°, but without head–neck offset abnormalities, the most appropriate surgical treatment would include a femoral derotation osteotomy [72, 75] (Fig. 11.4). Similarly, an elevated femoral anteversion would be protective or even adaptive [76] to acetabular retroversion. Final decision to perform adjunctive femoral osteotomy should be based on perioperative impingement-free range of motion of the hip.

11.5.3 Femoral Varus

In Legg–Calvé–Perthes-related deformity, it has been well established that the varus femoral neck, known as coxa vara, will increase the ease of impingement of the femoral head and greater trochanter on the superior anterior acetabular rim [75, 77]. This situation will be made even worse if retroversion is present [7]. Femoral varus defined as a neck–shaft angle of <125° is also common after childhood hip disease treated with varus intertrochanteric osteotomies (ITO) [77], after femoral neck fractures [78], and in patient with global overcoverage [38]. Thus, if the affected Perthes hip abduction is restricted

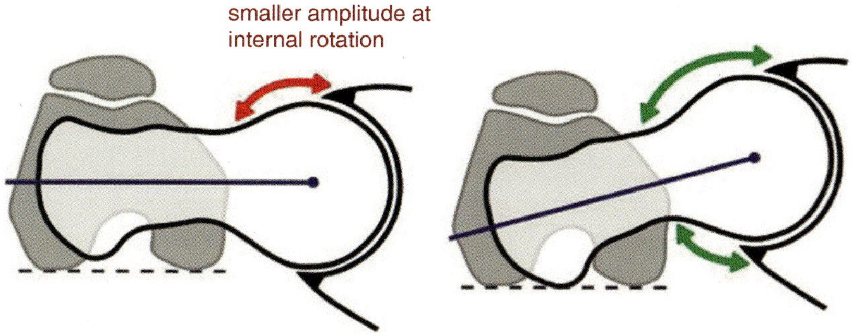

Fig. 11.4 Femoral retroversion has a direct effect on hip range of motion in internal rotation; *left* retroversion, *right* normal version (Figure adapted and reprinted with permission Sutter et al. [73])

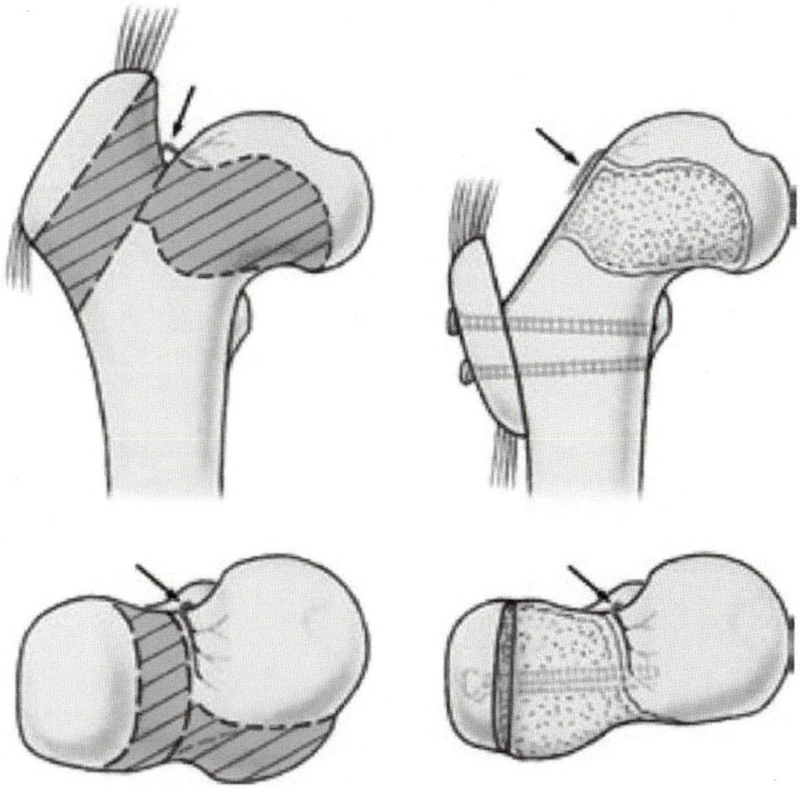

Fig. 11.5 During surgical dislocation of the hip, careful dissection of the retinacular soft tissue flap on the superior femoral neck allows for resection of the deepest segment of the greater trochanter remaining on femur. Once the femoral head–neck osteochondroplasty is completed and has reshaped the anterior part of the head, the greater trochanter fragment is mobilized distally and re-anchored with cortical screws (Figure reprinted with permission Tannast et al. [88])

to less than 20°, a proximal femoral osteotomy should be considered [77]. A final decision dictating whether a valgus-producing ITO [79, 80] or a relative femoral neck lengthening (RFNL) [81, 82] is most appropriate warrants evaluation if extra-articular impingement is present and if femoral offset is enough for adequate abductor muscle tension. The valgus ITO is designed to lateralize the femur to restore normal mechanical alignment of the hip joint [83] while facilitating femoroacetabular clearance. The RFNL procedure is intended to address both extra-articular impingement by advancement of the greater trochanter and intra-articular impingement by head–neck offset improvement via osteochondroplasty [84] (Fig. 11.5). In a study on femoral osteotomies in Perthes hips, Novais noted that 20 % of cases required a valgus-producing ITO, while 61 % underwent a RFNL procedure during the open FAI correcting surgery without increasing complication risks [85]. The overall hip comfort and function has been shown to improve postoperatively [85] with only one posttraumatic femoral neck fracture occurring postoperatively [82]. Midterm OA progression has been noted in 36–40% of cases with a conversion to a total hip replacement in 7–10% of cases [84, 86, 87]. Albers et al. have subsequently demonstrated, in a series of 41 isolated RFNL procedures for Perthes disease at a minimum of 5 years of follow-up, that the intervention can reduce pain and improve hip abduction and function [84].

11.6 Contemporary Open Surgical Techniques

The mainstay of any hip preservation surgery is the protection and maintenance of the vascular supply of the non-arthritic femoral head as well as the preservation of cartilage, labral, and capsular tissues in order to stop or slow the progression of early osteoarthritis [89]. The secondary goal is then to relieve the femoroacetabular impingement by improving hip clearance in the functional range of motion defined by the patient's anatomy and function in order to avoid a pathological cascade of injury to the hip joint to continue. One should aim at obtaining 110–115° of hip flexion [90] and a minimum of 20–30° of internal rotation with the hip at 90° of flexion [91] after surgical correction although no strict guideline has been published at this time. Surgical decision-making at the first clinical encounter with a patient with a complex hip morphologic abnormality warrants poised wisdom. Despite knowing that an intra-articular impingement secondary to anatomic causes is unlikely to respond to conservative management, surgical candidates should have undergone proper activity modification and/or physical therapy. The physical therapy is aimed at improving core stability and movement control, with strengthening hip external rotators and abductor for at least a 3-month period before considering a surgical intervention [92].

In addition to considering all the abovementioned diagnostic radiological parameters, the extent of articular cartilage damage must be evaluated. The posterior inferior joint space must be studied for joint space loss with the false profile view of Lequesne and de Sèze [93]. The posterior inferior joint space loss is an indirect measure and secondary sign via contrecoup of the extent of damage created by the lever effect of the pincer morphology [1, 4, 38, 94]. Moreover, an increased LCEA and the presence of a crossover sign have been associated with significant changes in cartilage health [58, 95], suggesting a relationship of these specific mechanical differences with evidence of early cartilage degeneration [96]. It remains unclear how hip pain at the initial clinical encounter can be a reliable predictor of future hip osteoarthritis [97]. The mere presence of more than one radiographic parameter describing pincer morphology may imply that the hip cartilage may be in a more fragile homeostasis than the remaining joint space width would suggest. Magnetic resonance imaging techniques can supplement radiographs and CT imaging to better characterize cartilage damage before undergoing surgery [71, 98–100].

Surgical candidates of *pincer-type* FAI thus will present failure to improve after a minimum 3-month course of conservative management and complete investigation highly suggestive that the pincer morphology is contributory. Most patients will have persistent anterior/anterolateral hip pain for a minimum of 6 months, restricted hip flexion (<105°), and/or internal rotation in 90° hip flexion (<15°), with a positive impingement maneuver on physical exam [101, 102]. Moreover, an adequate surgical candidate should have no or minimal articular damage with no signs of advanced degenerative joint disease (more than 2 mm of joint space) [103, 104].

11.7 Surgical Dislocation of the Hip

Detailed knowledge of the vascular anatomy of the proximal femur [105–107] has allowed surgeons to safely perform open surgical dislocation of the hip [108]. While there is no report of avascular necrosis in the literature, the complications associated with this technique are well known [109, 110]. The surgical hip dislocation technique (SDH) is a versatile approach providing 360° access to the femoral neck and acetabulum and allowing complex surgery to the proximal femur safely. This technique has been utilized in traumatology for open reduction and internal fixation of femoral head fragments [111, 112], posterior acetabular walls [113], and in tumor surgery for safe excision of juxta-articular benign tumors [114–117].

11.7.1 Indications

The main indication for SDH in pincer-type impingement is to address the acetabular rim resection and manage the resulting labral damage. Secondary intentions would include RFNL procedures and/or concomitant femoral redirection ITO. In cases of *global overcoverage*, a circumferential access to abnormal acetabular rim is required and is well addressed via SDH. In cases of *focal overcoverage*, isolated *cranial retroversion* can be well suited for the SDH for selected rim trimming. In *acetabular retroversion*, the SDH is indicated if the retroversion index is less than 30% or concomitantly to an anteverting periacetabular osteotomy in order to address proximal femoral anatomy such as in patients with sequel after Perthes disease.

11.7.2 Surgical Technique [108, 118]

The patient is positioned in lateral decubitus on the operating table with the operated leg free, disinfected from last ribs to toes, and draped accordingly. A 20 cm skin incision is made in line with the femoral longitudinal axis, centered on the greater trochanter. Subcutaneous fat is approached until proximal fascia lata is opened longitudinally along the anterior border of the gluteus maximus muscle as well as distally, centered on the femur, for the length of the skin incision. In muscular individuals, dissection is carried further anterior from the midpoint lateral and under the fascia lata, to free the hypertrophied gluteus maximus muscle fibers. This plane is further liberated proximally toward the iliac crest, in the interval between gluteus maximus and fascia lata in order to maximize exposure for later. Gluteus maximus muscle is then reclined posteriorly through gluteus medium fascial sheath, to expose the posterior border of the gluteus medius muscle and allow proper identification of piriformis and short external rotators. The posterior border of the proximal vastus lateralis muscle is elevated on a segment of 5 cm. Careful and precise dissection will allow protection of the inferior gluteal artery which runs along the piriformis muscle and tendon and is aiming to anastomose to the ramus profundus originating from the medial femoral circumflex artery [105]. The greater trochanteric osteotomy will leave a few muscle fibers from the most posterior aspect of the gluteus medius attached to the stable trochanter along with the insertion of the piriformis tendon to protect the extension of the gluteal tributaries to the ramus profundus. The osteotomy should be no greater than 1.5 cm deep and parallel to the leg when the knee is flexed at 90° and the hip in 20° internal rotation. The trochanteric osteotomy can be performed with a 6 mm step cut at its center, and with the saw blade excursion going from posterior to anterior, and just a few millimeter shy of breaking through anteriorly in order to obtain a triplanar trochanteric flip osteotomy [119] (Fig. 11.6). This simple modification from the original technique will allow for increased stability of the trochanteric fragment at closure and earlier weight bearing during recovery. This trochanteric osteotomy is elevated anteriorly (with gluteus medius, gluteus minimus, and vastus lateralis attached) to expose anterior capsule once the interval between gluteus minimus and the cranial border of the piriformis tendon is developed. Bringing the hip in slight flexion and external rotation will expose the joint capsule so a Z-shaped capsulotomy can be performed and the femoral head dislocated posterosuperiorly.

Complete dislocation requires section of the ligamentum teres with long curved scissors while taking care of avoiding acetabular or femoral head cartilage damage in the process. A bone hook placed on the femoral calcar may help in mobilizing the femur in external rotation and flexion to place the leg into a sterile bag on the opposite side of the table. Acetabular rim, labrum, and acetabular cartilage is, at this point, fully

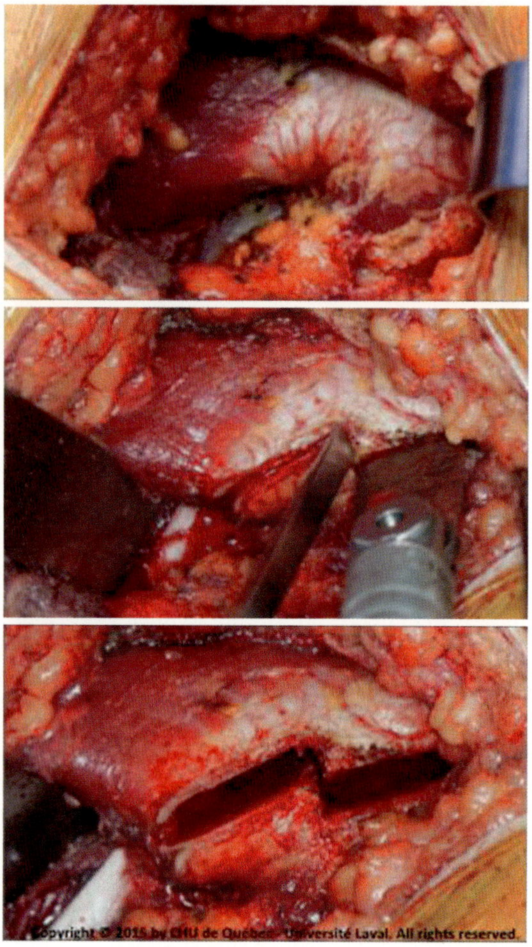

Fig. 11.6 Posterior view of a patient in a lateral decubitus position with the right hip exposed. (*Top image*) The greater trochanter is approached. (*Middle image*) On the right, the gluteus medius tendon is retracted to show the piriformis tendon. Once the posterior border of the vastus lateralis has been incised, the proximal osteotomy is performed with a slightly inclined pitch and leads to the distal osteotomy via a vertical limb created with a 6 mm straight osteotome. (*Bottom image*) The greater trochanter is then lifted off femur pediculated by both the gluteus medius and minimus, as well as vastus lateralis

accessible for surgical treatment [118, 120]. Labral and cartilage integrity is evaluated carefully. In cases of simple labral tears, labral base can be debrided down to bleeding bone for refixation using bone anchors. Suture knots are typically tied on the capsular outer surface of the labrum to avoid direct contact with the femoral cartilage. When overcoverage has been diagnosed, acetabular rim trimming with a curved osteotome and labral refixation has been described (Fig. 11.7). If the labrum attachment to the acetabular rim is intact, a sharp dissection is required to detach labral tissue for subsequent rim trimming. However, if labrum tissue has been damaged or avulsed, the degenerative labral base is debrided before refixation after appropriate rim trimming. When the labrum is severely damaged or ossified, over a given segment or its totality, and its functional integrity compromised, labral reconstruction has been recommended [121] using ligamentum teres autograft [122], iliotibial band autograft [123], or semitendinosus allograft [124]. Acetabular rim trimming should be conducted with attention to avoid over or under resection. Rim trimming would only be indicated if the lunate surface is oversized [67]; otherwise, it would render the weight-bearing surface smaller, thus increasing joint contact pressure or render the hip unstable [125].

Once the acetabular rim has been decompressed and labral lesions addressed, the residual focal acetabular cartilage injury can be addressed by debridement and microfracture techniques. On the femoral side, the lack of head–neck offset can be evaluated using transparent spherical templates to locate exactly where the head becomes out of sphericity and to guide how much osteochondroplasty is required. The zone of resection is delimited, and a sharp curved osteotome is used to initiate the bone resection from proximal to distal at the head–neck junction. Careful resection is dictated to avoid injury to the retinacular vessels on the superolateral femoral neck. Furthermore, over-resection is discouraged since it may lead to a break in the sealing function of the labrum as it rests onto the femoral head during hip flexion [126]. The femoral head cartilage can also be treated for central osteochondral defects [112, 127–129]. Upon finalization of acetabular rim trimming and femoral osteochondroplasty, a perioperative hip examination under direct visualization should confirm impingement-free full range of motion.

Capsular closure is performed loosely and the trigastric trochanteric osteotomy repositioned on

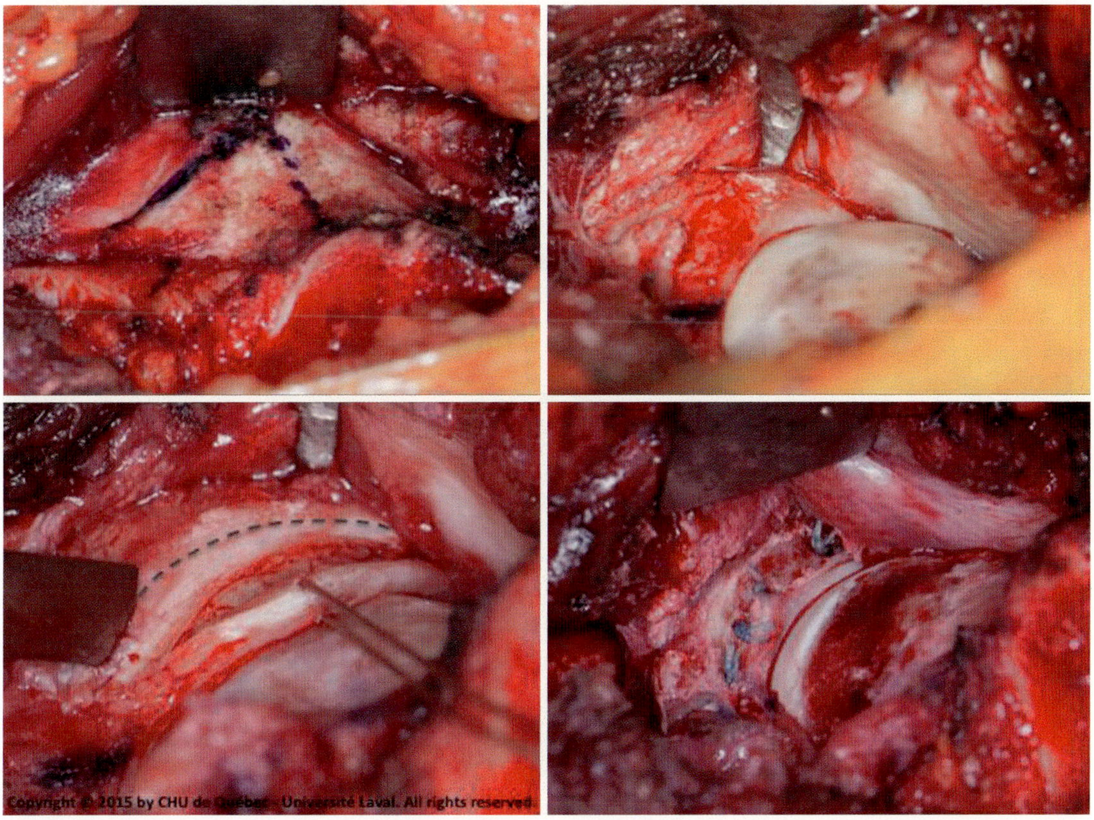

Fig. 11.7 Posterior view of a patient in a lateral decubitus position with the right hip exposed. (*Top left*) The Z-shaped capsulotomy allows for full anterior exposure of the hip joint. (*Top right*) Once the anterior capsular flap is retracted, the anterior pincer lesion is evaluated and good-quality labrum preserved. (*Bottom left*) Once the bone–labrum interval has been sharply developed, the labrum is retracted as rim trimming is performed along the dotted line. (*Bottom right*) After labral refixation using bony anchors and sutures, the hip joint is evaluated through full range of motion for labral seal quality as well as for residual CAM-type impingement

the stable trochanter for fixation with two 4.0 or 4.5 mm cortical screws oriented parallel to each other and toward the lesser trochanter. In cases where subsequent trochanteric distal mobilization, RFNL procedure, or femoral reorientation ITO are indicated, the trochanteric osteotomy would be performed flat to avoid the triplanar deformation at reattachment. Since the vastus lateralis can be safely dissected off the femur distally, surgical exposure for ITO is the same as described above with the addition of an extended skin incision. In rare cases of combined periacetabular osteotomy during the same surgical day, Ganz et al. suggest to perform the ischial osteotomy under direct visualization in a dissection window between inferior gemellus and obturator externus/quadratus femoris (Fig. 11.8).

At closure, the posterior aponeurosis of the vastus lateralis is closed. The fascia lata and subcutaneous tissue are meticulously closed. No drains are necessary. Postoperative mobilization is allowed with 25 % weight bearing, while hip flexion >80° is avoided as well as active abduction. Continuous passive motion of the hip from 0 to 70° has been recommended to avoid intra-articular adhesions for at least 48 hrs. Thromboprophylaxis should also be considered. Weight bearing on the operated leg is progressed when greater trochanter shows signs of healing at 6–8 weeks.

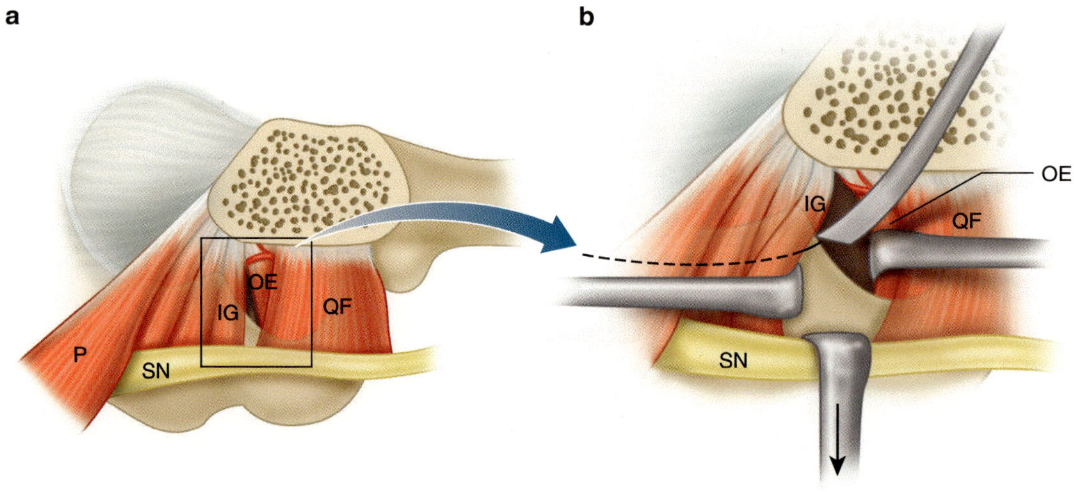

Fig. 11.8 (**a**) Illustration of the short external rotators during SDH focusing on the interval to dissect for completion of the ischial osteotomy before performing a periacetabular osteotomy; piriformis (*P*), sciatic nerve (*SN*), inferior gemellus (*IG*), obturator externus (*OE*), quadratus femoris (*QF*). (**b**) After splitting the interval between inferior gemellus and obturator externus/quadratus femoris, careful sciatic nerve retraction will allow for adequate visualization to complete the partial ischial osteotomy (Figure reprinted with permission Ganz et al. [77])

11.7.3 Outcomes

The complication rate for the SDH has been evaluated at 9 % in a retrospective multicenter study when SDH was the surgical approach of a multitude of hip FAI morphologies at 1 year of follow-up [110]. This rate was diminished to 4.8 % if heterotopic ossification was excluded. Of 355 SDH, one complete sciatic paralysis partially resolved, nine patients suffered trochanteric nonunion, one deep infection, and two deep vein thrombosis in the calf that resolved with medical therapy [110]. In the original publication by Ganz et al. on 213 patients, two cases of partial neurapraxia and three cases of trochanteric nonunion were reported. Other authors have subsequently published a 1–1.5 % rate of complications [130, 131].

In patients with overcoverage, the critical part of surgery is the acetabular rim trimming. Removal of an excessive amount of acetabular rim will render a deep socket into a dysplastic one. This complication has never been reported following SDH but has been seen after arthroscopic rim trimming that led to postoperative hip dislocation and the LCEA angle <23°[125, 132]. Steppacher et al. identified a higher failure rate of hips with excessive rim trimming (acetabular index >14°, LCEA <22°), osteoarthritis (OA), increased age (>40), or weight (BMI>30) at the 5-year mark [133]. There are no guidelines for acetabular bone resection. Preoperative planning is key while some have proposed a mathematical rule [ΔLCEA° = 1.8 + (0.64 × Δmm)] dictating that one millimeter of bony resection corresponds to a 2.4° decrease of the LCEA and five millimeters corresponds to 5°[134]. Others have debated the accuracy of this method and proposed an alternative formula [ΔLCEA°= 1.5 – (1.3 × Δmm)] by studying normal cadaveric hips [135]. The clinical validity and applicability of these calculation methods have not been evaluated to date.

When looking at revision FAI surgery, Ross et al. [136] noted that 13/50 patients presenting for recurrent FAI symptoms had a LCEA equal or greater than 40°. Another center reported on 152 hips undergoing revision FAI surgery, of which 3 had an isolated pincer and 74 had combined lesions [137]. Identified risk factors for revision surgery included female gender and younger age. Moreover, increased anteversion (>20°) was present in 30 %, while femoral retroversion (<5°) was present in 13 % in the revision patient cohort [137]. In a series of 93 hips undergoing SDH, undercorrection and persisting pincer impingement (LCEA >32°) was an important predictor of failure [138]. At the latest follow-up at 10 years, 80 % of patients avoided THA and OA progression, while 38 % had a persisting positive impingement sign.

Systematic reviews conclude that early evidence in the treatment of FAI has proven beneficial for hip function and hip pain with clinically good to excellent results in 68–96 % of the cases [139–141]. Current literature is limited concerning such evidence for *pincer-type* FAI treatment in isolation. Most of the studies reporting on FAI treatment do so by classifying pincer in combination with CAM lesions as mixed type or as pincer alone which represent typically 2–4 % of the total cohorts [139, 141]. SDH has shown improved function in 73 % of pediatric and adolescent patients with FAI where 31/71 hips had rim resection and labral reattachment. No femoral head osteonecrosis was observed at the average of 27 months of follow-up despite having 30 % of patient reoperated for hardware removal [142]. In patients with mixed FAI (CAM lesion and crossover sign), Hingsammer et al. evaluated the need for acetabular rim trimming during SDH according to intraoperative hip flexion of >100° and 20° of internal rotation at 90° flexion [143]. If this objective was obtained after the femoral osteochondroplasty, no rim trimming was performed. At a short (1.6 years) follow-up time, all patients achieved 90° hip flexion, there was no difference in patient-reported outcome measures, and half of the impingements sign resolved whether the rim trimming was performed or not. This finding supports Larson et al. [52] who reported on a high prevalence of the crossover sign and/or posterior wall sign in asymptomatic hips (37 %) suggesting that these radiological signs are not necessarily pathognomonic for *pincer-type* impingement. Contemporary research thus encourages a more conservative approach with surgical resections on the acetabular rim in the presence of cranial retroversion.

11.8 Anteverting Periacetabular Osteotomy

The extensive knowledge on pelvic osteotomy developed for developmental hip dysplasia has served hip preservation surgery well. The periacetabular osteotomy (PAO) technique can be slightly modified to reorient the acetabulum in order to decrease the femoral coverage. Such technique is regarded as reverse or anteverting PAO.

11.8.1 Indications

Anteverting PAO is indicated in overcoverage when the acetabulum would risk diminishing the size of its weight-bearing articular surface if adequate rim trimming is underdone. Hence, a reverse PAO would better serve *global overcoverage* with short, down-sloping acetabular sourcil or a negative acetabular index. As for *focal overcoverage*, the anteverting PAO is indicated in *acetabular retroversion* with a retroversion index of >30 % [144] or if one aims at a correction of at least 10–20° of anteversion [18]. In rare cases of total acetabular retroversion, the anteverting PAO is the only treatment option. If complicated acetabular reorientation revision surgery is required, one may consider the possibility of arterial compromise of the supra-acetabular arcades from previous surgeries and thus opt for a Tönnis-type triple pelvic osteotomy in order to avoid acetabular fragment osteonecrosis [10].

11.8.2 Surgical Technique [44, 145]

The modern PAO is performed through an abductor-sparing Smith–Peterson approach with the patient positioned supine on a radiolucent operating table [146]. A 5 cm skin incision is made obliquely from the anterior superior iliac spine (ASIS) to laterally over the iliac crest, and a longitudinal distal extension is made over the medial edge of the tensor fascia lata for 10 cm. Careful subcutaneous dissection is warranted to avoid injury to the lateral femoral cutaneous nerve. The sheath of the tensor fascia lata is opened longitudinally and entered in order to retract its muscle fibers laterally (see Fig. 11.9). The aponeurosis of the abdominal muscle, the inguinal ligament, and the sartorius muscle are surgically detached from the anterior third of the iliac crest. After mobilizing the iliacus muscle subperiosteally down the iliac bone, the hip is brought into flexion to relax tension on rectus femoris and iliopsoas muscle.

Deep dissection down the iliac crest to the anterior inferior iliac spine (AIIS) exposes the origin of the rectus tendon and its reflected head. Special attention must be brought to the cauterization of the ascending branches of the lateral femoral circumflex artery as they appear in the intermuscular interval between tensor and rectus femoris. From the AIIS, the rectus femoris is medially retracted in order to free the capsular attachment of the iliocapsularis muscle from lateral to medial. The iliocapsularis can then be mobilized medially to the rectus, en bloc with the iliopsoas/iliacus muscle complex (see Fig. 11.10). The origin of the rectus is only detached when intracapsular work is indicated which is mostly for femoral head–neck offset correction. Peters et al. have described a modification of the surgical approach that avoids the rectus takedown by approaching medial to rectus femoris and lateral to the iliocapsularis/iliopsoas/iliacus down to medial hip capsule [147].

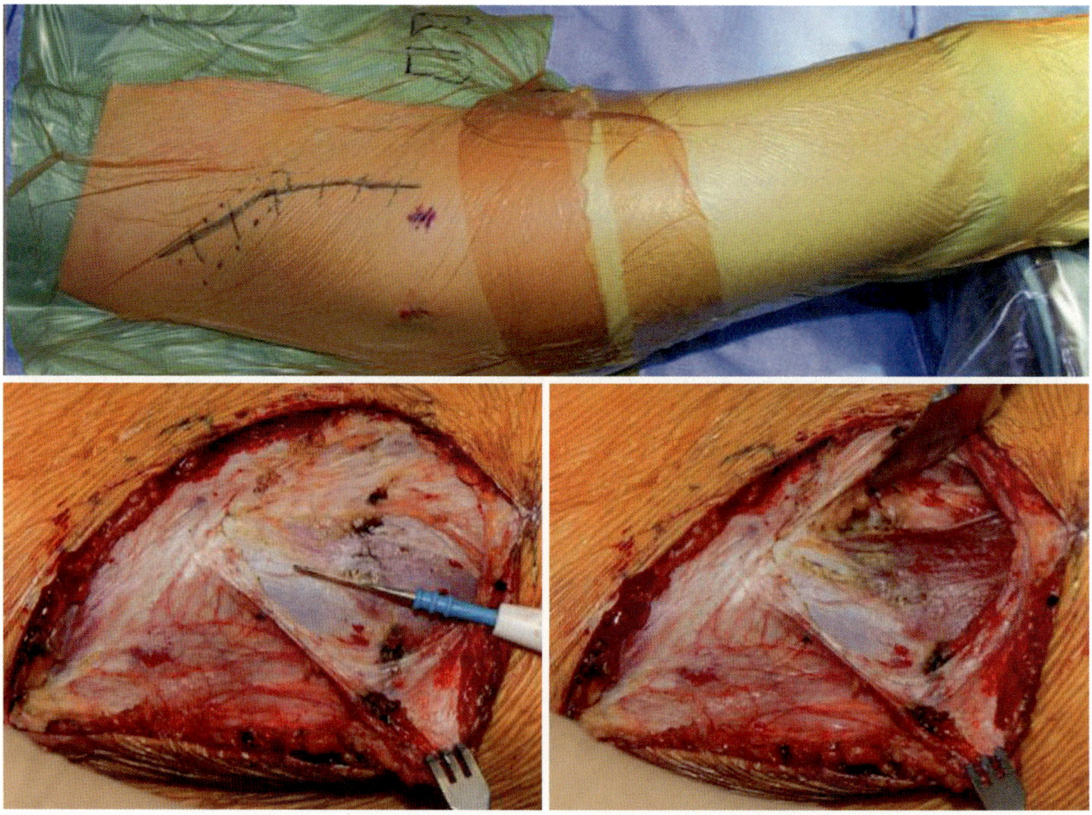

Fig. 11.9 Representation of a patient in a supine position with the right hip exposed. The iliac bone is drawn in a *dotted line* and the skin incision outlined by the continuous line. Puncture wounds from the intra-articular exploration via hip arthroscopy are seen. (*Bottom Left*) Once skin is incised, the superficial fascia of the TFL is open and the plane of dissection shown by the electrocautery tip. (*Bottom Right*) A Hohmann retractor is positioned medial to the descending iliac wing, below ASIS, and above AIIS and retracts the sartorius, while the TFL is exposed

At this point, the anterior ischium is accessible for the placement of a curved osteotome for the ischial osteotome after blunt dissection down into the infra-articular space between psoas and capsule. The superior pubic ramus is also accessible through this window after retraction of the iliopsoas medial to the iliopubic eminence. The preparation of the outer iliac bone can then be conducted by undergoing a subperiosteal dissection between ASIS and AIIS, in line toward the apex of the greater sciatic notch, for a very limited width to allow for saw motion and positioning. Then, medially over the pelvic brim and down the quadrilateral plate but avoiding the greater sciatic notch, a blunt subperiosteal dissection will allow free motion of osteotomes during the retroacetabular osteotomy.

The first osteotomy is usually the inferior ischial cut. This osteotomy can be performed blind by going medially into the lateral obturator foramen or under fluoroscopic guidance with a false profile view of the hemipelvis [146]. One aims at initiating the bone cut at a 1 cm distance inferior to the articulation and going 15–20 mm deep with the osteotome. Care must be taken to avoid a complete ischial bone cut in order to preserve the posterior ischium in full integrity with the posterior column. The second cut will be conducted at the pubic ramus and as close to the acetabulum as feasible and medial to the iliopubic

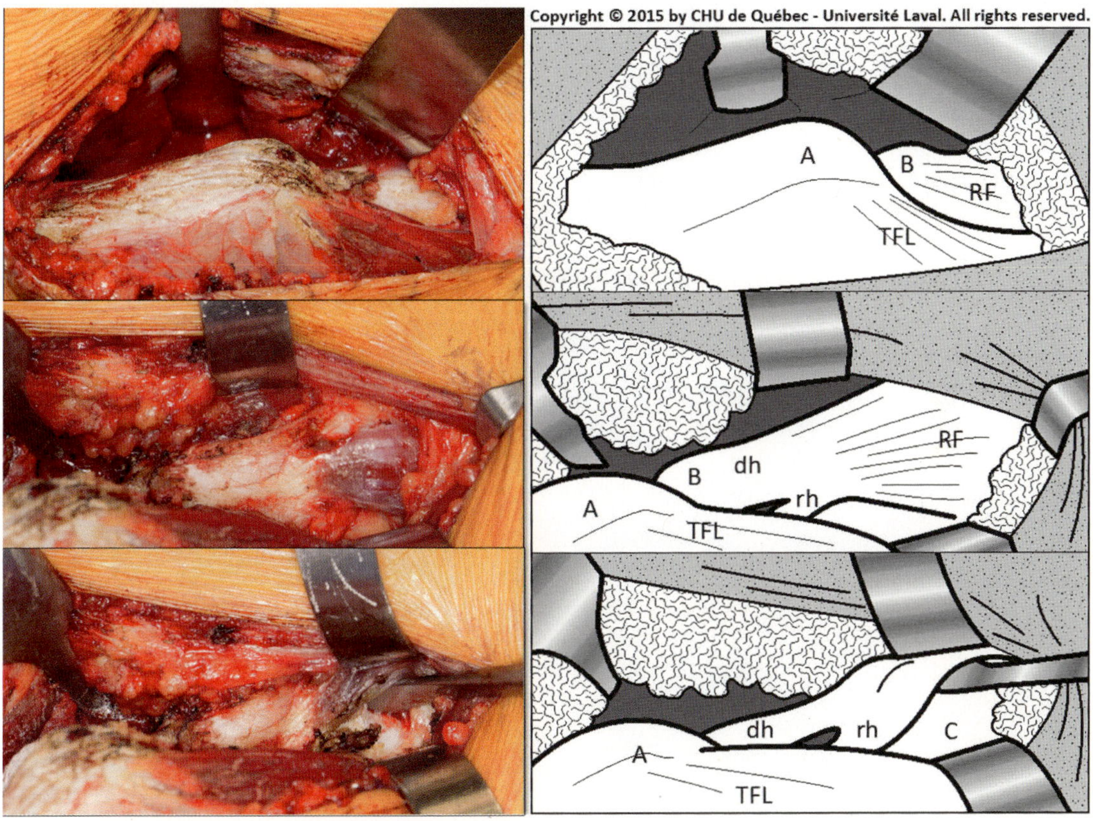

Fig. 11.10 (*Top images*) The ASIS (*A*) is center to the exposure with a Hohmann retractor on the pelvic brim and a Hibbs retractor mobilizes the iliopsoas muscle along with the sartorius, inguinal ligament, and abdominal wall. (*TFL* tensor fascia lata) (*Middle images*) The origin of the rectus femoris tendon (*RF*) is shown distal to the AIIS (*B*). (*dh* direct head, *rh* reflected head) (*Bottom images*) The muscular portion of the proximal rectus femoris muscle is elevated off the hip capsule with a Cobb (*C*) along with fibers of the iliocapsularis muscle. This dissection will allow for the safe development of the interval between rectus and iliopsoas muscles, distal to AIIS and medial to the hip capsule. Once detached laterally, the iliocapsularis muscle fibers mobilize much easily along with the iliopsoas muscle

eminence. The bone cut should be performed perpendicular to the longitudinal axis of the ramus to facilitate acetabular fragment motion. Retractors can be introduced in the superior obturator foramen to protect its content from osteotome injury. A sharp osteotome or a Gigli saw can be used for this osteotomy [146] (see Fig. 11.11).

The third osteotomy is the supra-acetabular osteotomy. It can be performed with an oscillating saw under direct vision while assuming proper muscle protection medially and laterally from the iliac bone. The starting point is just below the ASIS and aiming at the apex of the greater sciatic notch but should end 2 cm from the pelvic brim. At this point, the iliac bone osteotomy travels down the quadrilateral plate to become the retroacetabular osteotomy at equal distance from the greater sciatic notch and the acetabulum as visualized on the false profile view under fluoroscopy. Thus allowing the preservation of the pelvic integrity and safeguarding from intra-articular osteotome penetration. At completion, the retroacetabular osteotomy shall meet the ischial osteotomy to free the acetabular fragment. In very hard bone, a high-speed burr may help in cutting through the pelvic brim turn from the iliac osteotomy into the retroacetabular osteotomy.

Once the acetabular fragment is fully osteotomized, it can be manipulated using a Weber clamp on the pubic rami stump and a 5 mm Schanz screw positioned in the iliac bone, 15 mm above the superior articular line. Initial flexion of the fragment is aided with laminar spreaders and the Schanz screw to distract the iliac and retroacetabular osteotomy. Later, traction upward from the table, followed by rocking motion from medial to lateral with the Schanz screw, will free the residual retroacetabular bony attachments. Then, the acetabular fragment is extended and internally rotated to obtain the desired reorientation of the fragment (Fig. 11.12). In order to mobilize the acetabular

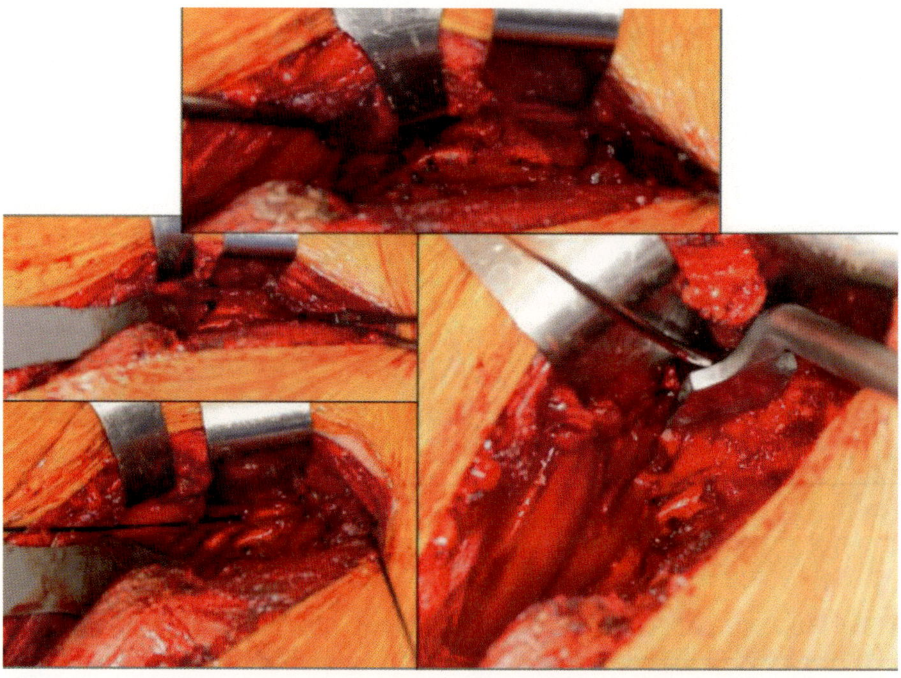

Fig. 11.11 (*Top center image*) Instruments develop an entry point at the superior and lateral corner of the obturator foramen allowing the passage for a Satinsky clamp (*middle left*) from distal to proximal. A Gigli saw can then be guided into place using a long 1-0 silk suture (*bottom left*). Others may elect to hold the retracted structure medial to the osteotomy site with a 2.4 mm K-wire unicortically fixed onto the pubic ramus and use a Ganz osteotome to perform the transverse pubic ramus cut (*bottom right*)

fragment into position to correct a retroverted socket, a bone wedge may have to be removed from the iliac bone to allow fragment motion proximally.

Before final fixation with bone screws running from the top of the iliac crest down into the fragment, K-wires stabilize the fragment (Fig. 11.13). A careful radiologic assessment is then required to judge the acetabular fragment position. One aims at obtaining a horizontal acetabular sourcil, appropriate anteversion with the disappearance of the crossover sign and the absence of a posterior wall sign. Moreover, overt medialization or lateralization of the femoral head should be avoided. The acetabular coverage should correspond to a LCEA of 23–33°. Upon finalization of acetabular fragment fixation, a perioperative hip exam under direct vision should confirm impingement-free full range of motion. Otherwise, a capsulotomy should be performed and osteochondroplasty undertaken accordingly.

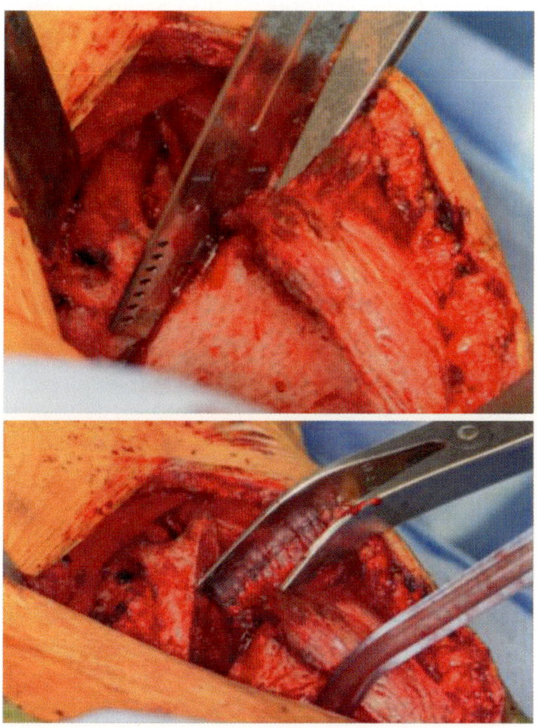

Fig. 11.12 This is a view of the surgical field from the head of the patient for a right hip. The iliac bone osteotomy is performed using a sagittal saw. Then, the acetabular bony fragment can be mobilized and freed using a laminar spreader

At closure, the sartorius, inguinal ligament, and abdominal musculature are reinserted with transosseous sutures on the iliac crest. Aponeuroses and subcutaneous planes are closed in layers, followed by skin, leaving a suction drain deep under the iliacus. After surgery, the patient remains partial weight bearing with crutches for 6 weeks postoperatively.

11.8.3 Outcomes

Anteverting PAOs are rare procedures and few publications have reported on their clinical results. Since the technical differences are few with the classical PAO performed on dysplastic hips, complication rates could probably be extrapolated from the more widely used procedure. Complications range from 6 to 37 % [148–151]. The major complication rate after PAO has been evaluated at 6 % in a prospective multicenter study of 205 hips at 1 year of follow-up [152]. Such major complications included venous thromboembolism, deep infection, acetabular fragment migration, intra-articular screw, posterior column nonunion requiring refixation, Brooker grade III heterotopic ossification, and a peroneal palsy.

In his study describing the acetabular retroversion as a cause of hip pain, Reynolds et al. presented 12 patients treated by anteverting PAO with promising results [18]. Siebenrock et al. have reported on 29 hips in 22 patients from their early series at 30 months of follow-up with 90 % good to excellent results [43]. More recently, a report at a mean of 10 years of follow-up on the same 29 hips revealed a cumulative survivorship of 100 % with no conversion to total arthroplasty [144]. Fourteen percent developed OA while another 14 % necessitated another FAI surgery. Over-correction and persisting impingement secondary to lack of femoral head–neck offset was an important predictor of failure.

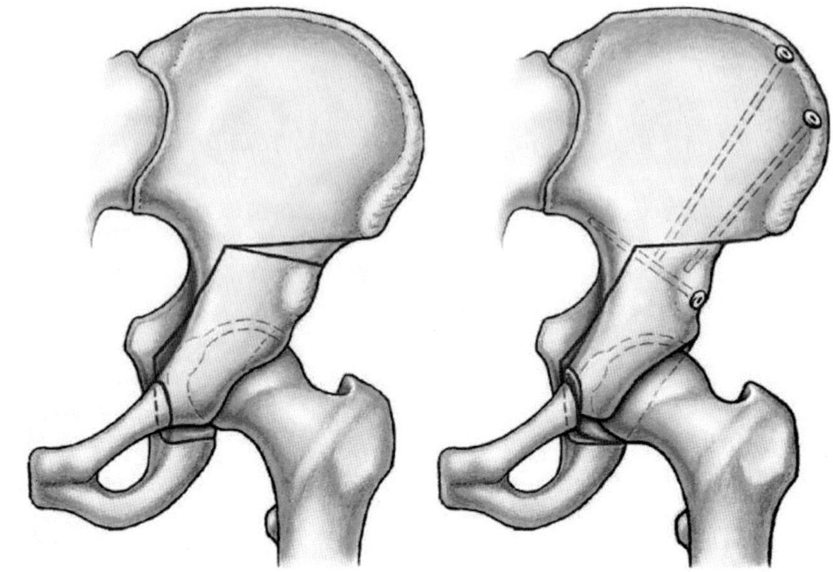

Fig. 11.13 Osteotomies around the acetabulum are the same as for periacetabular osteotomy for dysplastic hips (*left*). To allow acetabular fragment extension during an anteverting PAO, a supra-acetabular wedge resection of roughly 10° way be required prior to final fragment positioning (*right*) (Figure reprinted with permission Albers et al. [44])

Even though observational studies suggest early correction of acetabular retroversion improves hip pain after short-term follow-up [153], no long-term data exist to evaluate the longitudinal effects of such treatment on the progression to osteoarthritis.

11.9 Total Hip Arthroplasty

Arthroplasty for hip degenerative conditions is a very common procedure around the world. An experienced arthroplasty surgeon is versed in recognizing many different bony deformities and has been trained to address them skillfully. As the *pincer-type* hip deforms and undergoes joint degeneration, the labrum ossifies and medial migration may take place. Two different scenarios may render the primary THA more difficult. First, the ossification of the labrum will make the hip dislocation more challenging. This situation may require the ossification removal prior to femoral head dislocation in order to avoid an uncontrolled fracture of the acetabular rim. The second scenario is the severe protruded hip [83]. Hip dislocation may be impossible and thus necessitate in situ femoral neck osteotomy to gain access to the acetabulum with an optional piecemeal removal of the femoral head to avoid acetabular wall fractures. Once the acetabulum is exposed, medial bone grafting is advised to obtain a more lateralized acetabular cup positioning with final implant insertion to diminish the medial wall stresses [154]. A recent study on 206 THA in 155 patients from the Mayo Clinic registry reports a survival rate of the uncemented hemispherical acetabular components in hips with protrusio acetabuli of 94 % at 10 years and 89 % at 15 years [155]. The risk of aseptic cup revision increased by 24 % for every 1 mm, medial or lateral; the cup center of rotation missed the target native hip center of rotation as defined by the Ranawat triangle method [156].

When performing a total hip arthroplasty (HA) on a patient with acetabular retroversion, careful attention must be paid to avoid aligning the acetabular component with an insufficient posterior wall and thereby orient the cup in retroversion [7]. In cases of severe posterior wall insufficiency due to acetabular retroversion, acetabular cup positioning may be compromised. Alternative strategy to supplement cup fixation may include posterior wall reconstruction using transfer of the overhanging anterior wall and its

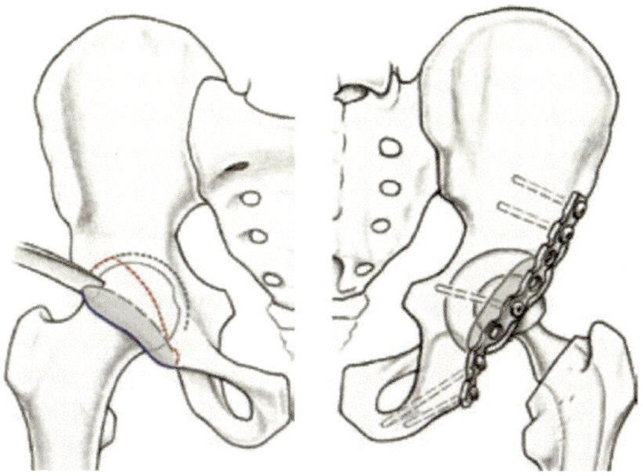

Fig. 11.14 In severe retroversion, the overhanging anterior wall can be transferred (*left*) to the posterior wall at the time of the total hip arthroplasty (*right*). This procedure avoids anterior extra-articular impingement between the anterior wall and the femoral stem while preserving bone stock for the deficient posterior wall

fixation with a reconstruction plate (Fig. 11.14) [10]. Other, more commonly used, strategies would be for the surgeon to opt for highly porous cups with multiple divergent screws or the addition of a reconstruction cage.

Conclusion

The hip joint preservation specialist must be prepared to recognize many different variants of the normal anatomy as well as the most problematic hip deformity. Proper analysis of clinical symptoms, physical signs, and hip joint imaging will lead to the recognition of *pincer-type* femoroacetabular impingement when present. The treatment of these patients is demanding since they symbolize a "triple threat" by representing a diagnostic challenge, undergoing technically difficult surgery, and by being a young and active group of patients with high expectations [157]. Large cohorts with longer-term results are needed to formulate specific evidence-based recommendations and to determine whether treatment for FAI alters its natural course [139]. Such prospective clinical trials will require the incorporation of advanced structural imaging in addition to validated patient-reported outcomes to better evaluate outcomes following hip FAI surgery [158].

Take-Home Points

1. Obtain standardized and properly performed Pelvis radiographs to avoid pelvic tilt or rotation when diagnosing pincer FAI.
2. A CT scan of the pelvis may help further describe the focal acetabular retroversion in relation to the antero-inferior iliac spine projection during pre-operative planning.
3. Aim to obtain 110 degres of flexion, and 20 degres of internal rotation with the hip in 90 degres of flexion after open pincer FAI surgery.
4. Acetabular rim trimming is only indicated if the acetabular lunate surface is oversized, ioatrogenic instability must be avoided.
5. Persisting impingement after acetabular re-orientation procedures can usually be resolved by femoral head-neck offset correction.

Key Evidence Related Sources

1. Ganz R, Parvizi J, Beck M, et al. Femoroacetabular impingement: a cause for osteoarthritis of the hip. Clin Orthop Relat Res. 2003;417:112–120. doi:10.1097/01.blo.0000096804.78689.c2.
2. Ezoe M, Naito M, Inoue T. The prevalence of acetabular retroversion among various disorders of the hip. J Bone Joint Surg Am. 2006;88:372–9. doi:10.2106/JBJS.D.02385.
3. Tannast M, Hanke MS, Zheng G, et al. What are the radiographic reference values for acetabular under- and overcoverage? Clin Orthop Relat Res. 2015;473:1234–46. doi:10.1007/s11999-014-4038-3.
4. Larson CM. Arthroscopic management of pincer-type impingement. Sports Med Arthrosc. 2010;18:100–7. doi:10.1097/JSA.0b013e3181dc652e.

5. Ganz R, Horowitz K, Leunig M. Algorithm for femoral and periacetabular osteotomies in complex hip deformities. Clin Orthop Relat Res. 2010;468:3168–80. doi:10.1007/s11999-010-1489-z.
6. Siebenrock KA, Schaller C, Tannast M, et al. Anteverting periacetabular osteotomy for symptomatic acetabular retroversion: results at ten years. J Bone Joint Surg. 2014;96:1785–92. doi:10.2106/JBJS.M.00842.

Acknowledgment The author would like to thank Mike Millis, MD; Young-Jo Kim, MD; Paul E Beaulé, MD; and Thomas E. Brown, MD, for their leadership, guidance, mentorship, and teaching.

References

1. Ganz R, Parvizi J, Beck M, et al. Femoroacetabular impingement: a cause for osteoarthritis of the hip. Clin Orthop Relat Res. 2003;417:112–120. doi:10.1097/01.blo.0000096804.78689.c2.
2. Rab GT. The geometry of slipped capital femoral epiphysis: implications for movement, impingement, and corrective osteotomy. J Pediatr Orthop. 1999; 19:419–24.
3. Leunig M, Casillas MM, Hamlet M, et al. Slipped capital femoral epiphysis: early mechanical damage to the acetabular cartilage by a prominent femoral metaphysis. Acta Orthop Scand. 2000;71:370–5. doi:10.1080/000164700317393367.
4. Beck M, Kalhor M, Leunig M, Ganz R. Hip morphology influences the pattern of damage to the acetabular cartilage: femoroacetabular impingement as a cause of early osteoarthritis of the hip. J Bone Joint Surg. 2005;87:1012–8. doi:10.1302/0301-620X.87B7.15203.
5. Dora C, Zurbach J, Hersche O, Ganz R. Pathomorphologic characteristics of posttraumatic acetabular dysplasia. J Orthop Trauma. 2000; 14:483–9.
6. Sankar WN, Schoenecker JG, Mayfield ME, et al. Acetabular retroversion in Down syndrome. J Pediatr Orthop. 2012;32:277–81. doi:10.1097/PO.0b013e31824b27fc.
7. Ezoe M, Naito M, Inoue T. The prevalence of acetabular retroversion among various disorders of the hip. J Bone Joint Surg Am. 2006;88:372–9. doi:10.2106/JBJS.D.02385.
8. Dora C, Mascard E, Mladenov K, Seringe R. Retroversion of the acetabular dome after Salter and triple pelvic osteotomy for congenital dislocation of the hip. J Pediatr Orthop B. 2002;11:34–40.
9. Myers SR, Eijer H, Ganz R. Anterior femoroacetabular impingement after periacetabular osteotomy. Clin Orthop Relat Res. 1999;363:93–99.
10. Tannast M, Pfander G, Steppacher SD, et al. Total acetabular retroversion following pelvic osteotomy: presentation, management, and outcome. Hip Int. 2013;23:14–26. doi:10.5301/hipint.5000089.
11. Khanna V, Beaule PE. Defining structural abnormalities of the hip joint at risk of degeneration. J Hip Preserv Surg. 2014;1:12–20. doi:10.1093/jhps/hnu004.
12. Nepple JJ, Lehmann CL, Ross JR, et al. Coxa profunda is not a useful radiographic parameter for diagnosing pincer-type femoroacetabular impingement. J Bone Joint Surg Am. 2013;95:417–23. doi:10.2106/JBJS.K.01664.
13. Anderson LA, Kapron AL, Aoki SK, Peters CL. Coxa profunda: is the deep acetabulum overcovered? Clin Orthop Relat Res. 2012;470:3375–82. doi:10.1007/s11999-012-2509-y.
14. Clohisy JC. A systematic approach to the plain radiographic evaluation of the young adult hip. J Bone Joint Surg Am. 2008;90:47. doi:10.2106/JBJS.H.00756.
15. Jamali AA, Mladenov K, Meyer DC, et al. Anteroposterior pelvic radiographs to assess acetabular retroversion: high validity of the “cross-over-sign.”. J Orthop Res. 2007;25:758–65. doi:10.1002/jor.20380.
16. Fujii M, Nakamura T, Hara T, et al. Does radiographic coxa profunda indicate increased acetabular coverage or depth in hip dysplasia? Clin Orthop Relat Res. 2015;473:2056–66. doi:10.1007/s11999-014-4084-x.
17. Siebenrock KA, Kalbermatten DF, Ganz R. Effect of pelvic tilt on acetabular retroversion: a study of pelves from cadavers. Clin Orthop Relat Res. 2003;407: 241–248. doi:10.1097/01.blo.0000030508.43495.79.
18. Reynolds D, Lucas J, Klaue K. Retroversion of the acetabulum. A cause of hip pain. J Bone Joint Surg Br. 1999;81:281–8.
19. Clohisy JC, Knaus ER, Hunt DM, et al. Clinical presentation of patients with symptomatic anterior hip impingement. Clin Orthop Relat Res. 2009;467:638–44. doi:10.1007/s11999-008-0680-y.
20. Kassarjian A, Belzile E. Femoroacetabular impingement: presentation, diagnosis, and management. Semin Musculoskelet Radiol. 2008;12:136–45. doi:10.1055/s-2008-1078701.
21. Yen Y-M, Kocher MS. Clinical and radiographic diagnosis of femoroacetabular impingement. J Pediatr Orthop. 2013;33 Suppl 1:S112–20. doi:10.1097/BPO.0b013e318288b450.
22. Tannast M, Siebenrock KA, Anderson SE. Femoroacetabular impingement: radiographic diagnosis – what the radiologist should know. AJR Am J Roentgenol. 2007;188:1540–52. doi:10.2214/AJR.06.0921.
23. Ganz R, Leunig M, Leunig-Ganz K, Harris WH. The etiology of osteoarthritis of the hip. Clin Orthop Relat Res. 2008;466:264–72. doi:10.1007/s11999-007-0060-z.
24. Stull JD, Philippon MJ, LaPrade RF. “At-risk” positioning and hip biomechanics of the Peewee ice hockey

sprint start. Am J Sports Med. 2011;39(Suppl):29S–35. doi:10.1177/0363546511414012.

25. Sink EL, Gralla J, Ryba A, Dayton M. Clinical presentation of femoroacetabular impingement in adolescents. J Pediatr Orthop. 2008;28:806–11. doi:10.1097/BPO.0b013e31818e194f.
26. Hack K, Di Primio G, Rakhra K, Beaulé PE. Prevalence of cam-type femoroacetabular impingement morphology in asymptomatic volunteers. J Bone Joint Surg Am. 2010;92:2436–44. doi:10.2106/JBJS.J.01280.
27. Gosvig KK, Jacobsen S, Sonne-Holm S, et al. Prevalence of malformations of the hip joint and their relationship to sex, groin pain, and risk of osteoarthritis: a population-based survey. J Bone Joint Surg Am. 2010;92:1162–9. doi:10.2106/JBJS.H.01674.
28. Laborie LB, Lehmann TG, Engesaeter IO, et al. Prevalence of radiographic findings thought to be associated with femoroacetabular impingement in a population-based cohort of 2081 healthy young adults. Radiology. 2011;260:494–502. doi:10.1148/radiol.11102354.
29. Dudda M, Kim Y-J, Zhang Y, et al. Morphologic differences between the hips of Chinese women and white women: could they account for the ethnic difference in the prevalence of hip osteoarthritis? Arthritis Rheum. 2011;63:2992–9. doi:10.1002/art.30472.
30. Kapron AL, Peters CL, Aoki SK, et al. The prevalence of radiographic findings of structural hip deformities in female collegiate athletes. Am J Sports Med. 2015;43:1324–30. doi:10.1177/0363546515576908.
31. Allen D, Beaule PE, Ramadan O, Doucette S. Prevalence of associated deformities and hip pain in patients with cam-type femoroacetabular impingement. J Bone Joint Surg. 2009;91:589–94. doi:10.1302/0301-620X.91B5.22028.
32. Kohl S, Hosalkar HS, Mainil-Varlet P, et al. Histology of damaged acetabular cartilage in symptomatic femoroacetabular impingement: an observational analysis. Hip Int. 2011;22(2):154–62. doi:10.5301/HIP.2011.6515.
33. Tannast M, Goricki D, Beck M, et al. Hip damage occurs at the zone of femoroacetabular impingement. Clin Orthop Relat Res. 2008;466:273–80. doi:10.1007/s11999-007-0061-y.
34. Corten K, Ganz R, Chosa E, Leunig M. Bone apposition of the acetabular rim in deep hips: a distinct finding of global pincer impingement. J Bone Joint Surg Am. 2011;93:10–6. doi:10.2106/JBJS.J.01799.
35. Kim WY, Hutchinson CE, Andrew JG, Allen PD. The relationship between acetabular retroversion and osteoarthritis of the hip. J Bone Joint Surg. 2006;88:727–9. doi:10.1302/0301-620X.88B6.17430.
36. Kassarjian A, Brisson M, Palmer WE. Femoroacetabular impingement. Eur J Radiol. 2007;63:29–35. doi:10.1016/j.ejrad.2007.03.020.
37. Pfirrmann CWA, Mengiardi B, Dora C, et al. Cam and pincer femoroacetabular impingement: characteristic MR arthrographic findings in 50 patients. Radiology. 2006;240:778–85. doi:10.1148/radiol.2403050767.
38. Leunig M, Nho SJ, Turchetto L, Ganz R. Protrusio acetabuli: new insights and experience with joint preservation. Clin Orthop Relat Res. 2009;467:2241–50. doi:10.1007/s11999-009-0853-3.
39. Wiberg G. Relation between congenital subluxation of the hip and arthritis deformans. Acta Orthop. 1939;10:351–71.
40. Tönnis D. Allgemeine Röntgendiagnostik des Hüftgelenks. In: Die angeborene Hüftdysplasie und Hüftluxation im kindes – und Erwachsenenalter Grundlagen, Diagnostik, konservative und operative Behandlung. Berlin/Heidelberg: Springer Berlin Heidelberg; 1984. p. 104–47.
41. Heyman CH, Herndon CH. Legg-perthes disease; a method for the measurement of the roentgenographic result. J Bone Joint Surg Am. 1950;32:767–78.
42. Nehme A, Trousdale R, Tannous Z, et al. Developmental dysplasia of the hip: Is acetabular retroversion a crucial factor? Orthop Traumatol Surg Res. 2009;95:511–9. doi:10.1016/j.otsr.2009.06.006.
43. Siebenrock KA, Schoeniger R, Ganz R. Anterior femoro-acetabular impingement due to acetabular retroversion. Treatment with periacetabular osteotomy. J Bone Joint Surg Am. 2003;85-A:278–86.
44. Albers CE, Steppacher SD, Tannast M, Siebenrock KA. Surgical technique: reverse periacetabular osteotomy. In: Nho SJ, Leunig M, Kelly BT, et al., editors. Hip arthroscopy and hip joint preservation surgery. New York: Springer New York; 2014. p. 1–17.
45. Werner CML, Copeland CE, Stromberg J, Ruckstuhl T. Correlation of the cross-over ratio of the cross-over sign on conventional pelvic radiographs with computed tomography retroversion measurements. Skeletal Radiol. 2010;39:655–60. doi:10.1007/s00256-009-0854-z.
46. Tannast M, Fritsch S, Zheng G, et al. Which radiographic hip parameters do not have to be corrected for pelvic rotation and tilt? Clin Orthop Relat Res. 2015;473:1255–66. doi:10.1007/s11999-014-3936-8.
47. Werner CML, Copeland CE, Ruckstuhl T, et al. Radiographic markers of acetabular retroversion: correlation of the cross-over sign, ischial spine sign and posterior wall sign. Acta Orthop Belg. 2010;76:166–73.
48. Kalberer F, Sierra RJ, Madan SS, et al. Ischial spine projection into the pelvis: a new sign for acetabular retroversion. Clin Orthop Relat Res. 2008;466:677–83. doi:10.1007/s11999-007-0058-6.
49. Tannast M, Hanke MS, Zheng G, et al. What are the radiographic reference values for acetabular under- and overcoverage? Clin Orthop Relat Res. 2015;473:1234–46. doi:10.1007/s11999-014-4038-3.
50. Larson CM. Arthroscopic management of pincer-type impingement. Sports Med Arthrosc. 2010;18:100–7. doi:10.1097/JSA.0b013e3181dc652e.
51. Armbuster TG, Guerra Jr J, Resnick D, et al. The adult hip: an anatomic study: part I: the bony landmarks 1. Radiology. 1978;128:1–10.
52. Larson CM, Moreau-Gaudry A, Kelly BT, et al. Are normal hips being labeled as pathologic? a CT-based method for defining normal acetabular coverage. Clin

Orthop Relat Res. 2015;473:1247–54. doi:10.1007/s11999-014-4055-2.
53. Tannenbaum E, Kopydlowski N, Smith M, et al. Gender and racial differences in focal and global acetabular version. J Arthroplasty. 2014;29:373–6. doi:10.1016/j.arth.2013.05.015.
54. Kopydlowski NJ, Tannenbaum EP, Bedi A, et al. An increase in cranial acetabular version with age: implications for femoroacetabular impingement. J Arthroplasty. 2014;29:1741–4. doi:10.1016/j.arth.2014.03.042.
55. Zaltz I, Kelly BT, Hetsroni I, Bedi A. The crossover sign overestimates acetabular retroversion. Clin Orthop Relat Res. 2012;471:2463–70. doi:10.1007/s11999-012-2689-5.
56. Cadet ER, Babatunde OM, Gorroochurn P, et al. Inter- and intra-observer agreement of femoroacetabular impingement (FAI) parameters comparing plain radiographs and advanced, 3D computed tomographic (CT)-generated hip models in a surgical patient cohort. Knee Surg Sports Traumatol Arthrosc. 2014. doi:10.1007/s00167-014-3315-8.
57. Enseki K, Harris-Hayes M, White DM, et al. Nonarthritic hip joint pain. J Orthop Sports Phys Ther. 2014;44:A1–32. doi:10.2519/jospt.2014.0302.
58. Giori NJ, Trousdale RT. Acetabular retroversion is associated with osteoarthritis of the hip. Clin Orthop Relat Res. 2003;417:263–9. doi:10.1097/01.blo.0000093014.90435.64.
59. Perreira AC, Hunter JC, Laird T, Jamali AA. Multilevel measurement of acetabular version using 3-D CT-generated models: implications for hip preservation surgery. Clin Orthop Relat Res. 2011;469:552–61. doi:10.1007/s11999-010-1567-2.
60. Nogier A, Bonin N, May O, Gedouin J. Descriptive epidemiology of mechanical hip pathology in adults under 50 years of age. Prospective series of 292 cases: Clinical and radiological aspects and physiopathological review. Orthop Traumatol Surg Res. 2010;96S:S53–8.
61. Li PLS, Ganz R. Morphologic features of congenital acetabular dysplasia. Clin Orthop Relat Res. 2003;416:245–53. doi:10.1097/01.blo.0000081934.75404.36.
62. Mast JW, Brunner RL, Zebrack J. Recognizing acetabular version in the radiographic presentation of hip dysplasia. Clin Orthop Relat Res. 2004;418:48–53.
63. Troelsen A, Rømer L, Jacobsen S, et al. Cranial acetabular retroversion is common in developmental dysplasia of the hip as assessed by the weight bearing position. Acta Orthop. 2010;81:436–41.
64. Fujii M, Nakashima Y, Yamamoto T, et al. Acetabular retroversion in developmental dysplasia of the hip. J Bone Joint Surg Am. 2010;92:895–903. doi:10.2106/JBJS.I.00046.
65. Dora C, Bühler M, Stover MD, et al. Morphologic characteristics of acetabular dysplasia in proximal femoral focal deficiency. J Pediatr Orthop B. 2004;13:81–7. doi:10.1097/01.bpb.0000091575.01531.06.
66. Köhnlein W, Ganz R, Impellizzeri FM, Leunig M. Acetabular morphology: implications for joint-preserving surgery. Clin Orthop Relat Res. 2009;467:682–91. doi:10.1007/s11999-008-0682-9.
67. Steppacher SD, Lerch TD, Gharanizadeh K, et al. Size and shape of the lunate surface in different types of pincer impingement: theoretical implications for surgical therapy. Osteoarthritis Cartilage. 2014;22:951–8. doi:10.1016/j.joca.2014.05.010.
68. Al-Moussa S, Moroz P, Beaulé PE. Effect of pelvic osteotomy in the skeletally immature on acetabular coverage. HSS J. 2012;8:235–9. doi:10.1007/s11420-012-9286-8.
69. Schenker M, Martin R, Weiland D, Philippon M. Current trends in hip arthroscopy: a review of injury diagnosis, techniques, and outcome scoring. Curr Opin Orthop. 2005;16:89.
70. Charbonnier C, Kolo FC, Duthon VB, et al. Assessment of congruence and impingement of the hip joint in professional ballet dancers: a motion capture study. Am J Sports Med. 2011;39:557–66. doi:10.1177/0363546510386002.
71. Duthon VB, Charbonnier C, Kolo FC, et al. Correlation of clinical and magnetic resonance imaging findings in hips of elite female ballet dancers. Arthroscopy. 2013;29:411–9. doi:10.1016/j.arthro.2012.10.012.
72. Bedi A, Dolan M, Leunig M, Kelly BT. Static and dynamic mechanical causes of hip pain. Arthroscopy. 2011;27:235–51. doi:10.1016/j.arthro.2010.07.022.
73. Sutter R, Dietrich TJ, Zingg PO, Pfirrmann CWA. Femoral antetorsion: comparing asymptomatic volunteers and patients with femoroacetabular impingement. Radiology. 2012;263:475–83. doi:10.1148/radiol.12111903.
74. Philippon MJ, Stubbs AJ, Schenker ML, et al. Arthroscopic management of femoroacetabular impingement: osteoplasty technique and literature review. Am J Sports Med. 2007;35:1571–80. doi:10.1177/0363546507300258.
75. Rebello G, Spencer S, Millis MB, Kim Y-J. Surgical dislocation in the management of pediatric and adolescent hip deformity. Clin Orthop Relat Res. 2009;467:724–31. doi:10.1007/s11999-008-0591-y.
76. Buller LT, Rosneck J, Monaco FM, et al. Relationship between proximal femoral and acetabular alignment in normal hip joints using 3-dimensional computed tomography. Am J Sports Med. 2012;40:367–75. doi:10.1177/0363546511424390.
77. Ganz R, Horowitz K, Leunig M. Algorithm for femoral and periacetabular osteotomies in complex hip deformities. Clin Orthop Relat Res. 2010;468:3168–80. doi:10.1007/s11999-010-1489-z.
78. Eijer H, Myers SR, Ganz R. Anterior femoroacetabular impingement after femoral neck fractures. J Orthop Trauma. 2001;15:475–81.
79. Pécasse GABM, Eijer H, Haverkamp D, Marti RK. Intertrochanteric osteotomy in young adults for sequelae of Legg-Calvé-Perthes' disease – a long term follow-up. Int Orthop. 2004;28:44–7. doi:10.1007/s00264-003-0513-2.
80. Clohisy JC, Nunley RM, Curry MC, Schoenecker PL. Periacetabular osteotomy for the treatment of acetabular dysplasia associated with major aspherical

femoral head deformities. J Bone Joint Surg Am. 2007;89:1417–23. doi:10.2106/JBJS.F.00493.
81. Eijer H, Podeszwa DA, Ganz R, Leunig M. Evaluation and treatment of young adults with femoro-acetabular impingement secondary to Perthes' disease. Hip Int. 2006;16:273–80.
82. Ganz R, Huff T, Leunig M. Extended retinacular soft-tissue flap for intra-articular hip surgery: surgical technique, indications, and results of application. Instr Course Lect. 2009;58:241.
83. McBride MT, Muldoon MP, Santore RF, et al. Protrusio acetabuli: diagnosis and treatment. J Am Acad Orthop Surg. 2001;9:79–88.
84. Albers CE, Steppacher SD, Schwab JM, et al. Relative femoral neck lengthening improves pain and hip function in proximal femoral deformities with a high-riding trochanter. Clin Orthop Relat Res. 2015;473:1212–23. doi:10.1007/s11999-014-4032-9.
85. Novais EN. Application of the surgical dislocation approach to residual hip deformity secondary to Legg-Calvé-Perthes disease. J Pediatr Orthop. 2013;33 Suppl1:S62–9.doi:10.1097/BPO.0b013e318281132d.
86. Shore BJ, Novais EN, Millis MB, Kim Y-J. Low early failure rates using a surgical dislocation approach in healed legg-calvé-perthes disease. Clin Orthop Relat Res. 2011;470:2441–9. doi:10.1007/s11999-011-2187-1.
87. Anderson LA, Erickson JA, Severson EP, Peters CL. Sequelae of Perthes disease: treatment with surgical hip dislocation and relative femoral neck lengthening. J Pediatr Orthop. 2010;30:758–66. doi:10.1097/BPO.0b013e3181fcbaaf.
88. Tannast M, MacIntyre N, Steppacher SD, et al. A systematic approach to analyse the sequelae of LCPD. Hip Int. 2013;23:61–70. doi:10.5301/hipint.5000071.
89. Tannast M, Leunig M, Session Participants. Report of breakout session: Coxa profunda/protrusio management. Clin Orthop Relat Res. 2012;470:3459–61. doi:10.1007/s11999-012-2572-4.
90. Guanche CA, Bare AA. Arthroscopic treatment of femoroacetabular impingement. Arthroscopy. 2006; 22:95–106. doi:10.1016/j.arthro.2005.10.018.
91. Nötzli HP, Wyss TF, Stoecklin CH, et al. The contour of the femoral head-neck junction as a predictor for the risk of anterior impingement. J Bone Joint Surg. 2002;84:556–60.
92. Wall PDH, Fernandez M, Griffin DR, Foster NE. Nonoperative treatment for femoroacetabular impingement: a systematic review of the literature. PM R. 2013;5:418–26. doi:10.1016/j.pmrj.2013.02.005.
93. Lequesne M, de Sèze S. False profile of the pelvis. A new radiographic incidence for the study of the hip. Its use in dysplasias and different coxopathies. Rev Rhum Mal Osteoartic. 1961;28:643–52.
94. Kiyama T, Naito M, Shiramizu K, Shinoda T. Postoperative acetabular retroversion causes posterior osteoarthritis of the hip. Int Orthop. 2007;33:625–31. doi:10.1007/s00264-007-0507-6.
95. Albers CE, Steppacher SD, Ganz R, et al. Impingement adversely affects 10-year survivorship after periacetabular osteotomy for DDH. Clin Orthop Relat Res. 2013;471:1602–14. doi:10.1007/s11999-013-2799-8.
96. Lansdown DA, Kumar D, Wyatt C, et al. Quantitative cartilage imaging and patient-reported outcome measures for four common findings of femoroacetabular impingement. Osteoarthr Cartil. 2014;22:S246–7.
97. Palmer AJR, Ayyar-Gupta V, Dutton SJ, et al. Protocol for the Femoroacetabular Impingement Trial (FAIT): a multi-centre randomised controlled trial comparing surgical and non-surgical management of femoroacetabular impingement. Bone Joint Res. 2014;3:321–7. doi:10.1302/2046-3758.311.2000336.
98. Nepple JJ, Prather H, Trousdale RT, et al. Diagnostic imaging of femoroacetabular impingement. J Am Acad Orthop Surg. 2013;21 Suppl 1:S20–6. doi:10.5435/JAAOS-21-07-S20.
99. Sur S, Mamisch TC, Hughes T, Kim Y-J. High resolution fast T1 mapping technique for dGEMRIC. J Magn Reson Imaging. 2009;30:896–900. doi:10.1002/jmri.21869.
100. Jessel RH, Zilkens C, Tiderius C, et al. Assessment of osteoarthritis in hips with femoroacetabular impingement using delayed gadolinium enhanced MRI of cartilage. J Magn Reson Imaging. 2009;30:1110–5. doi:10.1002/jmri.21830.
101. Clohisy JC, Zebala LP, Nepple JJ, Pashos G. Combined hip arthroscopy and limited open osteochondroplasty for anterior femoroacetabular impingement. J Bone Joint Surg Am. 2010;92:1697–706. doi:10.2106/JBJS.I.00326.
102. Collins JA, Ward JP, Youm T. Is prophylactic surgery for femoroacetabular impingement indicated? A systematic review. Am J Sports Med. 2014;42:3009–15. doi:10.1177/0363546513499227.
103. Philippon MJ, Schroder e Souza BG, Briggs KK. Hip arthroscopy for femoroacetabular impingement in patients aged 50 years or older. Arthroscopy. 2012;28:59–65. doi:10.1016/j.arthro.2011.07.004.
104. Larson CM, Giveans MR, Taylor M. Does arthroscopic FAI correction improve function with radiographic arthritis? Clin Orthop Relat Res. 2011;469:1667–76. doi:10.1007/s11999-010-1741-6.
105. Gautier E, Ganz K, Krügel N, et al. Anatomy of the medial femoral circumflex artery and its surgical implications. J Bone Joint Surg. 2000;82:679–83.
106. Lavigne M, Kalhor M, Beck M, et al. Distribution of vascular foramina around the femoral head and neck junction: relevance for conservative intracapsular procedures of the hip. Orthop Clin North Am. 36:171–6– viii. doi:10.1016/j.ocl.2005.02.002.
107. Nötzli HP, Siebenrock KA, Hempfing A, et al. Perfusion of the femoral head during surgical dislocation of the hip. Monitoring by laser Doppler flowmetry. J Bone Joint Surg Br. 2002;84:300–4.
108. Ganz R, Gill TJ, Gautier E, et al. Surgical dislocation of the adult hip a technique with full access to the femoral head and acetabulum without the risk of avascular necrosis. J Bone Joint Surg. 2001;83: 1119–24.
109. Beck M, Leunig M, Parvizi J, et al. Anterior femoroacetabular impingement: part II. Midterm results of surgical treatment. Clin Orthop Relat Res. 2004;418:67–73.

110. Sink EL. Multicenter study of complications following surgical dislocation of the hip. J Bone Joint Surg Am. 2011;93:1132–6. doi:10.2106/JBJS.J.00794.
111. Solberg BD, Moon CN, Franco DP. Use of a trochanteric flip osteotomy improves outcomes in Pipkin IV fractures. Clin Orthop Relat Res. 2009;467:929–33. doi:10.1007/s11999-008-0505-z.
112. Bastian JD, Büchler L, Meyer DC, et al. Surgical hip dislocation for osteochondral transplantation as a salvage procedure for a femoral head impaction fracture. J Orthop Trauma. 2010;24:e113–8. doi:10.1097/BOT.0b013e3181dfbb52.
113. Tannast M, Krüger A, Mack PW, et al. Surgical dislocation of the hip for the fixation of acetabular fractures. J Bone Joint Surg. 2010;92:842–52. doi:10.1302/0301-620X.92B6.22994.
114. de Los Santos O, Filomeno P, Rey R, Cúneo A. Acetabular osteoid osteoma excision by controlled hip dislocation: a case report. J Pediatr Orthop B. 2013;22:195–9. doi:10.1097/BPB.0b013e32835f57fc.
115. Fukui K, Kaneuji A, Kinoshita E, et al. Localized pigmented villonodular synovitis of the hip: sudden-onset pain caused by torsion of the tumor pedicle. Case Rep Orthop. 2013;2013:862935. doi:10.1155/2013/862935.
116. Li M, Luettringhaus T, Walker KR, Cole PA. Operative treatment of femoral neck osteochondroma through a digastric approach in a pediatric patient: a case report and review of the literature. J Pediatr Orthop B. 2012;21:230–4. doi:10.1097/BPB.0b013e3283524bc3.
117. Jellicoe P, Son-Hing J, Hopyan S, Thompson GH. Surgical hip dislocation for removal of intraarticular exostoses: report of two cases. J Pediatr Orthop. 2009;29:327–30. doi:10.1097/BPO.0b013e3181a56b4f.
118. Espinosa N, Beck M, Rothenfluh DA, et al. Treatment of femoro-acetabular impingement: preliminary results of labral refixation. Surgical technique. J Bone Joint Surg Am. 2007;89(Suppl 2 Pt 1):36–53. doi:10.2106/JBJS.F.01123.
119. Bastian JD, Wolf AT, Wyss TF, Nötzli HP. Stepped osteotomy of the trochanter for stable, anatomic refixation. Clin Orthop Relat Res. 2009;467:732–8. doi:10.1007/s11999-008-0649-x.
120. Lavigne M, Parvizi J, Beck M, et al. Anterior femoroacetabular impingement: part I. Techniques of joint preserving surgery. Clin Orthop Relat Res. 2004;61–66.
121. Ayeni OR, Alradwan H, de Sa D, Philippon MJ. The hip labrum reconstruction: indications and outcomes-a systematic review. Knee Surg Sports Traumatol Arthrosc. 2014;22:737–43. doi:10.1007/s00167-013-2804-5.
122. Sierra RJ, Trousdale RT. Labral reconstruction using the ligamentum teres capitis: report of a new technique. Clin Orthop Relat Res. 2009;467:753–9. doi:10.1007/s11999-008-0633-5.
123. Philippon MJ, Briggs KK, Hay CJ, et al. Arthroscopic labral reconstruction in the hip using iliotibial band autograft: technique and early outcomes. Arthroscopy. 2010;26(6):750–6. doi:10.1016/j.arthro.2009.10.016.
124. Costa Rocha P, Klingenstein G, Ganz R, et al. Circumferential reconstruction of severe acetabular labral damage using hamstring allograft: surgical technique and case series. Hip Int. 2013;23:42–53. doi:10.5301/HIP.2013.11662.
125. Matsuda DK. Acute iatrogenic dislocation following hip impingement arthroscopic surgery. Arthroscopy. 2009;25:400–4.
126. Ferguson SJ, Bryant JT, Ganz R, Ito K. An in vitro investigation of the acetabular labral seal in hip joint mechanics. J Biomech. 2003;36:171–8.
127. Khanna V, Tushinski DM, Drexler M, et al. Cartilage restoration of the hip using fresh osteochondral allograft: resurfacing the potholes. Bone Joint J. 2014;96-B:11–6. doi:10.1302/0301-620X.96B11.34734.
128. Mancini D, Fontana A. Five-year results of arthroscopic techniques for the treatment of acetabular chondral lesions in femoroacetabular impingement. Int Orthop. 2014;38:2057–64. doi:10.1007/s00264-014-2403-1.
129. Leunig M, Tibor LM, Naal FD, et al. Surgical technique: second-generation bone marrow stimulation via surgical dislocation to treat hip cartilage lesions. Clin Orthop Relat Res. 2012;470:3421–31. doi:10.1007/s11999-012-2466-5.
130. Peters CL, Erickson JA, Hines JL. Early results of the Bernese periacetabular osteotomy: the learning curve at an academic medical center. J Bone Joint Surg. 2006;88-A:1920–6.
131. Beaulé PE, Le Duff MJ, Zaragoza E. Quality of life following femoral head-neck osteochondroplasty for femoroacetabular impingement. J Bone Joint Surg Am. 2007;89:773–9. doi:10.2106/JBJS.F.00681.
132. Benali Y, Katthagen BD. Hip subluxation as a complication of arthroscopic debridement. Arthroscopy. 2009;25:405–7. doi:10.1016/j.arthro.2009.01.012.
133. Steppacher SD, Huemmer C, Schwab JM, et al. Surgical hip dislocation for treatment of femoroacetabular impingement: factors predicting 5-year survivorship. Clin Orthop Relat Res. 2014;472:337–48. doi:10.1007/s11999-013-3268-0.
134. Philippon MJ, Wolff AB, Briggs KK, et al. Acetabular rim reduction for the treatment of femoroacetabular impingement correlates with preoperative and postoperative center-edge angle. Arthroscopy. 2010;26:757–61. doi:10.1016/j.arthro.2009.11.003.
135. Colvin AC, Koehler SM, Bird J. Can the change in center-edge angle during pincer trimming be reliably predicted? Clin Orthop Relat Res. 2010;469:1071–4. doi:10.1007/s11999-010-1581-4.
136. Ross JR, Larson CM, Adeoyo O, et al. Residual deformity is the most common reason for revision hip arthroscopy: a three-dimensional CT study. Clin Orthop Relat Res. 2015;473:1388–95. doi:10.1007/s11999-014-4069-9.
137. Ricciardi BF, Fields K, Kelly BT, et al. Causes and risk factors for revision hip preservation surgery. Am J Sports Med. 2014;42:2627–33. doi:10.1177/0363546514545855.

138. Steppacher SD, Anwander H, Zurmühle CA, et al. Eighty percent of patients with surgical hip dislocation for femoroacetabular impingement have a good clinical result without osteoarthritis progression at 10 years. Clin Orthop Relat Res. 2015;473:1333–41. doi:10.1007/s11999-014-4025-8.
139. Ng VY, Arora N, Best TM, et al. Efficacy of surgery for femoroacetabular impingement: a systematic review. Am J Sports Med. 2010;38:2337–45. doi:10.1177/0363546510365530.
140. Bedi A, Chen N, Robertson W, Kelly BT. The management of labral tears and femoroacetabular impingement of the hip in the young, active patient. Arthroscopy. 2008;24:1135–45. doi:10.1016/j.arthro.2008.06.001.
141. Clohisy JC, St John LC, Schutz AL. Surgical treatment of femoroacetabular impingement: a systematic review of the literature. Clin Orthop Relat Res. 2010;468:555–64. doi:10.1007/s11999-009-1138-6.
142. Sink EL, Fabricant PD, Pan Z, et al. Results of treatment of femoroacetabular impingement in adolescents with a surgical hip dislocation approach. Clin Orthop Relat Res. 2013;471:2563–9. doi:10.1007/s11999-013-3004-9.
143. Hingsammer AM, Lee CB, LaReau J, et al. Is acetabular osteoplasty always required in mixed impingement? Eur J Orthop Surg Traumatol. 2015;25:331–8. doi:10.1007/s00590-014-1507-z.
144. Siebenrock KA, Schaller C, Tannast M, et al. Anteverting periacetabular osteotomy for symptomatic acetabular retroversion: results at ten years. J Bone Joint Surg. 2014;96:1785–92. doi:10.2106/JBJS.M.00842.
145. Ganz R, Klaue K, Vinh TS, Mast JW. A new periacetabular osteotomy for the treatment of hip dysplasias. Technique and preliminary results. Clin Orthop Relat Res. 1988;232:26–36.
146. Murphy SB, Millis MB. Periacetabular osteotomy without abductor dissection using direct anterior exposure. Clin Orthop Relat Res. 1999;364:92.
147. Peters CL, Erickson JA, Anderson MB, Anderson LA. Preservation of the rectus femoris origin during periacetabular osteotomy does not compromise acetabular reorientation. Clin Orthop Relat Res. 2015;473:608–14. doi:10.1007/s11999-014-3837-x.
148. Biedermann R, Donnan L, Gabriel A, et al. Complications and patient satisfaction after periacetabular pelvic osteotomy. Int Orthop. 2008;32:611–7. doi:10.1007/s00264-007-0372-3.
149. Davey JP, Santore RF. Complications of periacetabular osteotomy. Clin Orthop Relat Res. 1999;363:33–7.
150. Hussell JG, Rodriguez JA, Ganz R. Technical complications of the Bernese periacetabular osteotomy. Clin Orthop Relat Res. 1999;363:81–92.
151. Trousdale RT, Cabanela ME. Lessons learned after more than 250 periacetabular osteotomies. Acta Orthop. 2003;74:119–26. doi:10.1080/00016470310013824.
152. Zaltz I, Baca G, Kim Y-J, et al. Complications associated with the periacetabular osteotomy: a prospective multicenter study. J Bone Joint Surg. 2014;96:1967–74. doi:10.2106/JBJS.N.00113.
153. Millis MB, Kim Y-J. Rationale of osteotomy and related procedures for hip preservation: a review. Clin Orthop Relat Res. 2002;405:108–21.
154. Crowninshield RD, Brand RA, Pedersen DR. A stress analysis of acetabular reconstruction in protrusio acetabuli. J Bone Joint Surg Am. 1983;65:495–9.
155. Baghdadi YMK, Larson AN, Sierra RJ. Restoration of the hip center during THA performed for protrusio acetabuli is associated with better implant survival. Clin Orthop Relat Res. 2013;471:3251–9. doi:10.1007/s11999-013-3072-x.
156. Ranawat CS, Dorr LD, Inglis AE. Total hip arthroplasty in protrusio acetabuli of rheumatoid arthritis. J Bone Joint Surg Am. 1980;62:1059–65.
157. Tibor LM, Leunig M. The pathoanatomy and arthroscopic management of femoroacetabular impingement. Bone Joint Res. 2012;1:245–57. doi:10.1302/2046-3758.110.
158. Chu CR, Millis MB, Olson SA. Osteoarthritis: from palliation to prevention: AOA critical issues. J Bone Joint Surg. 2014;96:e130. doi:10.2106/JBJS.M.01209.

Treatment of Labral Tears in FAI Surgery

12

Marc J. Philippon and Karen K. Briggs

Contents

M.J. Philippon, MD (✉)
Orthopaedic Surgeon, Steadman Clinic and Steadman Philippon Research Institute, Vail, CO, USA
e-mail: mjp@sprivail.org

K.K. Briggs, MPH
Steadman Philippon Research Institute, Center for Outcomes-based Orthopaedic Research,
181 West Meadow Suite, Vail, CO 1000, USA
e-mail: Karen.briggs@sprivail.org

12.1 Introduction

In the last 10 years, femoroacetabular impingement (FAI) has been brought to the forefront of the current literature on hip arthroscopy. Most of literature has focused on diagnosis and treatment of the soft tissue and bony pathology involved with FAI [1–5]. As arthroscopic techniques and the tools available have advanced, the treatment of FAI and associated labral tears has been refined [2–4]. While labral debridement for labral tears was the initial standard of care in the early days of hip arthroscopy, treatment now is based on specific variations of the labral tear. The purpose of this chapter will be to present the current labral treatment algorithm and discuss the evidence that supports the algorithm.

12.2 The Labrum

The labrum augments the femoral head coverage within the acetabulum and provides a joint sealing effect that ensures adequate joint lubrication, contributing to cartilage nutrition, reducing joint friction (Song) and hip stability [6–8]. The labrum runs circumferentially around the bony acetabulum to the base of the fovea, where it is attached to the transverse ligament posteriorly and anteriorly. The apex of the labrum has free margins and is attached at its base to the acetabular bony rim. The mechanical role of the labrum

O.R. Ayeni et al. (eds.), *Diagnosis and Management of Femoroacetabular Impingement*,
DOI 10.1007/978-3-319-32000-7_12

is not completely understood but experimental studies have shown that the labrum provides a seal against fluid flow in and out of the intra-articular space as well as fluid flow out of the articular cartilage [7, 9]. It also provides a suction effect, thus further enhancing stability [10, 11]. In a recent study on joint kinematics, the disruption of the labrum led to decreased femoral stability in extreme range of hip motions [11]. The reduced stiffness of the injured labrum makes the joint susceptible to increased impact loading and repetitive microtrauma [11].

12.3 Nonsurgical Treatment

Typically, a trial of nonsurgical management, including relative rest, anti-inflammatory medications, and pain medications as necessary, combined with a focused physical therapy (PT) protocol for 6–8 weeks, is recommended for most patients with signs and symptoms of labral injury. Occasionally, it is necessary to restrict weight bearing in patients with acute or traumatic onset of symptoms. In cases of an infolded labrum or mechanically locked joint, delay of hip arthroscopy could result in additional damage to the labrum and joint cartilage. As such in these cases, arthroscopy should not be delayed. While nonoperative treatment may decrease pain with normal movement, pain with activities does not always improve. Furthermore, bony deformities such as FAI are commonly associated with labral pathology, and delay of treatment past the initial 6–8 weeks may increase the potential of damage caused by the bony impingement. There is also limited evidence supporting the use of nonsurgical treatment over surgical treatment for labral tears.

12.4 Labral Debridement

Most of the early literature focuses on labral debridement for the management of symptomatic labral tears. Labral tissue that was damaged was selectively removed from the joint; however, this led to less protective effect of the labrum and based on current understanding may have led to further alteration of hip mechanics and function. In another joint such as the knee, the prevalence of meniscus repairs has significantly increased, as tissue preservation has been appreciated, and it is likely that this will occur in the hip with better understanding of joint function [13]. Moreover, a recent basic science study showed that if a segment of the labrum was removed and the hip joint was loaded, the tissue that replaced the area of resection did not possess the circumferential fiber bundle characteristic of the normal labrum [14]. Abrams et al. did demonstrate spontaneous regrowth of the labrum after resection in a small case series; however, the biomechanical and histological properties of this regrowth are unknown [12].

A systematic review by Tibor et al. found good short-term results in both treatment groups: labral debridement and labral repair [15]. While follow-up was limited and the studies analyzed were a mixture of open and arthroscopic treatments, the results did support the conclusion that repair was better than debridement in the short term. In a study by Espinosa et al., progression of osteoarthrosis was noted to increase in the debridement group compared with labral repair [16]. As the function of the labrum has been better defined, the author's treatment of choice has shifted to labral repair when possible [17]. The clinical indications for labral debridement are limited to the hips presenting with simple peripheral tears (small flaps or fraying) in which the resection will allow enough remaining tissue for the labrum to maintain its physiological functions. Finally, two studies (on the overlapping patient population) by Larson et al. have demonstrated, in short and medium terms, that clinical outcomes are significantly improved in the labral repair group when compared to labral debridement [25, 26].

12.4.1 Labral Repair

Research has dramatically increased the current knowledge on the role of the labrum on hip joint function. The labrum's role in maintaining the joint seal, enhancing stability of the hip joint, and participation in nociception and proprioception is better understood. Likewise, basic science studies have further demonstrated the ability of the repaired labrum to heal. In an experimental study using an ovine model, healing was demonstrated in the arthroscopically repaired labrum. The repair appeared stable and grossly healed at 12 weeks via fibrovascular scarring or new bone formation [18].

Biomechanical studies have further demonstrated that the labrum provides a seal creating a hydrostatic fluid pressure [9]. Partial labral resection caused significant decrease in intra-articular pressure; meanwhile, labral repair restored the pressure mechanics again (ref). In a second part of this study, the researchers showed that labral resection decreased the distractive strength of the hip fluid seal [10]. Philippon et al. showed that labral repair resulted in significant improvement of the strength of the hip fluid seal [9, 10].

These studies, in addition to the studies on clinical outcome, have led to labral repair becoming the treatment of choice for most labral tears found at the time of surgery.

12.4.2 Technique

Hip arthroscopy is performed with the patient in the supine position with the use of general anesthesia and supplementary regional anesthesia [11]. The techniques used for traction and positioning have been described in the previous chapters (Fig. 12.1).

Accurate portal placement is essential for optimal visualization and enabling of accurate anchor placement. The tip of the greater trochanter and the soft area between sartorius and tensor musculature are used as anatomic landmarks. The anterolateral portal is placed 1 cm superior and 1 cm anterior to the tip of the greater trochanter. The mid-anterior portal is localized in the soft spot between the sartorius and tensor musculature approximately 7 cm distal and medial to the anterolateral portal on a 45° plane (Figure). These portal locations are meant to avoid the branches of the lateral femoral cutaneous nerve and minimize trauma to the hip flexors (rectus femoris).

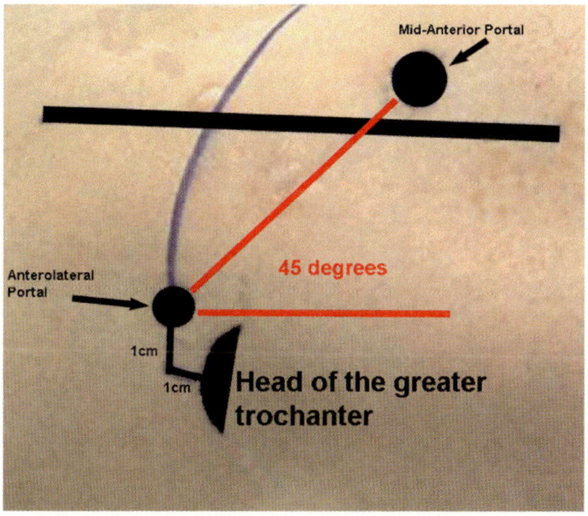

Fig. 12.1 Portal positioning for labral repair

An arthroscopic needle is placed into the hip joint through anterolateral incision first. Once the arthroscope is introduced into the hip joint through the anterolateral cannula, the anterior triangle where the mid-anterior portal will enter the joint is visualized. To decrease the risk of damaging the cartilage of the femoral head or piercing the labrum, the placement of the mid-anterior portal is visualized through the arthroscope.

A diagnostic examination of the hip is thereafter performed. All aspects of both the central and peripheral compartments should be inspected in addition to performing a dynamic examination to determine where bony conflicts occur. The chondrolabral junction is inspected. A probe is used to determine if the labrum has been separated from the acetabular rim and if the chondrolabral junction has been disrupted. Delamination of the acetabular cartilage at the chondrolabral junction is common with CAM-type impingement and usually occurs at the site of impingement and labral damage (Fig. 12.2). It is very important to thoroughly and carefully inspect the chondrolabral junction. If they are not addressed at the time of the initial surgery, they can be the source of recurrent pain and disability as the junction between the labrum and the delaminated cartilage can degenerate further [19].

To assess the labrum, the arthroscope is placed in the central compartment through the anterolateral portal. To improve visualization, a capsulot-

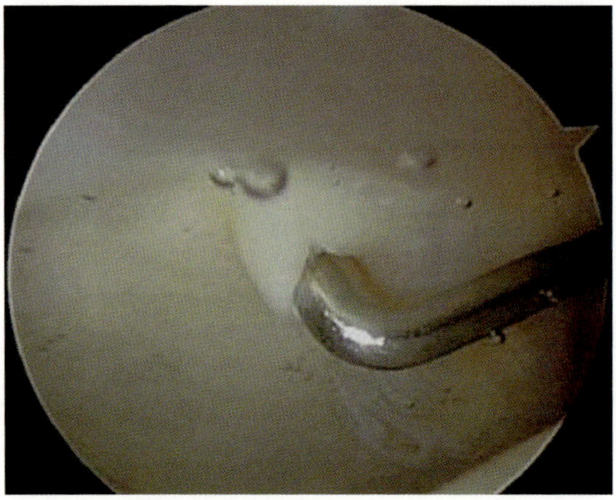

Fig. 12.2 Chondrolabral separation dysfunction with delaminated acetabular cartilage

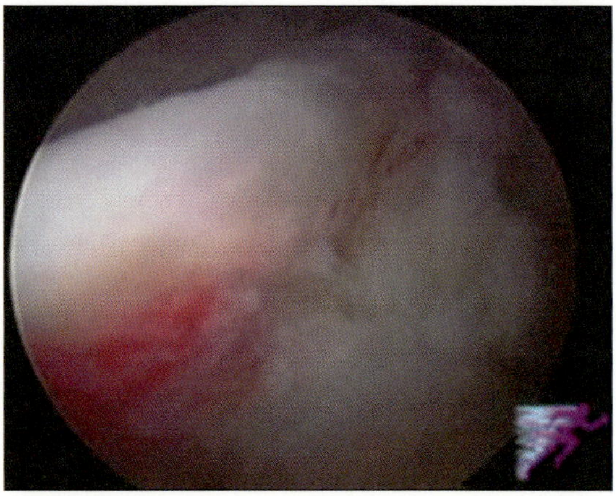

Fig. 12.3 Bruised acetabular labrum associated with pincer impingement

omy is performed. The capsulotomy connects the two portal sites in the capsule within the central compartment and should be kept as small as needed based on the need for visualization. In the peripheral compartment, visualization during the dynamic exam will evaluate the sealing function of the labrum and identify areas needing treatment. The bony abnormality of the femoral head-neck junction can be identified, and a CAM osteoplasty can be performed. The vessels of the femoral neck can also be identified in the peripheral compartment and protected during CAM resection. Once the CAM resection is complete, a dynamic examination is again performed to make sure the entire impingement lesion has been addressed.

The arthroscope is then returned to the central compartment. If pincer impingement exists, a rim trimming is performed (Fig. 12.3). Measuring the width of the acetabulum and comparing this to the center-edge angle (CE angle) can help avoid over-resection of the rim [20]. The labrum is detached from the acetabular rim, and the rim or pincer lesion is trimmed. The goal of the rim resection should be to remove this area of the bone and restore the normal anatomy and relative position of the acetabulum with respect to the pelvis and femoral neck. A 5.5-mm motorized burr is used to perform the rim trimming (Fig. 12.4). With the labrum detached and safely out of the way, the bone is slowly removed from the anterior superior margin of the acetabular rim.

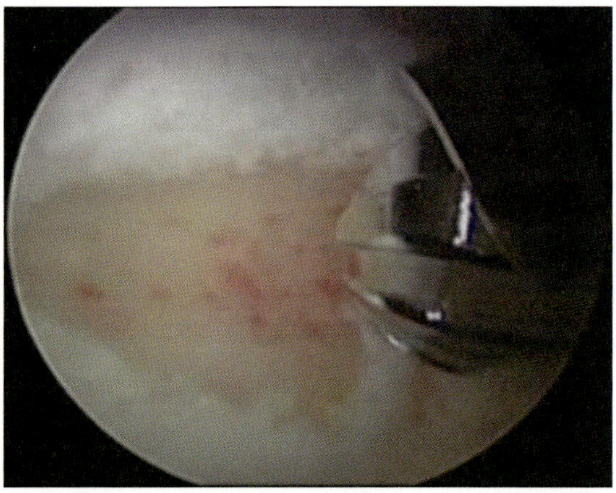

Fig. 12.4 Arthroscopic view of burring of pincer lesion. *A* acetabulum, *L* labrum

Proper reattachment of the labrum to the acetabular rim is critical to reestablish the seal for the hip joint, the proper tracking of the labrum on the femoral head cartilage, and increases the surface area for pressure distribution within the hip joint. Failure in any one of these three areas can lead to subsequent pain and potential instability.

If a rim trimming was not necessary, the acetabular rim should be prepared with limited

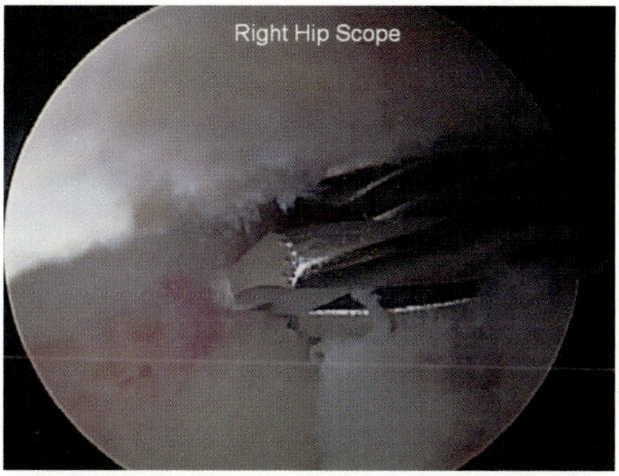

Fig. 12.5 Suture anchor guides device in place on the acetabular rim

decortication using a burr, for anchor placement and to improve the healing of the labrum to the acetabulum. The anchor should be placed perpendicular to the rim, and penetration of the acetabular surface must be avoided (Fig. 12.5). To help with the placement of the anchor, the acetabular rim angle should be determined for proper anchor placement [21]. The rim angle provides a safety margin when placing anchors and varies based on the location on the rim. Larger rim angles are seen with shorter drill depth and rim trimming. The smallest angle is at the 3-o'clock position [21]. The size of anchor and the type of suture are based on the location of fixation. A pierced suture, which goes through the body of the labrum, is used to invert the labrum when there is adequate tissue. A loop suture, which goes around the entire labrum, will typically cause the labrum to evert. The balanced use of the loop and through/intrasubstance sutures helps recreate the suction seal. For anchors in the 9-o'clock to 12-o'clock position, a 2.3 mm anchor is used with a pierced suture. At 12 o'clock, a 2.9 mm anchor with a loop suture is recommended. At 2–3 o'clock, a 1.7 mm anchor is used, and at greater than 3 o'clock, a 1.5 mm anchor is used with a pierced suture. Anchor size is based on the shape of the acetabulum as it varies based on the location. All knots are placed on the capsular side and buried in the drill hole to avoid contact with adjacent cartilage (Fig. 12.6).

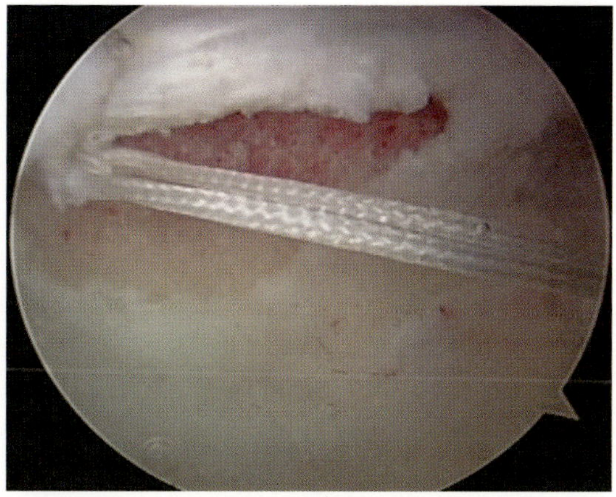

Fig. 12.6 Knots from the labral repair are recessed into the drill hole on the capsular side of the repair to avoid damage to the acetabular cartilage

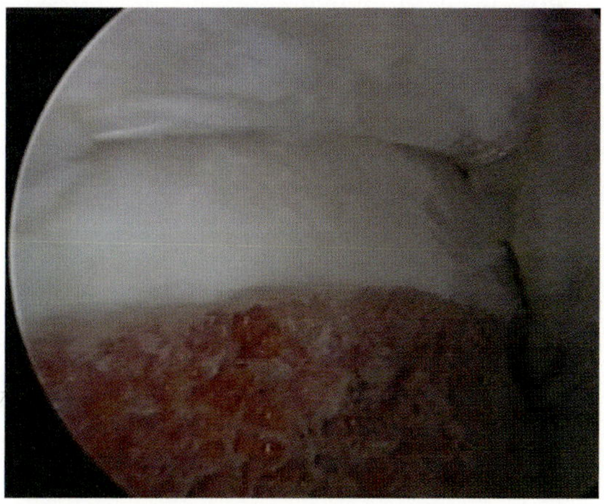

Fig. 12.7 Dynamic evaluation following labral repair, rim trimming, and osteochondroplasty showing normal tracking of the labrum with the femoral head

After completion of the labral repair, the traction is released and the arthroscope is moved into the peripheral compartment. A dynamic examination is performed to evaluate the repair (Fig. 12.7). The labrum should lie on the femoral head and recreate the seal as the hip is taken through a normal range of motion. For athletes who use their hip in extreme ranges, the athletic maneuver should be replicated to ensure that the labrum functions during the "at risk" motion. If the labrum appears unstable, additional sutures are used. Full decompression of pincer and CAM is also confirmed. If areas of conflict still exist, traction should be reestablished and additional osteoplasty performed as needed. If additional anchors are placed or further resection of the bone is performed, the dynamic examination should be undertaken again to ensure the labrum seals with the femoral head.

12.5 Postoperative Rehabilitation

Early postoperative rehabilitation is focused on preventing the formation of adhesions, protecting the repair, and regaining pain-free motion [22]. The prevention of adhesion formation consists of passive range-of-motion exercises for 4 weeks and circumduction exercises. Patients may also begin stationary biking as soon as tolerable. Abduction is restricted to 0–45° for 2 weeks. In order to protect the repaired labrum, a brace which limits extension is worn while ambulating for the first 21 postoperative days. Patients are restricted to flatfoot weight bearing with 20 lbs of pressure for 3 weeks. These are typical recommendations; however, specific recommendations vary for each patient and depend on the individual case.

12.6 Evidence and Outcomes

There are few reports discussing the long-term outcomes of hip arthroscopy for labral dysfunction and associated femoroacetabular impingement. Several studies have documented better outcomes following labral repair compared to labral debridement. A recent systematic review concluded labral repair results in superior outcomes when compared to labral debridement [23]. One level 1 study has been published. Krych et al. performed a randomized prospective study comparing labral repair to labral debridement [24]. Labral repairs averaged 3.1 anchors, and the debridement was performed while attempting to preserve stable labral tissue. At follow-up between 12 and 48 months, the labral repair group had significantly better functional and sports-specific scores compared to the labral debridement group.

Several other studies have compared repair to debridement. Larson et al. published two studies, one with short-term outcomes [25] and one with 3–5-year outcomes [26]. These retrospective cohort studies compared labral debridement to labral repair. With a minimum follow-up of 2 years, good-to-excellent results were found in 68 % of debridements and 92 % of labral repairs. Patients with labral repair had better Harris hip scores, VAS pain outcomes, and SF-12 general health. Another study also found similar results [27]. They showed significantly more improvement in modified Harris hip score in the labral repair group compared to the debridement group. Philippon et al. also found labral repair as a predictor of superior outcomes compared to labral debridement when treating FAI; however, the amount of joint space was the most important predictor of failure [28]. The current evidence includes one level 1 study and a limited number of level 2 or 3 studies. Most studies are case series or level 4 evidence. Such studies are noted to have biases (such selection) that limit one's ability to make definitive statements. Although the current evidence may be limited, there have been a large number of patients treated with labral repair showing positive longer-term results. Due to the possibility of poor results of labral debridement and available biomechanical rationale for repair over debridement, randomized controlled trials addressing this topic may be difficult to execute in the future.

12.7 Complications

A recent systematic review by Gupta et al. of 81 studies found the rate for major complications of 0.41 and 4.1 % for minor complications following hip arthroscopy FAI surgery [29]. In addition, they found a revision rate of 4 %. The most common complication was postoperative neuropraxia followed by the development of heterotopic ossification. The most common major complication was abdominal fluid extravasation; however, this was only seen in 5 % of patients. Although on specific to labral repair or debridement, labral tissue injury was often managed concurrently with FAI.

In an internal review of the senior author's patient series, the most common complication after labral surgery has been postoperative tendonitis of the hip flexor. This will typically start to cause anterior groin pain with hip flexion approximately 6 weeks after surgery. Two interventions have been made to decrease the frequency of this complication. First, the position of the senior author's anterior portal was changed to move further away from the mid substance of hip flexor musculature. The mid-anterior portal allows excellent visualization and is further lateral than the anterior portal and thus further from the hip flexors. Since the use of this portal, a dramatic decrease in hip flexor tendonitis has been seen. Secondly, multiple adjustments to the postoperative rehabilitation with respect to the hip flexors have been made. By limiting active flexion for the first 2–3 weeks, patients have noted less subjective pinching in the anterior groin postoperatively.

Capsulolabral adhesions are also a common complication seen in hip arthroscopy patients. By changing the rehabilitation protocol, Willimon et al. noted a significant decrease in the presence of capsulolabral adhesions [30]. Adhesions reduce hip motion, creating a vicious cycle of reduced motion, pain, deconditioning of the hip musculature, and further reductions of motion. The use of circumduction exercises postoperatively has limited the occurrence of postoperative adhesions [30]. Patients who did not receive circumduction therapy were 4.1 times more likely to have adhesions compared to those who performed circumduction exercises [95 % CI: 1.25–11.0]. This exercise is now a standard in senior author's hip rehabilitation program. Finally, anecdotal use of the addition of platelet-rich plasma by the senior author may also be beneficial with respect to limiting the formation of adhesions. The hemostatic properties of this PRP injection, directly at the site of the head and neck resection, may reduce the formation of adhesions following hip arthroscopy; however, further prospectively designed trials are needed to evaluate the full efficacy of this additional intervention in preventing adhesions.

There have been other complications pertaining to hip arthroscopy described in the literature. These include perineal numbness, transient neurological symptoms, both motor and sensory, impotence, and bruising of the genitalia. Proper attention to detail during the setup of the operative theater is very important to avoid these complications. Close attention to the amount of traction time, with frequent release of traction during arthroscopy, is very effective in reducing these complications.

Conclusions

Treatment of labral tears is commonly dictated by the type of tear and the quality of labral tissue. Several studies have shown that labral repair results in superior results as compared to labral debridement. In addition, several biomechanical studies have shown the importance of reestablishing the labral seal for fluid mechanics and hip stability.

Take-Home Points

1. The labrum plays a critical role in the suction seal of hip.
2. Reestablishment of the labral seal is critical to the health of the hip, maintaining the proper environment for cartilage health and stability of the hip.
3. Labral debridement removes critical tissue and may lead to a deficient labrum in cases of small labral or extensive debridements.
4. Labral repair has shown superior results compared to labral debridement in several studies.
5. Midterm data has shown that labral repair can provide years of relief of patient's symptoms.

Key Evidence Related Sources

1. Ayeni OR, Adamich J, Farrokhyar F, Simunovic N, Crouch S, Philippon MJ, Bhandari M. Surgical management of labral tears during femoroacetabular impingement surgery: a systematic review. Knee Surg Sports Traumatol Arthrosc. 2014;22:756–62. (Level 3)
2. Krych AJ, Thompson M, Knutson Z, Scoon J, Coleman SH. Arthroscopic labral repair versus selective labral debridement in female patients with femoroacetabular impingement: a prospective randomized study. Arthroscopy. 2013;29:46–53. (Level 1)
3. Philippon MJ, Stubbs AJ, Schenker ML, Maxwell RB, Ganz R, Leunig M. Arthroscopic management of femoroacetabular impingement: Osteoplasty technique and literature review. Am J Sports Med. 2007;35:1571–80. (Level V)
4. Philippon MJ, Briggs KK, Yen YM, Kuppersmith DA. Outcomes following hip arthroscopy for femoroacetabular impingement with associated chondrolabral dysfunction: minimum 2 year follow-up. J Bone Joint Surg Br. 2009;91:16–23. (Level 4)
5. Tibor LM, Leunig M. Labral Resection or Preservation During FAI Treatment? A Systematic Review. HSS J. 2012;8: 225–9. (Level 3)

References

1. Beck M, Kalhor M, Leunig M, Ganz R. Hip morphology influences the pattern of damage to the acetabular cartilage: femoroacetabular impingement as a cause of early osteoarthritis of the hip. J Bone Joint Surg Br. 2005;87:1012–8.
2. Philippon hilippon MJ, Maxwell RB, Johnston TL, Schenker M, Briggs KK. Clinical presentation of femoroacetabular impingement. Knee Surg Sports Traumatol Arthrosc. 2007;15:1041–7.
3. Philippon MJ, Stubbs AJ, Schenker ML, Maxwell RB, Ganz R, Leunig M. Arthroscopic management of femoroacetabular impingement: osteoplasty technique and literature review. Am J Sports Med. 2007;35:1571–80.
4. Philippon MJ, Schroder eSouza BG, Briggs KK. Labrum: resection, repair and reconstruction sports medicine and arthroscopy review. Sports Med Arthrosc. 2010;18:76–82.
5. Tannast M, Goricki D, Beck M, Murphy SB, Siebenrock KA. Hip damage occurs at the zone of femoroacetabular impingement. Clin Orthop Relat Res. 2008;466:273–80.
6. Ferguson SJ, Bryant JT, Ganz R, Ito K. The acetabular labrum seal: a poroelastic finite element model. Clin Biomech. 2000;15:463–8.
7. Ferguson SJ, Bryant JT, Ganz R, Ito K. An in vitro investigation of the acetabular labral seal in hip joint mechanics. J Biomech. 2003;36:171–8.
8. Ferguson SJ, Bryant JT, Ganz R, Ito K. The influence of the acetabular labrum on hip joint cartilage consolidation: a poroelastic finite element model. J Biomech. 2000;33:953–60.
9. Philippon MJ, Nepple JJ, Campbell KJ, Dornan GJ, Jansson KS, LaPrade RF, Wijdicks CA. The hip fluid seal–part I: the effect of an acetabular labral tear, repair, resection, and reconstruction on hip fluid pressurization. Knee Surg Sports Traumatol Arthrosc. 2014;22:722–9.
10. Nepple JJ, Philippon MJ, Campbell KJ, Dornan GJ, Jansson KS, LaPrade RF, Wijdicks CA. The hip fluid seal–part II: the effect of an acetabular labral tear, repair, resection, and reconstruction on hip stability to distraction. Knee Surg Sports Traumatol Arthrosc. 2014;22:730–6.
11. Crawford MJ, Dy CJ, Alexander JW, Thompson M, Schroder SJ, Vega CE, Patel RV, Miller AR, McCarthy JC, Lowe WR, Noble PC. The 2007 Frank Stinchfield Award. The biomechanics of the hip labrum and the stability of the hip. Clin Orthop Relat Res. 2007;465:16–22.
12. Abrams GD, Safran MR, Sadri H. Spontaneous hip labrum regrowth after initial surgical debridement. Clin Orthop Relat Res. 2013;471(8):2504–8. doi:10.1007/s11999-013-2914-x.
13. Abrams GD, Frank RM, Gupta AK, Harris JD, McCormick FM, Cole BJ. Trends in meniscus repair and meniscectomy in the United States, 2005–2011. Am J Sports Med. 2013;41:2333–9.
14. Miozzari HH, Celia M, Clark JM, Werlen S, Naal FD, Nötzli HP. No regeneration of the human acetabular labrum after excision to bone. Clin Orthop Relat Res. 2014;473(4):1349–57.
15. Tibor LM, Leunig M. Labral resection or preservation during FAI treatment? A systematic review. HSS J. 2012;8:225–9.
16. Espinosa N, Beck M, Rothenfluh DA, Ganz R, Leunig M. Treatment of femoro-acetabular impingement: preliminary results of labral refixation. Surgical technique. J Bone Joint Surg Am. 2007;89(Suppl 2 Pt 1):36–53.
17. Skendzel JG, Philippon MJ. Management of labral tears of the hip in young patients. Orthop Clin North Am. 2013;44:477–87.
18. Philippon MJ, Arnoczky SP, Torrie A. Arthroscopic repair of the acetabular labrum: a histologic assessment of healing in an ovine model. Arthroscopy. 2007;23:376–80.

19. Philippon MJ, Schenker ML, Briggs KK, Kuppersmith DA, Maxwell RB, Stubbs AJ. Revision hip arthroscopy. Am J Sports Med. 2007;35:1918–21.
20. Philippon MJ, Wolff AB, Briggs KK, Zehms CT, Kuppersmith DA. Acetabular rim reduction for the treatment of femoroacetabular impingement correlates with preoperative and postoperative center-edge angle. Arthroscopy. 2010;26:757–61.
21. Lertwanich P, Ejnisman L, Torry MR, Giphart JE, Philippon MJ. Defining a safety margin for labral suture anchor insertion using the acetabular rim angle. Am J Sports Med. 2011;39(Suppl):111S–6.
22. Wahoff M, Ryan M. Rehabilitation after hip femoroacetabular impingement arthroscopy. Clin Sports Med. 2011;30:463–82.
23. Ayeni OR, Adamich J, Farrokhyar F, Simunovic N, Crouch S, Philippon MJ, Bhandari M. Surgical management of labral tears during femoroacetabular impingement surgery: a systematic review. Knee Surg Sports Traumatol Arthrosc. 2014;22:756–62.
24. Krych AJ, Thompson M, Knutson Z, Scoon J, Coleman SH. Arthroscopic labral repair versus selective labral debridement in female patients with femoroacetabular impingement: a prospective randomized study. Arthroscopy. 2013;29:46–53.
25. Larson CM, Giveans MR. Arthroscopic debridement versus refixation of the acetabular labrum associated with femoroacetabular impingement. Arthroscopy. 2009;25:369–76.
26. Larson CM, Giveans MR, Stone RM. Arthroscopic debridement versus refixation of the acetabular labrum associated with femoroacetabular impingement: mean 3.5-year follow-up. Am J Sports Med. 2012;40:1015–21.
27. Schilders E, Dimitrakopoulou A, Bismil Q, Marchant P, Cooke C. Arthroscopic treatment of labral tears in femoroacetabular impingement: a comparative study of refixation and resection with a minimum two-year follow-up. J Bone Joint Surg Br. 2011;93:1027–32.
28. Philippon MJ, Briggs KK, Yen YM, Kuppersmith DA. Outcomes following hip arthroscopy for femoroacetabular impingement with associated chondrolabral dysfunction: minimum two-year follow-up. J Bone Joint Surg Br. 2009;91:16–23.
29. Gupta A, Redmond JM, Hammarstedt JE, Schwindel L, Domb BG. Safety measures in hip arthroscopy and their efficacy in minimizing complications: a systematic review of the evidence. Arthroscopy. 2014;30:1342–8.
30. Willimon SC, Briggs KK, Philippon MJ. Intra-articular adhesions following hip arthroscopy: a risk factor analysis. Knee Surg Sports Traumatol Arthrosc. 2014;22:822–5.

Reconstructive Techniques in FAI Surgery

13

Marc J. Philippon and Karen K. Briggs

Contents

13.1 Introduction

As the understanding of the hip has advanced, more severe disease states are being treated with hip arthroscopy. This includes the deficient labrum, the absent ligamentum teres, and the deficient hip capsule. Techniques have been developed to treat these pathologies arthroscopically; however, since most of these techniques are relatively new, the literature on outcomes is sparse [1–9]. While there is limited evidence, the purpose of this chapter is to describe the techniques and provide supporting information and best available evidence.

M.J. Philippon, MD (✉)
Orthopaedic Surgeon, Steadman Clinic and Steadman Philippon Research Institute, Vail, CO, USA
e-mail: drphilippon@sprivail.org

K.K. Briggs, MPH
Center for Outcomes-based Orthopaedic Research, Steadman Philippon Research Institute, 181 West Meadow Suite 1000, Vail, CO, USA
e-mail: Karen.briggs@sprivail.org

13.2 Labral Reconstruction

Research in the past few years have detailed the detrimental effects of the loss of labral tissue and loss of function [10–15]. The intact labrum deepens the socket which limits femoral head translation [16, 17]. In addition, the labrum provides a fluid seal to maintain the hydrostatic fluid pressure within the joint [18, 19]. This fluid seal protects the cartilage with the diffusion of nutrients to chondrocytes and also reduces cartilage consolidation by helping to distribute forces throughout the joint [9]. Loss of labral function can lead to overloading of the articular cartilage of the hip and may be a precursor of osteoarthritis [11, 15, 17].

Loss of labral tissue can also change the fluid mechanics, the seal between the femoral head and acetabulum (Fig. 13.1), and hip stability. Ferguson and Ganz demonstrated that after labral resection, fluid pressurization in the central compartment was markedly lowered and the cartilage consolidation was greater in the labral deficient

O.R. Ayeni et al. (eds.), *Diagnosis and Management of Femoroacetabular Impingement*,
DOI 10.1007/978-3-319-32000-7_13

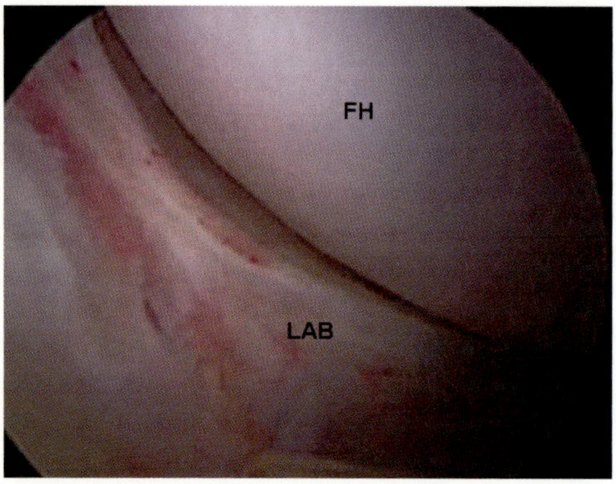

Fig. 13.1 View of deficient labrum (*LAB*) which does not maintain the seal with the femoral head (*FH*)

group than the intact group [20]. In a study by Philippon et al., labral partial resection had a 47 % decrease in intra-articular fluid pressurization, and a complete resection had 76 % decrease in intra-articular pressurization [13]. When a labral reconstruction was performed, the pressurization increased by 110 % compared with the intact state. The pressurization was significantly improved in the reconstruction compared to the partial resection group. In a follow-up study by Nepple et al., the resistance of the hip fluid seal to distraction was 29 % in a hip after partial resection and 27 % for complete labral resection [12]. When a labral reconstruction was performed, the resistance improved by 37 % compared to a partial labral resection.

Loss of labral tissue may also result in microinstability, which is a state of subtle instability of hip that may cause pain. Meyers et al. studied hip stability and the role of the labrum and the iliofemoral ligament [21]. That study reported that when the labrum was resected, there was increased anterior translation compared with the intact state. Benali et al. reported a case study where gross instability resulting in hip subluxation occurred after debridement of the acetabular labrum [22]. When the labrum is deficient, the amount of strain on the remaining labrum also puts the hip at risk for instability [14]. Smith et al. have also demonstrated that labral strain increases as the circumferential tear is enlarged, and with removal of 2 cm or more of the labrum, hip stability decreases [14]. Greaves et al. measured articular cartilage strain in cadaveric hips under a compressive load using 7 T MRI [23]. They found no significant effect of a labral tear compared with the intact state, but did find a 4–6 % decrease in cartilage strain associated with labral repair compared to labral resection [11]. These studies provide some evidence that a deficient labrum may initiate the process of degeneration in the hip joint.

Labral deficiency is most commonly seen in the case of revision hip arthroscopy following prior labral debridement. In addition, adhesions, or arthrofibrosis, can result in an entrapped labrum. Arthrofibrosis can frequently form after injury or as a sequela of hip surgery [24, 25]. Adhesions in the hip are commonly found at the site of the femoral neck osteoplasty and between the labrum and capsule. Occasionally, the hip capsule can adhere to the labrum effectively elevating the labrum and disrupting the contact between the labrum and femoral heal. This results in an area of deficiency in the biomechanical function of the labrum. Despite careful separation of these adhesions, the remaining tissue is either of insufficient volume or has poor quality, thereby creating a labral deficiency [24]. In cases of primary hip arthroscopy, the labrum can be torn in a complex manner, which cannot be repaired, and if the tissue was debrided, the labrum would not function adequately without labral reconstruction.

The goals of reconstruction are to reestablish the acetabular seal by replacing areas of deficient labrum to improve the fluid mechanics in the central compartment and reduce shear forces on the acetabular cartilage. Labral reconstruction is indicated when there is either a deficient labrum or a complex tear that completely disrupts the longitudinal fibers and cannot be repaired. The decision to reconstruct the labrum is often made at the time of arthroscopic examination.

13.2.1 Arthroscopic Technique

Patients are placed in the supine position and traction is placed with the operative hip. Standard arthroscopic portals are established as has been described in a previous chapter.

A diagnostic arthroscopy is performed and an interportal capsulotomy is routinely performed. The labrum is examined to determine if a labral reconstruction is necessary. The quality and stability of the remaining labral tissue are examined. A dynamic examination is performed to assess the suction seal between the injured labrum and the femoral head. The damaged section of the labrum is identified and removed with shavers, leaving healthy tissue at each end. The healthy labral tissue is needed at each end in order to attach the labral graft to the native labrum. After removal of the labral tissue, rim trimming and treatment of the articular cartilage during labral reconstruction are facilitated for improved visualization.

The autograft tissue currently used is the iliotibial band (ITB). The traction is released, and the graft is harvested with the leg in extension through a longitudinal incision centered over the greater trochanter, just distal to the anterolateral portal. At the junction of the anterior 2/3 and posterior 1/3 of the ITB, a rectangular piece of tissue 15–20 mm wide and 30–40 % longer than the measured defect is used. The ITB defect is not closed if there is no significant herniation of muscle or if excessive tension in the ITB occurs with attempted closure. The graft is cleaned of any soft tissue. At each end, #2 Vicryl sutures are placed and tied with locking knots. The graft is tubularized with 2-0 Vicryl. The thicker end of the graft gets a loop suture which will facilitate intra-articular maneuverability.

For placement of the graft, a suture anchor is placed at the most anterior aspect of the defect. One limb of the suture is passed through the graft extracorporeally, and the knot is pushed to introduce the graft to the joint via the mid-anterior portal through a 5.5 mm cannula (Fig. 13.2). The second suture limb is used for a side to side anastomosis with the healthy tissue at each end of the defect. A suture anchor is then placed at the posterior aspect of the defect and the graft is secured. Suture anchors are then placed along the graft to ensure stability of the graft (Fig. 13.3a). Combinations of two types of suture anchors are used to restore the seal. The loop suture, which goes around the graft tissue, tends to evert the labrum (Fig. 13.3b). The pierced suture, which goes through the graft tissue, tends to invert the labrum tissue (Fig. 13.3c). Using a combination of these sutures to manage the position of the graft results in better restoration of the suction seal. Sutures are placed until the autograft is stable. If the graft is unstable at certain positions, then additional sutures are added. Traction is released and a dynamic exam is performed to ensure the suction seal has been restored. The dynamic examination should include moving the hip through full range of motion to ensure adequate seal (Fig. 13.4). If the graft appears unstable, additional suture anchors can be placed. In addition, any CAM or pincer impingement that may further damage the new graft can be identified and resected during the hip arthroscopy examination. If necessary, further burring of the femoral neck can be performed at this time. The graft should resemble the native labrum and should recreate the suction seal of the hip joint. A flexible radiofrequency device can now be used to make the graft and the native labrum smooth by removing frayed edges to ensure good visualization.

Postoperative rehabilitation protocols are the same for labral repair and labral reconstruction. Patients ride a stationary bike with no resistance

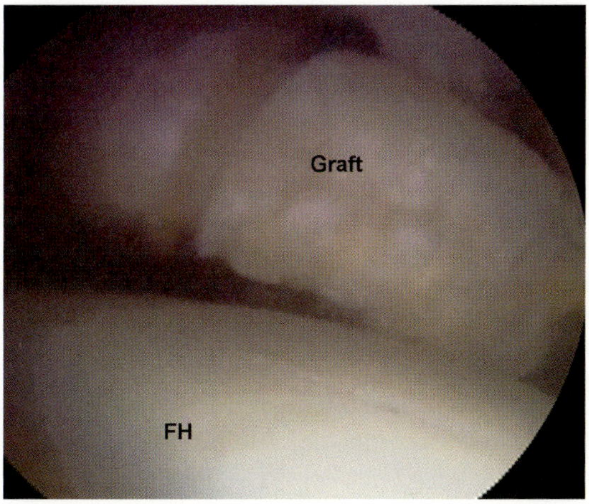

Fig. 13.2 Graft entering the joint through a large cannula with a suture pulling the graft toward the anterior aspect of the defect (*FH* femoral head)

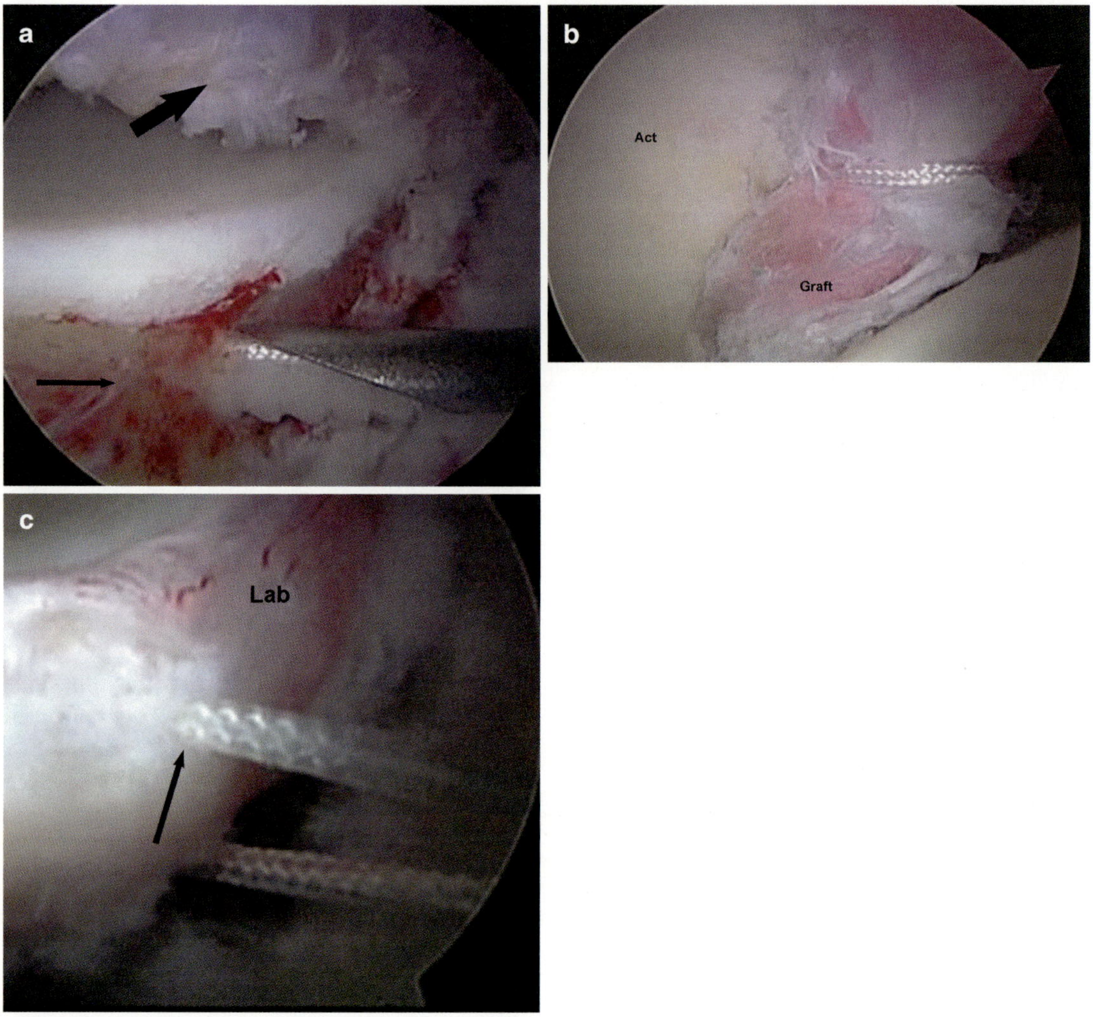

Fig. 13.3 (**a**) Suture anchors placed along the acetabular rim (*small arrow*) to stabilize the graft (*large arrow*). (**b**) Loop suture goes around the graft and tends to evert the labral graft (*Act* acetabulum). (**c**) Pierced suture (*arrow*) goes through labrum (Lab) and tends to invert the labral graft

within 4 h after surgery and use a continuous passive motion (CPM) machine immediately following surgery until 2–3 weeks postoperatively. They are kept at 9 kg of flat foot weight bearing for 2–3 weeks as well. This time is increased to 8 weeks if a microfracture procedure was performed. Patients are advised to wear an anti-rotational bolster and a hip brace to prevent stress on the repaired capsule. The goal of rehabilitation in the first 2–3 weeks is to prevent adhesions, especially in those patients with prior adhesions, and protect the repair. Early rehabilitation will help the patient regain pain-free motion while protecting the new labral graft. Of note, other graft choices include autograft (gracilis tendon) and allograft (gracilis tendon, tibialis tendon).

13.2.2 Outcomes

Since the description of the labral reconstruction techniques, there have been numerous studies describing the technique and clinical outcomes [1–5, 26–29]. A systematic review by Ayeni et al. reviewed the literature on FAI and labral reconstruction [26]. The review included 5 studies and

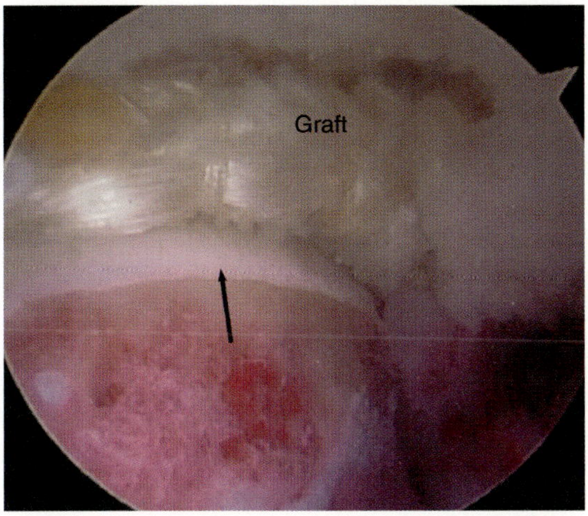

Fig. 13.4 Dynamic exam showing the labral graft reestablishing the seal with the femoral head (*arrow*)

128 patients. The authors documented improvement in outcomes and a conversion rate to total hip arthroplasty of 20 %. This systematic review concluded that labral reconstruction is a new technique that shows short-term improvement in terms of symptoms and function.

A cohort study by Domb et al. compared 11 reconstructions to 22 resections [29]. The reconstruction group was younger and showed greater improvement for all outcome scores. Similar findings were reported in another cohort study comparing 8 reconstructions to 46 labral refixations [2]. The reconstruction group showed greater improvement. However, the reconstruction group was older. In a large case series, Geyer et al. reported significant improvement in average modified Harris Hip score, HOS-ADL, and HOS sport score in 77 patients who underwent labral reconstructions [1]. Conversion to total hip arthroplasty was documented in 23 % of the patients, and these patients were older at time of reconstruction. In addition, limited joint space (2 mm or less) was a predictor of conversion to arthroplasty. At 3 years, 46 % of patients with 2 mm or less joint space survived with no joint replacement. This study emphasized the need for proper patient selection to achieve good results.

Labral reconstruction has also been shown to be effective in returning the elite athlete to the playing field. In a study by Boykin et al., 89 % of top-level athletes returned to play following labral reconstruction [27].

In addition to clinical studies, several biomechanics studies have also shown that labral reconstruction can improve the hip environment. In a study by Lee et al., labral resection decreased contact area, and labral reconstruction partially restored acetabular contact areas and pressures [30].

13.3 Capsular Reconstruction

The hip capsule consists of the iliofemoral ligament, the ilioischial ligament, the pubofemoral ligament, and the zona orbicularis. These ligaments that make up the capsule complex provide a critical component for maintaining stability in the hip. While the hip is considered a relatively stable joint due to the seating of the femoral head in the acetabulum, and vast soft tissue envelope, injuries to the hip capsule may result in hip instability [31]. Although traumatic injuries to the hip, such as dislocation, may be rare, chronic or repetitive injuries occur in activities or sports that require rotation around the hip. In addition, management of capsulotomies during hip arthroscopy have varied, including leaving the capsulotomy open. This has led to cases of deficient capsules that no longer provide the needed stability in certain cases [22]. A study by Bayne et al. demonstrated that following capsulotomy there was increased translation and rotation of the femoral head [32]. Indication for capsular reconstruction includes patient-reported instability, pain, and deficient capsule on radiographic and arthroscopic evaluation [6].

13.3.1 Technique

After other pathologies have been treated, the capsular defect is measured using an arthroscopic ruler. An iliotibial allograft is currently the graft used for reconstruction [6]. A large piece of allograft is folded three times so it is comparable to the thickness of the native hip capsule (Fig. 13.5). The graft is sized for the capsular deficiency. The

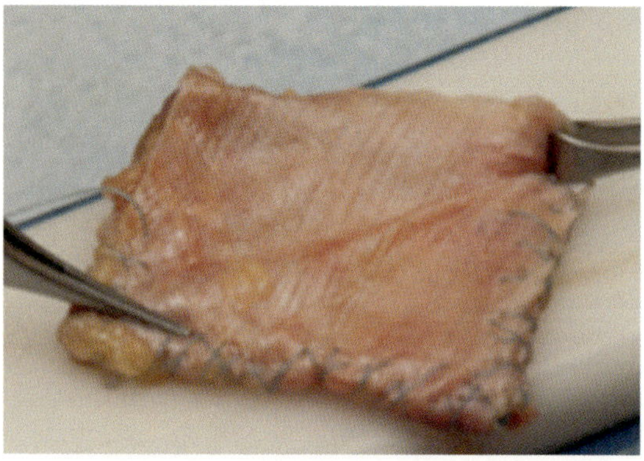

Fig. 13.5 The allograft tissue folded and the edges sutured to approximate the size and thickness of the native capsule

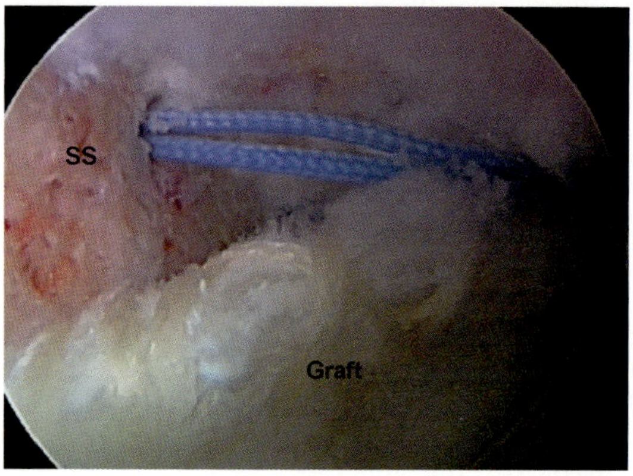

Fig. 13.6 Suture anchors placed on the subspinal region of the acetabulum (SS), with one medial and one more laterally, for attachment of the capsular graft (graft)

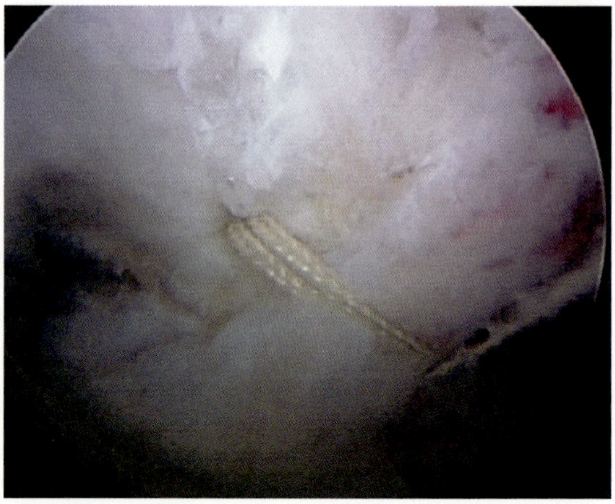

Fig. 13.7 Capsular graft sutured to the native capsule

edges of the rectangular graft are sutured, and on each corner, a loop is made for easier manipulation of the graft in the joint. Two suture anchors are placed in the subspinal region of the acetabulum, based on the location of the capsule deficiency and the normal anatomic insertion of the capsule (Fig. 13.6). The graft is pulled into the joint through a 5.5 mm cannula. After the graft is positioned, it is secured with the suture anchors previously placed (Fig. 13.7). Traction is released and the hip is placed in flexion and internal rotation. The graft is then secured to the native capsule. Postoperatively, the patient is limited to flat foot weight bearing for 21 days and then can wean off crutches at day 22. Continuous passive motion is recommended for 4 weeks, 6–8 h per day. Range of motion setting for the first week is 0 to 60°, 0–70° for the second week, and 0–80° for the fourth week. A brace is worn for 21 days. For the first 2 weeks, abduction is restricted to 0–45° and extension greater than 0 is allowed after 21 days. Hip flexion at 90° is avoided for the first 2 weeks. A key rehabilitation exercise to avoid adhesions is hip circumduction, which is done in 70° of flexion.

13.4 Ligamentum Teres Reconstruction

For many years, the ligamentum teres (LT) was viewed as a vestigial structure in the adult. There has been a growing body of literature that suggests the ligamentum teres plays an important role in hip biomechanics [33–38]. A study by Wenger et al. on porcine models demonstrated LT possesses tensile strength similar to ACL [38]. Recently in a cadaveric study by Kivlan et al., it was shown that the LT formed a "sling-like" structure to support the femoral head inferiorly as the hip joint was moved into squat position [34]. The LT appeared to prevent anterior/inferior subluxation of femoral head. The LT is tightest when the hip is flexed, adducted, and externally rotated [34].

LT reconstruction has been used as an adjunct to open relocation of congenital dislocated hip in children [39]. The LT was sacrificed for the open relocation and this led to a propensity for early re-dislocation. Wenger, et al., concluded that the LT provided additional stability [39]. With the increase of hip arthroscopy, it has noted that ligamentum teres ruptures are often associated with hip instability during activities.

In a systematic review by de Sa et al., nine studies were identified to determine treatment options and indications for arthroscopy for ligamentum teres injury [40]. The analysis showed that there is limited evidence showing debridement with the addition of capsular plication is superior to LT debridement or reconstruction without capsular plication. This study concluded that in patients who fail conservative management with partial tears, debridement is indicated. In patients with complete tears, where debridement failed or was not achievable, then LT reconstruction is indicated.

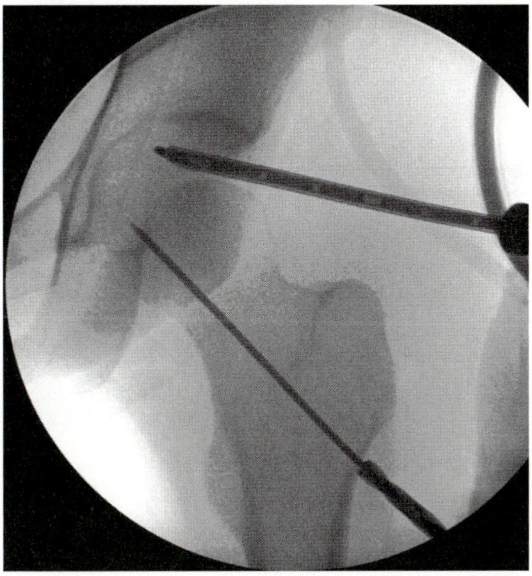

Fig. 13.8 Fluoroscopy view of a guidewire in the femoral neck exiting the fovea capitis

13.4.1 Technique

Following diagnostic arthroscopy and treatment of other intra-articular pathologies, the ligamentum teres is visualized and the graft is harvested. A graft measuring approximately 50 mm by 15 mm is taken from the middle third of the iliotibial band. The graft is tubularized similar to the labral reconstruction graft. In a retrograde fashion, a guidewire is passed through the femoral neck exiting the fovea capitis under fluoroscopy guidance (Fig. 13.8). Using an 8 mm reamer over the guidewire, a femoral tunnel is created. A suture anchor is placed at the footprint of the ligamentum teres on the cotyloid fossa (Fig. 13.9). The suture limbs are passed through the end of the graft, and the graft is then placed in the joint through a large 5.5 mm cannula. The graft is secured to the cotyloid fossa with the sutures and the other end is placed into the femoral tunnel. Approximately 2.5 cm of the graft is left in the joint with the hip in extension and external rotation (Fig. 13.10). The distal portion is secured in the tunnel with an interference screw, and bone graft from the drilling is put into the tunnel [7]. The capsulotomy is closed when the procedure is completed.

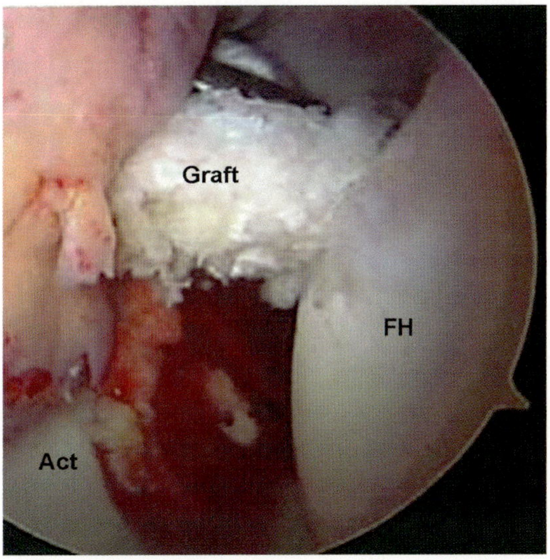

Fig. 13.9 The ligamentum teres graft sutured to the footprint of the native ligamentum teres on the cotyloid fossa (*Act* acetabulum, *FH* femoral head)

13.4.2 Outcomes

The reported outcomes following LT reconstruction have been limited to small case reports or series [7–9]. One case described a female dancer, and Simpson et al. reported the patient

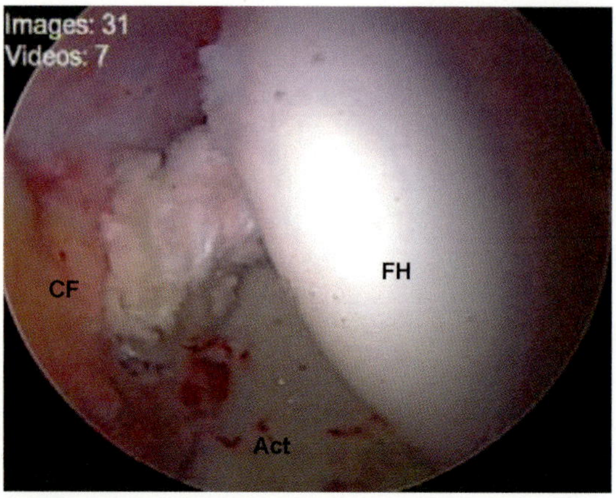

Fig. 13.10 The graft in the joint following attachment. Approximately 2.5 cm is left in the joint (*FH* femoral head, *Act* acetabulum, *CF* cotyloid fossa)

had improved at 8 months following reconstruction [8]. In a case report by Amenabar et al., an LT reconstruction was performed on a female patient with a complete tear using a double-stranded semitendinosus graft [9]. The patient showed improvement at 12 months, but at repeat arthroscopy at 15 months, the graft had resorbed. In the largest series, four patients underwent LT reconstruction using an iliotibial graft [7]. In this study by Philippon et al., all patients showed functional improvement at 1 year; however, one patient required a hip replacement by 2 years. More research is needed to identify strict guidelines for patient selection for LT reconstruction.

Take-Home Points

1. Advanced procedures have a longer learning curve than conventional techniques. Educational courses and practice on cadavers are important for good technique.
2. Adequate joint space (greater than 2 mm on x ray) is important for any advanced procedure.
3. Patients need to be educated that return to full activity may take longer for these more advanced procedures. While some procedures allow the patient to return to full activity at 3–6 months, return to activity in these advanced procedures may take 6–12 months, depending on the individual patient.
4. Outcomes have shown that patients who undergo labral reconstruction can expect reduction of symptoms and return to sporting activities at the same level as before their injury. In a study of professional athletes, 81 % returned to their previous level of competition [19].
5. Only early outcomes are available for LT and capsular reconstruction. While early results are promising, long-term outcomes are not known.

Key Evidence Related Sources

1. Ayeni OR, Alradwan H, de Sa D, Philippon MJ. The hip labrum reconstruction: indications and outcomes – a systematic review. Knee Surg Sports Traumatol Arthrosc. 2014;22(4):737–43.
2. Geyer MR, Philippon MJ, Fagrelius TS, Briggs KK. Acetabular labral reconstruction with an iliotibial band autograft: outcome and survivorship analysis at minimum 3-year follow-up. Am J Sports Med. 2013;41(8):1750–6.
3. Trindade CA, Sawyer GA, Fukui K, Briggs KK, Philippon MJ. Arthroscopic capsule reconstruction in the hip using iliotibial band allograft. Arthrosc Tech. 2015;4(1):e71–4.
4. de Sa D, Phillips M, Philippon MJ, Letkemann S, Simunovic N, Ayeni OR. Ligamentum teres injuries of the hip: a systematic review examining surgical indications, treatment options, and outcomes. Arthroscopy. 2014;30(12):1634–41.
5. Philippon MJ, Pennock A, Gaskill TR. Arthroscopic reconstruction of the ligamentum teres: technique and early outcomes. J Bone Joint Surg Br. 2012;94(11):1494–8.

References

1. Geyer MR, Philippon MJ, Fagrelius TS, Briggs KK. Acetabular labral reconstruction with an iliotibial band autograft: outcome and survivorship analysis at minimum 3-year follow-up. Am J Sports Med. 2013;41(8):1750–6.
2. Matsuda DK, Burchette RJ. Arthroscopic hip labral reconstruction with a gracilis autograft versus labral refixation: 2-year minimum outcomes. Am J Sports Med. 2013;41(5):980–7.
3. Philippon MJ, Briggs KK, Hay CJ, Kuppersmith DA, Dewing CB, Huang MJ. Arthroscopic labral reconstruction in the hip using iliotibial band autograft: technique and early outcomes. Arthroscopy. 2010;26(6):750–6.
4. Sierra RJ, Trousdale RT. Labral reconstruction using the ligamentum teres capitis: report of a new technique. Clin Orthop Relat Res. 2009;467(3):753–9.
5. Walker JA, Pagnotto M, Trousdale RT, Sierra RJ. Preliminary pain and function after labral reconstruction during femoroacetabular impingement surgery. Clin Orthop Relat Res. 2012;470(12):3414–20.
6. Trindade CA, Sawyer GA, Fukui K, Briggs KK, Philippon MJ. Arthroscopic capsule reconstruction in the hip using iliotibial band allograft. Arthrosc Tech. 2015;4(1):e71–4.
7. Philippon MJ, Pennock A, Gaskill TR. Arthroscopic reconstruction of the ligamentum teres: technique and early outcomes. J Bone Joint Surg Br. 2012;94(11):1494–8.
8. Simpson JM, Field RE, Villar RN. Arthroscopic reconstruction of the ligamentum teres. Arthroscopy. 2011;27(3):436–41.
9. Amenabar T, O'Donnell J. Arthroscopic ligamentum teres reconstruction using semitendinosus tendon: surgical technique and an unusual outcome. Arthrosc Tech. 2012;1(2):e169–74.
10. Cadet ER, Chan AK, Vorys GC, Gardner T, Yin B. Investigation of the preservation of the fluid seal effect in the repaired, partially resected, and reconstructed acetabular labrum in a cadaveric hip model. Am J Sports Med. 2012;40(10):2218–23.
11. Greaves LL, Gilbart MK, Yung AC, Kozlowski P, Wilson DR. Effect of acetabular labral tears, repair and resection on hip cartilage strain: a 7T MR study. J Biomech. 2010;43(5):858–63.
12. Nepple JJ, Philippon MJ, Campbell KJ, Dornan GJ, Jansson KS, LaPrade RF, Wijdicks CA. The hip fluid seal – part II: the effect of an acetabular labral tear, repair, resection, and reconstruction on hip stability to distraction. Knee Surg Sports Traumatol Arthrosc. 2014;22(4):730–6.
13. Philippon MJ, Nepple JJ, Campbell KJ, Dornan GJ, Jansson KS, LaPrade RF, Wijdicks CA. The hip fluid seal – part I: the effect of an acetabular labral tear, repair, resection, and reconstruction on hip fluid pressurization. Knee Surg Sports Traumatol Arthrosc. 2014;22(4):722–9.
14. Smith MV, Panchal HB, Ruberte Thiele RA, Sekiya JK. Effect of acetabular labrum tears on hip stability and labral strain in a joint compression model. Am J Sports Med. 2010;39(Suppl):103S–10.
15. Song Y, Ito H, Kourtis L, Safran MR, Carter DR, Giori NJ. Articular cartilage friction increases in hip joints after the removal of acetabular labrum. J Biomech. 2012;45(3):524–30.
16. Ferguson SJ, Bryant JT, Ganz R, Ito K. The acetabular labrum seal: a poroelastic finite element model. Clin Biomech. 2000;15(6):463–8.
17. Tan V, Seldes RM, Katz MA, Freedhand AM, Klimkiewicz JJ, Fitzgerald RH. Contribution of acetabular labrum to articulating surface area and femoral head coverage in adult hip joints: an anatomic study in a cadaver. Am J Sports Med. 2001;30(11):809–12.
18. Ferguson SJ, Bryant JT, Ganz R, Ito K. An in vitro investigation of the acetabular labral seal in hip joint mechanics. J Biomech. 2003;36(2):171–8.
19. Dwyer MK, Jones HL, Hogan MG, Field RE, McCarthy JC, Noble PC. The acetabular labrum regulates fluid circulation of the hip joint during functional activities. Am J Sports Med. 2014;42(4):812–9.
20. Ferguson SJ, Bryant JT, Ganz R, Ito K. The influence of the acetabular labrum on hip joint cartilage consolidation: a poroelastic finite element model. J Biomech. 2000;33:953–60.
21. Myers CA, Register BC, Lertwanich P, Ejnisman L, Pennington WW, Giphart JE, LaPrade RF, Philippon MJ. Role of the acetabular labrum and the iliofemoral ligament in hip stability: an in vitro biplane fluoroscopy study. Am J Sports Med. 2011;39(Suppl):85S–91.
22. Benali Y, Katthagen BD. Hip subluxation as a complication of arthroscopic debridement. Arthroscopy. 2009;25(4):405–7.
23. Greaves LL, Gilbart MK, Yung A, Kozlowski P, Wilson DR. Deformation and recovery of cartilage in the intact hip under physiological loads using 7T MRI. J Biomech. 2009;42(3):349–54.
24. Philippon MJ, Schenker ML, Briggs KK, Kuppersmith DA, Maxwell RB, Stubbs AJ. Revision hip arthroscopy. Am J Sports Med. 2007;35(11):1918–21.
25. Ward JP, Rogers P, Youm T. Failed hip arthroscopy: causes and treatment options. Orthopedics. 2012; 35(7):612–7.
26. Ayeni OR, Alradwan H, de Sa D, Philippon MJ. The hip labrum reconstruction: indications and outcomes – a systematic review. Knee Surg Sports Traumatol Arthrosc. 2014;22(4):737–43.
27. Boykin RE, Patterson D, Briggs KK, Dee A, Philippon MJ. Results of arthroscopic labral reconstruction of the hip in elite athletes. Am J Sports Med. 2013;41(10):2296–301.
28. Costa Rocha P, Klingenstein G, Ganz R, Kelly BT, Leunig M. Circumferential reconstruction of severe acetabular labral damage using hamstring allograft: surgical technique and case series. Hip Int. 2013;23 Suppl 9:S42–53.
29. Domb BG, El Bitar YF, Stake CE, Trenga AP, Jackson TJ, Lindner D. Arthroscopic labral reconstruction is superior to segmental resection for irreparable labral

tears in the hip: a matched-pair controlled study with minimum 2-year follow-up. Am J Sports Med. 2014;42(1):122–30.
30. Lee S, Wuerz TH, Shewman E, McCormick FM, Salata MJ, Philippon MJ, Nho SJ. Labral reconstruction with iliotibial band autografts and semitendinosus allografts improves hip joint contact area and contact pressure: an in vitro analysis. Am J Sports Med. 2015;43(1):98–104.
31. Domb BG, Philippon MJ, Giordano BD. Arthroscopic capsulotomy, capsular repair, and capsular plication of the hip: relation to atraumatic instability. Arthroscopy. 2013;29(1):162–73.
32. Bayne CO, Stanley R, Simon P, Espinoza-Orias A, Salata MJ, Bush-Joseph CA, Inoue N, Nho SJ. Effect of capsulotomy on hip stability-a consideration during hip arthroscopy. Am J Orthop. 2014;43(4):160–5.
33. Bardakos NV, Villar RN. The ligamentum teres of the adult hip. J Bone Joint Surg Br. 2009;91(1):8–15.
34. Kivlan BR, Richard Clemente F, Martin RL, Martin HD. Function of the ligamentum teres during multiplanar movement of the hip joint. Knee Surg Sports Traumatol Arthrosc. 2013;21(7):1664–8.
35. Martin HD, Hatem MA, Kivlan BR, Martin RL. Function of the ligamentum teres in limiting hip rotation: a cadaveric study. Arthroscopy. 2014;30(9):1085–91.
36. Martin RL, Kivlan BR, Clemente FR. A cadaveric model for ligamentum teres function: a pilot study. Knee Surg Sports Traumatol Arthrosc. 2013;21(7):1689–93.
37. Martin RL, Palmer I, Martin HD. Ligamentum teres: a functional description and potential clinical relevance. Knee Surg Sports Traumatol Arthrosc. 2012;20(6):1209–14.
38. Wenger D, Miyanji F, Mahar A, Oka R. The mechanical properties of the ligamentum teres: a pilot study to assess its potential for improving stability in children's hip surgery. J Pediatr Orthop. 2007;27(4):408–10.
39. Wenger DR, Mubarak SJ, Henderson PC, Miyanji F. Ligamentum teres maintenance and transfer as a stabilizer in open reduction for pediatric hip dislocation: surgical technique and early clinical results. J Child Orthop. 2008;2(3):177–85.
40. de Sa D, Phillips M, Philippon MJ, Letkemann S, Simunovic N, Ayeni OR. Ligamentum teres injuries of the hip: a systematic review examining surgical indications, treatment options, and outcomes. Arthroscopy. 2014;30(12):1634–41.

The Evidence for the Treatment of Cartilage Injuries in FAI Surgery

14

A Summary of Techniques and Outcomes of Cartilage Injury Management

Mats Brittberg and Marc Tey

Contents

M. Brittberg (✉)
Cartilage Research Unit, University of Gothenburg, Region Halland Orthopaedics, Kungsbacka Hospital, Kungsbacka S-434 80, Sweden
e-mail: mats.brittberg@telia.com

M. Tey
ICATME, Hospital Universitari Dexeus, C/ Sabino de Arana 19, Barcelona, Spain

14.1 Introduction

Articular hyaline cartilage provides the articular joints with a low friction surface for smooth movements and is difficult to repair when damaged. The poor ability to heal after injury is due to the lack of blood vessels, nerves and the low cell to matrix quota.

Cartilage damage in a hip joint could be seen as three different variants:

- Direct cartilage injury after trauma
- Indirect cartilage damage after a labral injury
- The direct combination of both direct cartilage injury and damage of the labrum

To study cartilage injuries in the hip, one needs to understand more the weight-bearing properties of cartilage on both the femoral head and in the acetabulum and the relation to the labrum and its injury pattern.

The femoral head forms 2/3 of a sphere being covered by a cartilaginous layer except at the ligamentum teres insertion into the fovea at the anteromedial part of the head. Furthermore, the articular cartilage is thickest at the anterolateral (AL) part of the femoral head [39]. It is possible to visualize 80 % of the femoral head cartilage using a 70°arthroscope [13, 14].

The acetabulum with its lunate surface, mostly described by surgeons as a horseshoe-shaped structure, encircles the acetabulum fossa and is

O.R. Ayeni et al. (eds.), *Diagnosis and Management of Femoroacetabular Impingement*,
DOI 10.1007/978-3-319-32000-7_14

divided into superior and posterior parts as well as anterior and posterior parts. In the acetabulum the thickest cartilage is found in the anterosuperior quadrant [39].

Today with an arthroscopy including the central compartment plus peripheral and pertrochanteric compartments, the surgeons can evaluate more than 90 % of the hip joint. It is only the most posteromedial regions that are difficult to reach.

The hip labrum consists of dense fibrocartilaginous tissue that is mainly of type 1 collagen. The labrum is about 2–3 mm thick and outlines the acetabular socket attaching to the bony rim of the acetabulum. Most of the labrum is avascular with only the peripheral third being supplied by the arteries. The superior and inferior portions are innervated [30]. The labrum is like the meniscus a shock absorber and contributes to the lubrication of the joint as well the distribution of joint pressure. It resists lateral and vertical motion within the acetabulum along with aiding in stability [28, 43].

The acetabular labrum subsequently appears to maintain a low friction milieu, possibly by sealing the joint from fluid exudation. The innervation of the labrum is important in the maintenance of proprioception [30]. Even focal labrectomy may result in increased joint friction and altered proprioception with instability, a condition that may be detrimental to articular cartilage and lead to osteoarthritis [56].

Furthermore, studies on pressure film techniques show that cartilage does not distribute the applied loads evenly. Afoke et al. studying cadaveric hips found a special area of high pressure, present in the three test positions in all of the specimens, in the anterosuperior segment of the joint [1].

One part of the labrum's stability function is the maintenance of a negative intra-articular pressure creating a suction-seal effect between the femoral head and the rim of acetabulum and by such a seal establishing a secondary stability effect. When the labrum is partly damaged, the joint contact pressure is diminished and the cartilage surface may be negatively influenced due to higher loading leading finally to OA [21].

14.2 The Lesions

Injured hip joint cartilage can be caused by trauma (localized lesions) and be caused by a generalized loss of cartilage as seen in osteoarthritis. The lesions can be located on either the femoral head or in the acetabulum. Diseases in the subchondral bone as seen after different types of osteonecrosis may also involve the cartilage surface with a collapse of the surface into the necrotic area.

Lesions on the femoral head are also seen after different degrees of hip instability and dislocations with a mixture of axial loads and shearing forces violating the cartilage surface and underlying subchondral bone. A direct lateral trauma to the trochanter area may also produce cartilage injuries [13, 14].

Lesions seen after shear force application include injuries such as chondral delamination, degrees of cartilage fissuring and chondral flaps. One may also see osteochondral fractures after impaction injuries. As these lesions progress to an advanced-stage degenerative condition, they often lose their defining characteristics.

Most common are the cartilage lesions found on the acetabulum. Such lesions can be found in the anterosuperior weight-bearing zone of the acetabular rim most often associated with femoro-acetabular impingement (FAI).

FAI consists of two types of lesions: either CAM or pincer lesion or coexisting both of the types [4, 26, 49]. A CAM lesion exists when the anterior femoral head/neck junction has an abnormal protrusion causing impingement on the anterior acetabulum. Such a lesion may then cause chondral damage to the anterior acetabulum near the chondro-labral junction. With a pincer deformity impingement occurs because extra bone extends out over the normal rim of the acetabulum. The labrum can be impinged under the prominent rim of the acetabulum and with time becomes damaged. FAI is a common cause of labral injury, and FAI with or without labral injury has been identified as an early cause of hip osteoarthritis [26].

To treat patients with cartilage lesions due to FAI means that not only the cartilage lesions need a treatment but one had also to address the

CAM and Pincer lesions and repair a damaged labrum. Treatment of cartilage lesions in the hip is subsequently mostly a combined treatment.

14.2.1 Frequency

Register et al. [53] found using magnetic resonance images of asymptomatic participants that abnormalities could be seen in 73 % of hips, with labral tears being identified in 69 % of the joints. Khanna et al. [37] found that traumatic injuries of the hip result in substantial intra-articular pathologic findings, including loose bodies, labral tears, joint surface step deformities and osteochondral lesions. They stated that arthroscopy is a powerful tool in identifying these injuries. Plain radiographs and CT scans appear to underestimate the true incidence of loose bodies and step deformities within the joint when compared with hip arthroscopy after a traumatic injury of the hip.

14.3 Diagnosis

14.3.1 Symptoms

Symptoms typical for cartilage injuries elsewhere are also seen in the hip with catching and locking phenomena, localized pain mainly as groin pain. The patients often cup the anterolateral hip with the thumb and forefinger in the shape of a "C," termed the C sign [13, 14].

14.3.2 Imaging

14.3.2.1 Plain X-Rays

Start with plain-standing radiographs for the evaluation of the hip after physical examination. Describe any degree of osteoarthritis using the Tönnis grading [62–64], see Table 14.1).

An anteroposterior (AP) view of the pelvis evaluates the hips for osteoarthritis and other findings including:

- The acetabulum for dysplasia, overhang or degrees of retroversion
- The femoral head for osteonecrosis or remodelling or pistol grip deformity
- The sacroiliac joints for arthritis
- The lower lumbar spine

Because standard AP and lateral views of the hip can miss important abnormalities in patients with FAI, axial Lauenstein view radiography [11, 40], in which the hip is flexed 90° and abducted 20°, should be ordered. An axial Lauenstein view is about comparable to a 45° axial Dunn view [17, 35].

Gdalevitch et al. [25] studied delamination cysts seen on the preoperative anteroposterior and/or frog lateral radiographs of the hip and found that they accurately predicted acetabular cartilage delamination, especially in hips with non-traumatic labrum tears. Such delamination cysts have been previously unrecognized as radiographic signs useful for the preoperative identification of acetabular cartilage delamination in patients with labrum tears. Finding such cysts may help to facilitate the selection of the right type of surgery and also determining prognosis [25].

Furthermore, patients with CAM-type FAI with an alpha angle of 65° or more are associated with an increased risk of cartilage injury but a concomitant increasing acetabular coverage appears to have a protective effect [5]. The alpha angle is measured on axial views between two lines from the centre of the femoral head through the middle of the femoral neck and through a point where the contour of the femoral head-neck junction exceeds the radius of the femoral head

Table 14.1 Tönnis hip OA grading

Grade 0	No signs of OA
Grade 1	Mild OA: Increased sclerosis, minimal joint space narrowing, no or minimal loss of head sphericity
Grade 2	Moderate OA: Small cysts, moderate joint space narrowing, moderate loss of head sphericity
Grade 3	Severe OA: Large cysts, severe joint space narrowing, severe deformity of the head

Tönnis [62]
Tönnis [63]
Tönnis and Heinecke [64]

[48]. An angle exceeding 50° is an indicator of an abnormally shaped femoral head-neck contour [60] increasing the risk for CAM impingement. One may also measure the anterior offset, which has been defined as the difference in radius between the anterior femoral head and the anterior femoral neck on a cross-table axial view of the proximal femur. Tannast et al. [60] have suggested that as a general rule for clinical practice, an anterior offset less than 10 mm is a strong indicator for CAM-type impingement.

14.3.2.2 CT

CT is useful for the detection of bone cysts in the acetabulum and in the femoral neck. In a recent paper by Sahin et al. [55], CT arthrography seemed to have an equal sensitivity and a higher specificity than MR arthrography for the detection of labral pathology. MR arthrography was better, but not statistically significant, in demonstrating acetabular and femoral cartilage pathology [55]. One may also use 3D CT to assess CAM morphology and to assess anteroinferior iliac spine (AIIS) for subspinous impingement.

14.3.2.3 MRI

In a recent study Sutter et al. [59] showed that MR arthrography was superior to conventional MRI for detecting labral tears and acetabular cartilage defects and showed a higher interobserver agreement. For femoral cartilage lesions, both modalities yielded comparable results. The use of specific cartilage protocols like delayed gadolinium-enhanced magnetic resonance imaging of cartilage (dGEMRIC) and T2 mapping is suggested. The limitation of the dGEMRIC technique is the need to do an intra-articular injection followed by letting the patient exercise before the scanning.

14.3.2.4 Arthroscopy

It is possible to use the ICRS classification system to describe hip cartilage lesions. The advantage of such a system in terms of local lesions is the depth description related to the post-operative follow-up of a cartilage repair. The classification could then also be used for MRI evaluation of lesion fill post-surgery [12]. See Table 14.2.

Konan et al. have developed a classification system for the acetabulum: grade 0, normal articular cartilage lesions; grade 1, softening or wave sign; grade 2, cleavage lesion; grade 3, delamination; and grade 4, exposed bone. The site of the lesion is further classed as A, B or C based on whether the lesion is less than one-third of the distance from the acetabular rim to the cotyloid fossa, one-third to two-thirds of the same distance and greater than two-thirds of the distance, respectively [38].

Outerbridge classification is a system originally developed for the evaluation of chondromalacia of the patellae. It has been used by many surgeons to describe cartilage lesions at all different sites. It does not take any consideration of the cartilage depth related to the grading of severity (see Table 14.2). Beck's classification [6, 7, 18] describes more the appearance of the traumatized cartilage tissue and has a similarity to the American Hip Institute's ALAD classification (http://www.americanhipinstitute.org/references/content/acetabular-cartilage-damage-alad-classification). See Table 14.2.

The authors suggest that when describing the lesions the ICRS classification could be used together with either the Beck's or ALAD's classification. An ALAD 3 could be a mixture of an ICRS II and III. An ALAD 4 could be from ICRS II–IV, while a Beck's full-thickness defect is either an ICRS 3 or 4. Furthermore, of interest to use is also the Multicenter Arthroscopy of the Hip Outcomes Research Network (MAHORN) classification that provides a useful system for describing labral and chondral injuries with precise assessment of the types of lesions and its location within the hip joint [54] See Table 14.2.

14.3.3 Outcome Scores

Thorborg et al. [61] have recently done a review on patient-reported outcome (PRO) scores for patients with hip and groin pain. They suggested that HAGOS, HOS, IHOT-12 and IHOT-33 can all be recommended for assessment of young-aged to middle-aged adults with pain related to the hip joint, undergoing non-surgical treatment

Table 14.2 Hip cartilage classifications

Outerbridge classification:	ICRS Classification	Beck's Hip Cartilage Classification:	Acetabular Cartilage Damage—the ALAD classification	MA HORN Classification of Acetabular Rim Articular Cartilage Lesions
Grade 0: Normal cartilage *Grade I*: Cartilage with softening and swelling: *Grade II*: A partial- thickness detect with fissures on the surface that do not reach subchondral bone or exceed 1.5 cm in diameter *Grade III*: Fissuring to the level of subchondral bone in an area with a diameter more than 15 cm *Grade IV*: Exposed subchondral bone	*Grade 0*: Normal cartilage *Grade I*: Lesions are superficial fissures and cracks *Grade II*: Lesions down to less than 50 % cartilage depth *Grade III*: Lesions that extend through >50 % of the cartilage thickness are classified as ICRS 3a–d *Grade IV*: Lesions extending through the subchondral bone	*Articular cartilage* *0. Normal* Macroscopically sound cartilage *1. Softening. Malacia* Roughening of surface, fibrillation *2. Pitting malacia* Roughening. partially thinning and full-thickness defects or deep fissuring to bone 3. Debonding Loss of fixation to the subchondral bone, macroscopically sound cartilage, caipet phenomenon 4. Cleavage Loss of fixation to tie subchondral bone: frayed edges, thinning of cartilage, flap 5. Defect Full-thickness defect	ALADO: Normal cartilage ALAD 1: Softening of tie adj acent cartilage ALAD2 Early peal of the cartilage (caipet delamination) ALAD 3: Large flap of the cartilage ALAD 4; Loss of cartilage	Softening of cartilage (Focal defect Extensive) -with la bral-chondral separation -without labral-chondral separation Bubble: cartilage detached from bone with an intact periphery -with la bral-chondral separation -without labral-chondral separation Pocket: cartilage detach ed from bone with free/open edge Flap: cartilage detached from bone with more than one edge free Exposed bone/no coverage; MA HORN j M ulticenter Arthroscopic Hip Outcomes Research Network
Outerbridge. J Bone Joint Surg Br. 1961 Nov:43-B:752–7	Brittberg Winalski. J Bans Joint Surf Am. 2003; 85-A Suppl 2:58–69	Back et al. Clin Orthop Relat Res 2004:413: 67–73 Beck et al. J Bona Joint Juts Br. 2005:87(7): 1012–1013 El Bitar et al., J Am Acad Orthop Sag. 2014 Jan: 22(1): 46–56	http://www.amencanhipinstitute.org/references/content/acetabular-cartilage-damage- alad-classification)	Safran MR, Hariri S: Hip Arthroscopy Assessment Toolsand Outcomes OPERATIVE TECHNIQUES IN ORTHOPAEDICS 20(4): 264–277, 2010

or hip arthroscopy [61]. However, in another recent review, Ramisetty and colleagues [52] found that iHOT-33 scored the best of all the PRO tools and was their choice out of the different hip outcome scores recommended for future use in hip preservation surgery.

14.4 Treatment Options

All cartilage lesions can be treated as related to cartilage lesions in other joints. The treatment choices are:

- Refixation of chondral flaps (more unique for the hip, not normally done in other joints)
- Bone marrow stimulation techniques
- Augmented bone marrow stimulation techniques
- Chondrogenic tissue-based implants (auto- and allo-osteochondral grafts)
- Chondrogenic cell-based implants (chondrocyte or mesenchymal stem cells grafts)
- Synthetic implants
- Mini-metal implants

For very large defects with large bone loss, still open surgery remains an important option. However, this chapter is related to patients with FAI meaning that the techniques described in this chapter are mainly the arthroscopic alternatives.

Unfortunately, very little evidence exists to tell which technology would be the best alternative and no RCTs exist so far.

14.4.1 Debridement and/or Refixation of Chondral Flaps

In general, as for other joints, the alternatives to do only debridement of injured cartilage exist. Fontana et al. carried out a controlled retrospective study of 30 patients affected by a post-traumatic hip chondropathy of the third or fourth degree, according to the Outerbridge classification, measuring 2 cm^2 in area or more. Of these patients, 15 underwent arthroscopic autologous chondrocyte implantation, whereas the other 15 underwent arthroscopic debridement. In both groups the mean follow-up was approximately 74 months (range, 72–76 months). The mean size of the defect was 2.6 cm^2. The patients who underwent ACI (group A) improved significantly more compared with the group that underwent debridement alone (group B).

However, in contrary to other joints, several surgeons are trying to preserve a healthy chondral flap by microfracturing of the underlying bone and completing a refixation of the chondral flap with fibrin glue. In the largest study on articular cartilage repair of the hip, Stafford et al. [57] used fibrin glue/adhesive to treat 43 patients with delaminated articular cartilage. The average follow-up was 28 months. The authors reported significant improvement in the modified Harris hip score (MHHS) pain subscale, with an average score of 21.8 preoperatively and an average score of 35.8 post-operatively.

They concluded that this type of articular cartilage repair is appropriate only for small lesions of delaminated cartilage. However, Hariri et al. [31] found that those chondral flaps are more dead than alive with a cell viability of less than 32 % and showing an abnormal biochemistry. The flaps may function as scaffolds but they are pieces of dead tissue.

14.4.2 Bone Marrow Stimulation Techniques, Simple or Augmented

14.4.2.1 Microfracture (MFX) or Deep Nano-Drilling with Curved Power Drills

The indication for using microfracture technique in the hip is lesions with size less than 2 cm^2. The MFX technique is same as for other joints. A debridement is first performed in order to produce a defect with vertical walls and a clean bony bottom. Insertions of the instruments are aided by the use of a slotted cannula. Higher degree angle-tipped awls (i.e. up to 90°) are used. Holes are prepared to 2–4 mm depth and 3–5 mm apart.

Recently, a modification of the microfracture technique has been presented where 1 mm thick needles are used to be drilled deeper down in the subchondral bone. The technique is called nano-drilling or nano-fracture and the depth will be down to 9 mm and otherwise same management as with simple microfracture technique [10]. In defects between 2 and 3 cm or after failed simple bone marrow stimulation, an augmented bone marrow stimulation technique may be used.

14.4.2.2 Reports on Microfracture Technique in Hip Surgeries

Karthikeyan et al. [36] report that 20 patients who underwent arthroscopic surgery for FAI had a localized full-thickness acetabular chondral defect treated by microfracture and then underwent a later second-look hip arthroscopic procedure. The size of the full-thickness defect was measured at the primary arthroscopic procedure. At an average follow-up of 17 months, 19 of the 20 patients had a mean fill of 96 ± 7 % with macroscopically good-quality repair tissue. One patient had only a 25 % fill with poor quality repair tissue. Histologically, the tissue was found to be composed of primarily fibrocartilage with some staining for type II collagen in the region closest to the bone. Philippon et al. [51] studied nine patients that underwent revision hip arthroscopy for a variety of procedures after undergoing microfracture for treatment of a full-thickness chondral defect of the acetabulum at primary arthroscopy. The size of the chondral defect was measured during primary arthroscopy, and the percent fill of the defect and repair grade were noted at revision hip arthroscopy. Eight of the nine patients had 95–100 % coverage of an isolated acetabular chondral lesion or acetabular lesion associated with a femoral head lesion, with grade 1 or 2 appearance of the repair product at an average of 20 months follow-up.

14.4.2.3 Autologous Matrix-Induced Chondrogenesis (AMIC)

The bone marrow stimulation area is covered with a collagen membrane or a hyaluronic acid membrane [23, 42]. Leunig et al. [42] treated six patients with AMIC in the hip between 2009 and 2010. Post-operative Oxford hip scores ranged from 13 to 17, UCLA activity scores ranged from 5 to 10, and MOCART scores ranged from 55 to 75. Also PLGA/polydioxanone membranes have been tested as a possible clinical application [24].

14.4.2.4 Blood Clot Enhancement

The bone marrow stimulation area is filled with a thermo-stabilizing gel acting as an enhancement of the normal blood clot formation attracting the ingrowth of bone marrow cells. [58]. See also section with the description of operative technique.

14.4.2.5 Scaffolds for Enhancement of Bone Marrow Cell Ingrowth

Carbon fibres may be used to improve the strength of the ingrowing repair tissue [16]. Carbon rods can be introduced arthroscopically. The carbon rods are an alternative when the lesions are surrounded by thin cartilage as seen in an early osteoarthritis. No published results exist with the carbon implants regarding hip implantations.

Other synthetic porous scaffolds may be used with similar purpose.

14.4.2.6 Mosaicplasty and Osteochondral Allografts

Mosaicplasty is a technique typically reserved for open surgery of the hip. There are opportunities to use mosaicplasties when there are very large ostochondral defects.

Girard et al. [27] treated 10 patients for femoral cartilage damage by an osteochondral mosaicplasty of the femoral head through a trochanteric flap with surgical dislocation of the hip. At a mean follow-up of 29.2 months, the autograft plugs were well incorporated at the site of osteochondroplasty in the femoral head with intact cartilage over them and smooth interfaces between articulating bony surface. Similarly Meyers [46] has shown the efficacy of allograft use in the hip for large osteochondral defects and osteonecrosis in young patients.

14.4.2.7 Autologous Chondrocyte Implantation

A few case reports exist on autologous chondrocyte implantation with first- and second-generation ACI. Those reports have been on open surgery [2, 47]. Murakibhavi et al. [47] concluded that the short-term results of ACI for osteochondral lesions of the hip suggest that if good early results are obtained, they are observed to continue for at least 5 years. They also found that there is a high failure rate in those with preoperative cyst formation in the hip.

However, hip cartilage lesion treatment with the 3rd-generation ACI with cell scaffolds like MACI or with cell-seeded grafts like Hyalograft can be completed arthroscopically. Mancini and Fontana [45] reviewed 57 consecutive patients that were treated with the MACI ($n=26$) or AMIC ($n=31$) technique. Patients were assessed preoperatively and up to 5 years using the MHHS to compare outcomes. The modified Harris hip score continued to improve up to 3 years postoperatively and remained stable over time until the final 5-year follow-up. Statistically significant differences between the groups were not observed. The authors suggest that both arthroscopic MACI and AMIC are relevant procedures to repair medium-sized chondral defects on the acetabular side of the hip found during treatment of femoro-acetabular impingement. Being a one-stage procedure and less expensive, AMIC seemed to be a preferable technique compared to ACI. However, the study was not randomized and the lesions were medium sized.

The 4th-Generation ACI s are one-stage procedures that we will see more of in the future. One such technique is the CAIS (cartilage autograft implantation system) where autologous fragments of cartilage are placed in fibrin glue and spread out on a resorbable membrane [15]. This membrane may be implanted arthroscopically into the hip joint. The CAIS technology may also be used similarly with allograft fragments [19]. Another 4th-generation ACI is when chondrocytes are isolated during the surgery in the OR and then mixed with a stem cell mixture aspirated from the iliac crest. The two cell types are seeded together on a restorable membrane for a final arthroscopic implantation [8].

14.4.2.8 Synthetic Implants

Field et al. [22] have described the grafting of chondral defects and subchondral cysts of the acetabular socket using a synthetic osteochondral plug. Computed tomography and MRI at 6 months confirmed the stability of the osteochondral plugs and on-going healing. Vundelinckx et al. [65] reported a short-term 6-month follow-up of synthetic plug implantation of caput femoris osteochondral lesions. The HOOS score improved and the patient was satisfied after those short months. No long-term results have been published.

14.4.2.9 Mini-Metal Implants

HemiCAP (Contoured Articular Prosthetic) hip resurfacing system has been used in young patients with osteochondral lesions of the caput femoris. However, no long-term results are available [34, 41].

14.5 Example of an Emerging Arthroscopic Cartilage Repair Technique

Here we describe an example of a cartilage repair method for the hip where the technique could be used for several of above-mentioned methods. We have used BST-CarGel to illustrate the possibilities for local repair of hip cartilage defects. It is a soluble polymer scaffold containing the polysaccharide chitosan, which is dispersed throughout uncoagulated whole blood in the OR and then delivered to a surgically prepared cartilage lesion.

The gel allows normal clot formation, reinforces the clot, impedes retraction, increases adhesivity and ensures prolonged residency of both the clot and critical tissue repair factors [58]. The soluble and physiological characteristics of this chitosan polymer solution permit its combination with freshly drawn autologous whole blood to form a hybrid polymer-blood mixture. This mixture can be applied to cartilage and bone surfaces of prepared lesions, regardless of its geometry and size, to which it adheres and solidifies as a polymer-stabilized hybrid clot [32].

14.5.1 One-Stage Implantation of a Bone Marrow Augmentation Gel

Hip arthroscopic surgery is performed with the patient placed in supine position on a traction table. Hip joint is distracted and standard anterolateral portal is used as viewing portal. Distal mid-anterior (DMA) and distal lateral (DL) portals are used as working portals (Fig. 14.1). An image intensifier is used to evaluate distraction and to guide accurate portal placement. Prepositioning of the anterolateral portal is performed with a 15 cm, 18G arthroscopic needle. DMA and DL portals are created under arthroscopic view control, and the integrity of the articular cartilage is then further assessed using a probe (Fig. 14.2). The irrigation pressure is set at 40–60 mmHg with the use of an arthroscopy pump.

Chondral debridement of delaminated cartilage is performed around the area of labral detachment using curettes and motorized shavers, in order to completely remove damaged cartilage and to obtain well defined, stable margins between the healthy cartilage and the cartilage defect (Fig. 14.3). If there is an associated labral detachment (usually found in CAM type of FAI cases), curettes can be inserted below the labrum in order to properly debride the most peripheral lesion. Healthy and stable margins of the defect must be obtained. The eventual parts of remaining calcified layer are then carefully removed in order to expose the subchondral bone while preserving its integrity (Fig. 14.4). In order to achieve a complete resection without damaging the subchondral bone, mechanical debridement is recommended, avoiding use of motorized bone burs. The exposed area is then microfractured with 60–90° hip arthroscopic awls as per the standard procedure, penetrating the subchondral bone approximately 4–9 mm depth and every 3–4 mm until covering the entire surface (Fig. 14.5). Observing bone marrow bleeding and/or fat droplets from the microfractured holes after reduction of the irrigation pressure can assess adequate penetration of the subchondral bone.

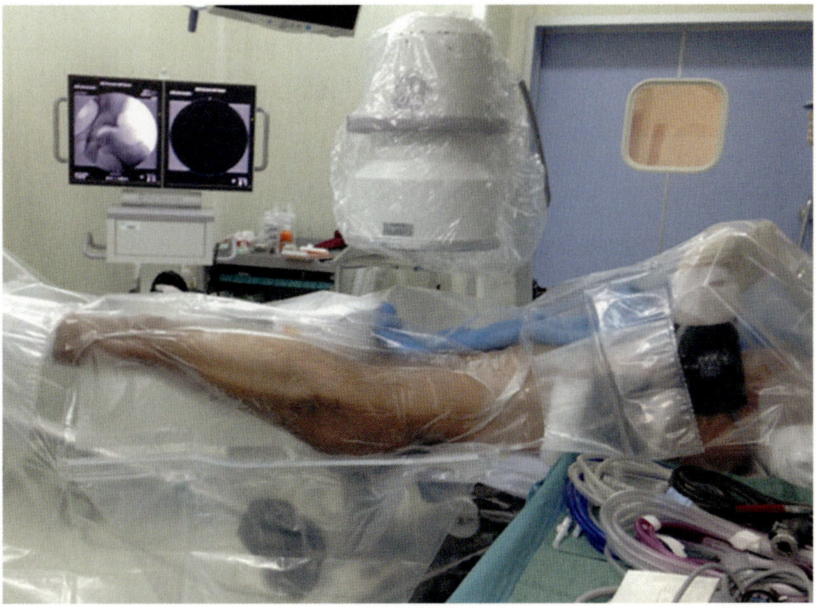

Fig. 14.1 Supine position in a traction table. Greater trochanter and anterosuperior iliac spine are the landmarks for portal placement; transparent draping allows proper identification

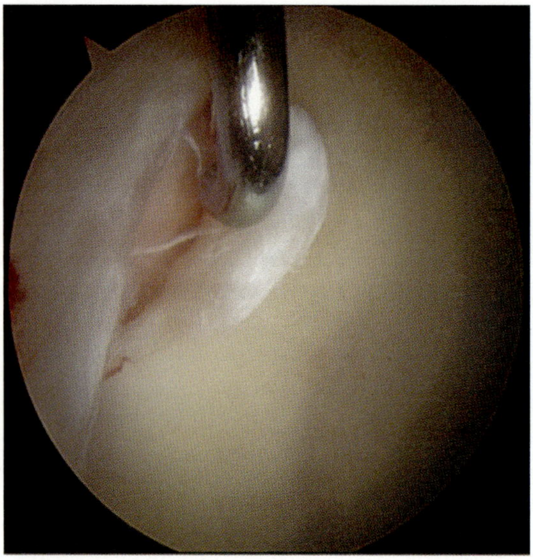

Fig. 14.2 Chondral delamination associated to CAM-type FAI identification. It is grade IV of the ICRS classification

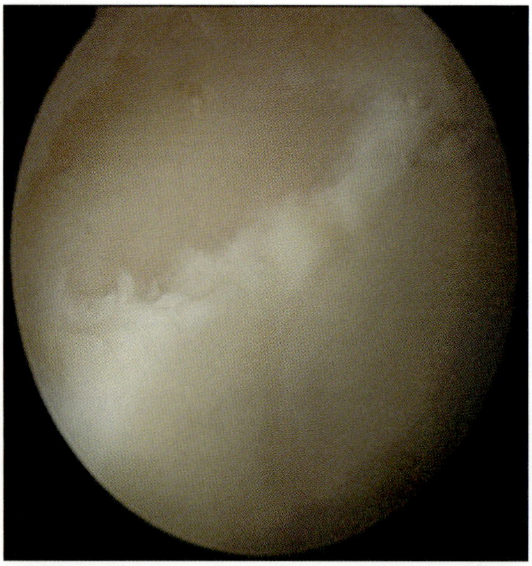

Fig. 14.3 Debridement of damaged cartilage with currettes until stable and healthy

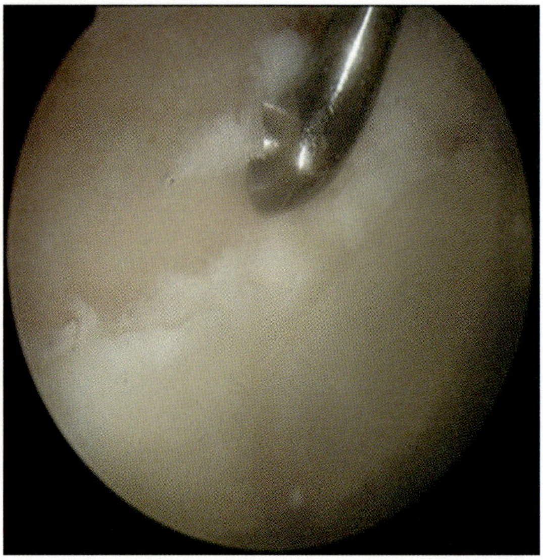

Fig. 14.4 It is important to ensure that the calcified layer is properly debrided without violation of subchondral bone

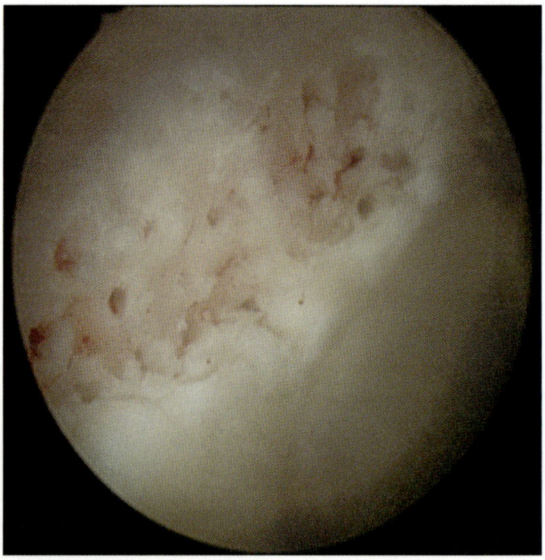

Fig. 14.5 Microfracture holes made 3–4 mm apart covering the entire damaged area

Labral reattachment is performed using suture anchors, prior to implant delivery, to ensure contention of the chondral lesion. Holes for labral anchors are drilled every 5 mm and 2–3 mm lateral to the bone edge of the acetabular rim. It is recommended to drill all the holes before attaching the labrum in order to be sure that all of them are in the right location (Fig. 14.6). In most cases 3–4 suture anchors are needed.

Once labral reattachment is performed, CAM deformity can be addressed. Release of traction to treat CAM lesions may help to avoid long

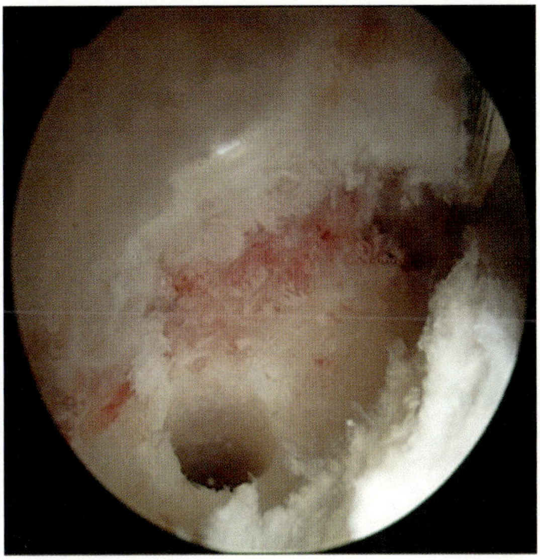

Fig. 14.6 Bone drill to labral reatachment close to the acetabular edge to ensure contention of the cartilage lesion

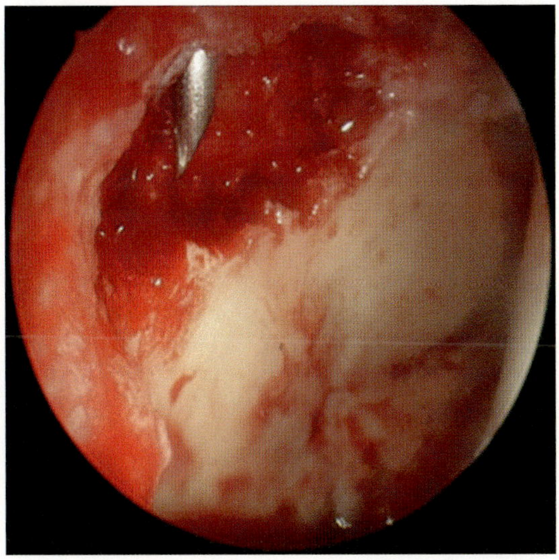

Fig. 14.7 The first layer of BST-CarGel is applied in a drop-wise manner using large 18G needles. Note that lesion is in the anterior acetabulum, so it is in an antigravitatory situation

traction time. However, it will increase soft tissue infiltration of arthroscopic liquid, preventing subsequent drying of the joint. In certain cases, CAM lesion can be addressed after BST-CarGel® application since release of traction will protect the implant while work is done in the peripheral compartment. If femoral head deformity is addressed before implant delivery, closure of the capsulotomy, especially if a T-capsulotomy has been performed, is strongly recommended before traction is reapplied to access the central compartment again.

BST-CarGel® is prepared by combining two components — a chitosan solution and a buffer. Chitosan is derived from chitin. One starts by dissolving the chitosan solution in an aqueous glycerophosphate buffer. The resulting solution is then manually mixed with fresh, autologous whole peripheral blood at a ratio 3:1 (blood: BST-CarGel). That mixture can be prepared 15–25 min before the implantation time, in order to achieve the optimal physical and mechanical properties of the product for a delivery to a vertically oriented wall like the acetabulum. Prior to its application, irrigation is stopped and the joint is completely drained of irrigation fluid. There is the use of an 18G arthroscopic needle through the posterolateral portal connected to a suction system, while the trocar faucet without any connection is opened to achieve a proper airflow that will help to dry the chondral lesion surface. Small gauze pad can help to completely dry the treatment surface. The first layer of the mixture is then delivered in a drop-wise manner using large 18G needles and without overfilling. Needles can be bended or inserted through the base of the labrum to ensure full contact with the chondral lesion and to facilitate BST-CarGel delivery (Fig. 14.7). This first layer, even if it is in the antigravitatory area, will stick in place due to its adhesive properties, sealing completely the damaged region. After that, the clot is constructed by delivering the remaining BST-CarGel until the damaged area is completely covered (Fig. 14.8). The mixture volume used per patient varied according to the lesion size. After delivery, the implant clotted in place during the required fifteen-minute waiting period in order to fully stabilize the implant. A step by step summary is indicated in Table 14.3.

It is also possible to use carbon dioxide during the final part of the arthroscopy, instead of stopping the irrigation to completely drain the joint from fluid. Without fluid in the joint, the capsule

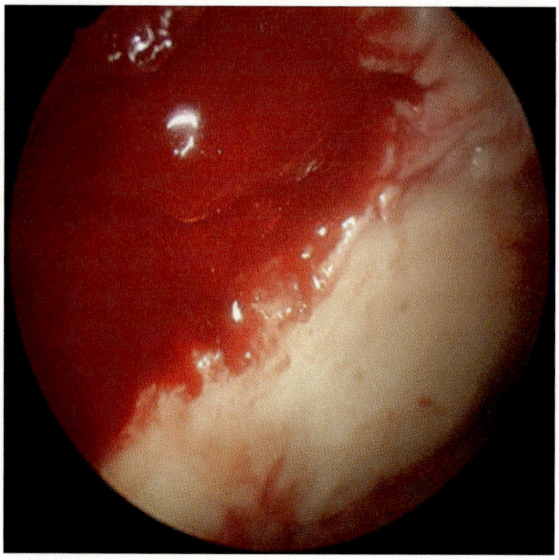

Fig. 14.8 View of the completed clot construction after BST-CarGel application

Table 14.3 Step-by-step summary of arthroscopic treatment of hip chondral defects with microfracture and BST-CarGel

Step	Description
1	*Patient position*: supine decubitus in a traction table
2	*Portals*: AL portal as viewing portal. DMA DL as working portals
3	*Instrumentation*: 70° arthroscope and hip arthoscopic set
4	*Joint evaluation* without fluid and case confirmation for chondral treatment
5	Set *fluid irrigation* pressure at 40–60 mmHg with an irrigation pump
6	*Chondral lesion preparation*:
	(a) Debridement of unstable or pathologic cartilage
	(b) Debridement of mineralized layer
	(c) Microfracture
7	*Labral reconstruction*:
	(a) Pincer resection
	(b) Acetabular rim trim
	(c) Drill bone tunnels for labral reatachment
	(d) Labral reatachment
8	*Osteoplasty for CAM lesion*:
	(a) Release of traction
	(b) T capsulotomy to access CAM deformity
	(c) Access to medial and lateral plica as usual edges of classic deformities
	(d) Osteochondroplasty
	(e) Suture of capsulotomy
9	*Apply traction* to access the central compartment
10	*Stop fluid irrigation* and aspiration of articular fluid
11	*18G needle placement* through posterolateral portal connected to suction system and free open
12	*Complete drying of the chondral defect* with small swabs
13	*Release of BST-CarGel with bended 18G* needles units cover the lesion
14	*Wait 15 min* before releasing traction

may collapse with less good arthroscopic visibility for gel implantation. With the carbon dioxide, the capsule will be distended and the joint will be dry facilitating gel implantation.

Passive motion starts day 1 and 6 weeks of partial weight bearing (less than 20 kg) assisted by crutches and is recommended in the postoperative period. Non- to partial weight bearing is the formal protocol in the knee, but it is not recommended to treat hip lesions since compression forces increase due to muscle forces [29, 44]. Low contact physical activities can be initiated at the third month, while high-impact sports must be avoided during the first year after surgery. BST-CarGel® has been used mainly for the knee joint and tested in a randomized trial with significant better outcomes regarding histology and MRI of repair in comparison with microfracture technique [58]. The use of BST-CarGel® in the hip is still experimental and under clinical study.

14.6 Summary and Conclusion

The literature is still not sufficiently strong to draw firm conclusions in terms of the best practice for chondral defects in the hip. Additional research is needed to expand the knowledge and to develop guidelines for the management of chondral injuries of the hip.

We know that surgical treatment for FAI reliably improves patient-related symptoms in the majority of patients without advanced osteoarthritis or chondral damage. Ng et al. [50] reviewed 970 patients after FAI surgery and found that patients with Outerbridge grade III or IV cartilage damage or with preoperative radiographs showing greater than Tönnis grade I osteoarthritis had worse outcomes after treatment of FAI.

Recently, one study showed that middle-aged people with hip cartilage labral lesions could benefit from surgery [9]. Further, arthroscopic management of FAI and labral repair in patients more than 50 years without significant arthritis (Tönnis grade 1 or less) were associated with significant improvement in outcome. Because of the potential importance of the labrum for long-term hip joint preservation, the authors suggested repair of the labrum in patients aged older than 50 years whenever possible.

There is not enough evidence to tell if repairing a local cartilage defect in the hip joint will prevent the progression into osteoarthritis. As in other joints, the indications for a repair are pain and functional disability. However, as the cartilage lesions are most often found in conjunction with CAM and/or pincer lesions and labral tears, the evidence treating such concomitant pathologies should be mentioned.

Ayeni et al. [3] showed in a recent review that based on the current available evidence, hip labrum reconstructions show short-term improvement in patient-reported outcomes and functional scores post-operatively. The main indication for reconstruction was a deficient labrum due to previous surgical excision or irreparable tears in young patients with no significant arthritis. Fayad et al. [20] found that arthroscopic corrections of structural abnormalities are increasingly becoming the standard treatment for FAI; however there is a paucity of high-level evidence comparing open and arthroscopic techniques in patients with similar FAI morphology and degree of associated articular cartilage damage.

Further research is needed to develop an understanding of the natural course of FAI and the definitive indications for surgery related to cartilage lesions and the outcomes.

Related to the treatment of hip cartilage lesions, we believe that we will see more treatments like:

Take-Home Points

1. Arthroscopic repair of isolated cartilage defects in the hip due to small-to-medium-sized defects with bone marrow stimulation techniques, simple or augmented
2. Arthroscopic repair of isolated cartilage defects in the hip with large chondral or osteochondral defects with 3rd- or 4th-generation autologous chondrocyte implantation with or without concomitant bone grafting
3. Arthroscopic repair of labral defects in combination with either alternative 1 or 2
4. Open repair of very large bipolar cartilage and/or labral lesions in young patients using alternative 1 or 2

Key Evidence Related Sources

1. Beck M, Kalhor M, Leunig M, Ganz R. Hip morphology influences the pattern of damage to the acetabular cartilage: femoroacetabular impingement as a cause of early osteoarthritis of the hip. J Bone Joint Surg Br. 2005;87(7):1012–8.
2. Brittberg M, Winalski CS. Evaluation of cartilage injuries and repair. J Bone Joint Surg Am. 2003;85-A Suppl 2:58–69.
3. El Bitar YF, Lindner D, Jackson TJ, Domb BG. Joint-preserving surgical options for management of chondral injuries of the hip. J Am Acad Orthop Surg. 2014;22(1):46–56.
4. Fontana A, Bistolfi A, Crova M, Rosso F, Massazza G. Arthroscopic treatment of hip chondral defects: autologous chondrocyte transplantation versus simple debridement – a pilot study. Arthroscopy. 2012;28(3):322–9.
5. Hariri S, Truntzer J, Smith RL, Safran MR. Biochemical and cellular assessment of acetabular chondral flaps identified during hip arthroscopy. J Arthrosc Relat Surg. Accepted for publication 2014.

6. Stanish WD, McCormack R, Forriol F, Mohtadi N, Pelet S, Desnoyers J, Restrepo A, Shive MS. Novel scaffold-based BST-CarGel treatment results in superior cartilage repair compared with microfracture in a randomized controlled trial. J Bone Joint Surg Am. 2013;95(18):1640–50.

References

1. Afoke NY, Byers PD, Hutton WC. Contact pressures in the human hip joint. J Bone Joint Surg Br. 1987;69(4):536–41.
2. Akimau P, Bhosale A, Harrison PE, Roberts S, McCall IW, Richardson JB, Ashton BA. Autologous chondrocyte implantation with bone grafting for osteochondral defect due to posttraumatic osteonecrosis of the hip – a case report. Acta Orthop. 2006;77(2):333–6.
3. Ayeni OR, Alradwan H, de Sa D, Philippon MJ. The hip labrum reconstruction: indications and outcomes – a systematic review. Knee Surg Sports Traumatol Arthrosc. 2014;22(4):737–43. doi:10.1007/s00167-013-2804-5. Epub 2013 Dec 7.
4. Banerjee P, McLean CR. Femoroacetabular impingement: a review of diagnosis and management. Curr Rev Musculoskelet Med. 2011;4(1):23–32.
5. Beaulé PE, Hynes K, Parker G, Kemp KA. Can the alpha angle assessment of cam impingement predict acetabular cartilage delamination? Clin Orthop Relat Res. 2012;470(12):3361–7.
6. Beck M, Leunig M, Parvizi J, Boutier V, Wyss D, Ganz R. Anterior femoroacetabular impingement: mid-term results of surgical treatment. Clin Orthop. 2004;418:67–73.
7. Beck M, Kalhor M, Leunig M, Ganz R. Hip morphology influences the pattern of damage to the acetabular cartilage: femoroacetabular impingement as a cause of early osteoarthritis of the hip. J Bone Joint Surg Br. 2005;87(7):1012–8.
8. Bekkers JE, Tsuchida AI, van Rijen MH, Vonk LA, Dhert WJ, Creemers LB, Saris DB. Single-stage cell-based cartilage regeneration using a combination of chondrons and mesenchymal stromal cells: comparison with microfracture. Am J Sports Med. 2013;41(9):2158–66.
9. Ben Tov T, Amar E, Shapira A, Steinberg E, Atoun E, Rath E. Clinical and functional outcome after acetabular labral repair in patients aged older than 50 years. Arthroscopy. 2014;30(3):305–10.
10. Benthien JP, Behrens P. Reviewing subchondral cartilage surgery: considerations for standardised and outcome predictable cartilage remodelling: a technical note. Int Orthop. 2013;37(11):2139–45.
11. Billing L, Bogren HG, Wallin J. Reliable X-ray diagnosis of slipped capital femoral epiphysis by combining the conventional and a new simplified geometrical method. Pediatr Radiol. 2002;32(6):423–30.
12. Brittberg M, Winalski CS. Evaluation of cartilage injuries and repair. J Bone Joint Surg Am. 2003;85-A Suppl 2:58–69.
13. Byrd JWT. Physical examination. In: Operative hip arthroscopy. New York: Springer; 2005. p. 36–50.
14. Byrd JWT. Hip arthroscopy, the supine approach: technique and anatomy of the intraarticular and peripheral compartments. Tech Orthop. 2005;20: 17–31.
15. Cole BJ, Farr J, Winalski CS, Hosea T, Richmond J, Mandelbaum B, De Deyne PG. Outcomes after a single-stage procedure for cell-based cartilage repair: a prospective clinical safety trial with 2-year follow-up. Am J Sports Med. 2011;39(6):1170–9.
16. de Windt TS, Concaro S, Lindahl A, Saris DB, Brittberg M. Strategies for patient profiling in articular cartilage repair of the knee: a prospective cohort of patients treated by one experienced cartilage surgeon. Knee Surg Sports Traumatol Arthrosc. 2012;20(11):2225–32.
17. Dunn DM. Anteversion of the neck of the femur; a method of measurement. J Bone Joint Surg Br. 1952;34-B(2):181–6.
18. El Bitar YF, Lindner D, Jackson TJ, Domb BG. Joint-preserving surgical options for management of chondral injuries of the hip. J Am Acad Orthop Surg. 2014;22(1):46–56.
19. Farr J, Cole BJ, Sherman S, Karas V. Particulated articular cartilage: CAIS and DeNovo NT. J Knee Surg. 2012;25(1):23–9.
20. Fayad TE, Khan MA, Haddad FS. Femoroacetabular impingement: an arthroscopic solution. Bone Joint J. 2013;95-B(11 Suppl A):26–30.
21. Ferguson SJ, Bryant JT, Ganz R, Ito K. An in vitro investigation of the acetabular labral seal in hip joint mechanisms. J Biomech. 2003;36(2):171–8.
22. Field RE, Rajakulendran K, Strambi F. Arthroscopic grafting of chondral defects and subchondral cysts of the acetabulum. Hip Int. 2011;21(4):479–86.
23. Fontana A, Bistolfi A, Crova M, Rosso F, Massazza G. Arthroscopic treatment of hip chondral defects: autologous chondrocyte transplantation versus simple debridement – a pilot study. Arthroscopy. 2012;28(3): 322–9.
24. Fontana A, Bistolfi A, Crova M, Massazza G. Primary stability of a PGLA/polydioxanone membrane for potential autologous chondrocyte implantation in the hip joint. A cadaveric study. Hip Int. 2013;23(3): 337–42.
25. Gdalevitch M, Smith K, Tanzer M. Delamination cysts: a predictor of acetabular cartilage delamination in hips with a labral tear. Clin Orthop Relat Res. 2009;467(4):985–91.

26. Ganz R, Parvizi J, Beck M, Leunig M, Notzli H, Siebenrock KA. Femoroacetabular impingement: a cause for osteoarthritis of the hip. Clin Orthop Relat Res. 2003;417:112–20.
27. Girard J, Roumazeille T, Sakr M, Migaud H. Osteochondral mosaicplasty of the femoral head. Hip Int. 2011;21(5):542–8.
28. Groh MM, Herrera J. A comprehensive review of hip labral tears. Curr Rev Musculoskeletal Med. 2009;2: 105–17.
29. Gosnell WC, Butcher MT, Maie T, Blob RW. Femoral loading mechanics in the Virginia opossum, Didelphis virginiana: torsion and mediolateral bending in mammalian locomotion. J Exp Biol. 2011;214(Pt 20):3455–66.
30. Grant AD, Sala DA, Davidovitch RI. The labrum: structure, function, and injury with femoro-acetabular impingement. J Child Orthop. 2012;6(5):357–72.
31. Hariri S, Truntzer J, Smith RL, Safran MR. Biochemical and cellular assessment of acetabular chondral flaps identified during hip arthroscopy. J Arthrosc Relat Surg. Accepted for publication 2014.
32. Hoemann CD, Hurtig M, Rossomacha E, Sun J, Chevrier A, Shive MS, Buschmann MD. Chitosan-glycerol phosphate/blood implants improve hyaline cartilage repair in ovine microfracture defects. J Bone Joint Surg Am. 2005;87(12):2671–86.
33. http://www.americanhipinstitute.org/references/content/acetabular-cartilage-damage-alad-classification
34. Jäger M, Begg MJ, Krauspe R. Partial hemi-resurfacing of the hip joint – a new approach to treat local osteochondral defects? Biomed Tech (Berl). 2006;51(5–6):371–6.
35. Kappe T, Kocak T, Bieger R, Reichel H, Fraitzl CR. Radiographic risk factors for labral lesions in femoroacetabular impingement. Clin Orthop Relat Res. 2011;469(11):3241–7.
36. Karthikeyan S, Roberts S, Griffin D. Chondrogeneic tissue based implants: microfracture for acetabular chondral defects in patients with femoroacetabular impingement: results at second-look arthroscopic surgery. Am J Sports Med. 2012;40(12):2725–30.
37. Khanna V, Harris A, Farrokhyar F, Choudur HN, Wong IH. Hip arthroscopy: prevalence of intra-articular pathologic findings after traumatic injury of the hip. Arthroscopy. 2014;30(3):299–304.
38. Konan S, Rayan F, Meermans G, Witt J, Haddad FS. Validation of the classification system for acetabular chondral lesions identified at arthroscopy in patients with femoroacetabular impingement. J Bone Joint Surg Br. 2011;93(3):332–6.
39. Kurrat HJ, Oberlander W. The thickness of the cartilage in the hip joint. J Anat. 1978;126:145–55.
40. Lauenstein C. Nachweis der Kocher'schen Verbiegung des Schenkelhalses bei der Coxa Vara durch Röntgen-Strahlen. Beitr Klin Chirurg. 1901;28:61–4 (In German).
41. Lea MA, Barkatali B, Porter ML, Board TN. Osteochondral lesion of the hip treated with partial femoral head resurfacing. Case report and six-year follow-up. Hip Int. 2014;24(4):417–20.
42. Leunig M, Tibor LM, Naal FD, Ganz R, Steinwachs MR. Surgical technique: second-generation bone marrow stimulation via surgical dislocation to treat hip cartilage lesions. Clin Orthop Relat Res. 2012;470(12):3421–31.
43. Lewis C, Sahrmann S. Acetabular labral tears. Phys Ther. 2006;86(1):110–21. 25.
44. Lewis CL, Sahrmann SA, Moran DW. Anterior hip joint force increases with hip extension, decreased gluteal force, or decreased iliopsoas force. J Biomech. 2007;40(16):3725–31.
45. Mancini D, Fontana A. Five-year results of arthroscopic techniques for the treatment of acetabular chondral lesions in femoroacetabular impingement. Int Orthop. 2014;38(10):2057–64.
46. Meyers MH. Resurfacing of the femoral head with fresh osteochondral allografts. Long-term results. Clin Orthop Relat Res. 1985;197:111–4.
47. Murakibhavi V, Ahmed N, Raj V, Richardson J. Early results of autologous chondrocyte implantation. J Bone Joint Surg Br. 2010; 92-B(Supp IV): 526.
48. Nötzli HP, Wyss TF, Stoecklin CH, Schmid MR, Treiber K, Hodler J. The contour of the femoral head-neck junction as a predictor for the risk of anterior impingement. J Bone Joint Surg Br. 2002;84(4):556–60.
49. Myers SR, Eijer H, Ganz R. Anterior femoroacetabular impingement after periacetabular osteotomy. Clin Orthop Relat Res. 1999;363:93–9.
50. Ng VY, Arora N, Best TM, Pan X, Ellis TJ. Efficacy of surgery for femoroacetabular impingement: a systematic review. Am J Sports Med. 2010;38(11):2337–45.
51. Philippon MJ, Schenker ML, Briggs KK, Maxwell RB. Can microfracture produce repair tissue in acetabular chondral defects? Arthroscopy. 2008;24(1):46–50.
52. Ramisetty N, Kwon Y, Mohtadi N. Patient-reported outcome measures for hip preservation surgery—a systematic review of the literature. J Hip Preserv Surg. 2015;2(1):1–13.
53. Register B, Pennock AT, Ho CP, Strickland CD, Lawand A, Philippon MJ. Prevalence of abnormal hip findings in asymptomatic participants: a prospective, blinded study. Am J Sports Med. 2012;40(12): 2720–4.
54. Safran MR, Hariri S. Hip arthroscopy assessment: tools and outcomes. Oper Techn Orthop. 2010;20(4): 264–77.
55. Sahin M, Calisir C, Omeroglu H, Inan U, Mutlu F, Kaya T. Evaluation of labral pathology and hip articular cartilage in patients with femoroacetabular impingement (FAI): comparison of multidetector CT arthrography and MR arthrography. Pol J Radiol. 2014;79:374–80.
56. Song Y, Ito H, Kourtis L, Safran MR, Carter DR, Giori NJ. Articular cartilage friction increases in hip joints after the removal of acetabular labrum. J Biomech. 2012;45(3):524–30.

57. Stafford GH, Bunn JR, Villar RN. Arthroscopic repair of delaminated acetabular articular cartilage using fibrin adhesive: results at one to three years. Hip Int. 2011;21(6):744–50.
58. Stanish WD, McCormack R, Forriol F, Mohtadi N, Pelet S, Desnoyers J, Restrepo A, Shive MS. Novel scaffold-based BST-CarGel treatment results in superior cartilage repair compared with microfracture in a randomized controlled trial. J Bone Joint Surg Am. 2013;95(18):1640–50.
59. Sutter R, Zubler V, Hoffmann A, Mamisch-Saupe N, Dora C, Kalberer F, Zanetti M, Hodler J, Pfirrmann CW. Hip MRI: how useful is intraarticular contrast material for evaluating surgically proven lesions of the labrum and articular cartilage? AJR Am J Roentgenol. 2014;202(1):160–9.
60. Tannast M, Siebenrock KA, Anderson SE. Femoroacetabular impingement: radiographic diagnosis – what the radiologist should know. AJR Am J Roentgenol. 2007;188(6):1540–52.
61. Thorborg K, Tijssen M, Habets B, Bartels EM, Roos EM, Kemp J, Crossley KM, Hölmich P. Patient-reported outcome (PRO) questionnaires for young to middle-aged adults with hip and groin disability: a systematic review of the clinimetric evidence. Br J Sports Med. 2015. pii: bjsports-2014-094224.
62. Tönnis D. Die angeborene Huftdysplasie und Huftluxation im Kindes- und Erwachsenenalter. Berlin/Heidelberg: Springer; 1984.
63. Tönnis D. Congenital dysplasia and dislocation of the hip in children and adults. Berlin/Heidelberg/New York: Springer; 1987.
64. Tönnis D, Heinecke A. Acetabular and femoral anteversion: relationship with osteoarthritis of the hip. J Bone Joint Surg Am. 1999;81(12):1747–70.
65. Vundelinckx B, De Mulder K, De Schepper J. Osteochondral defect in femoral head: Trufit implantation under fluoroscopic and arthroscopic control. Acta Orthop Belg. 2012;78(6):796–9.

Management of Extra-articular Hip Conditions in Patients with Concurrent FAI

15

Nolan S. Horner, Uffe Jorgensen, Darren de SA, and Olufemi R. Ayeni

Contents

15.1 Rationale/Introduction

Groin pain is an increasingly common condition in athletes, particularly those involved in cutting sports or sports involving frequent acceleration and deceleration. The differential diagnosis for groin pain in athletes is vast and often poses a significant diagnostic challenge for physicians. Among athletes, femoroacetabular impingement (FAI) is a relatively common source of intra-articular groin pain. Hammoud et al. [23] suggested that the reduced functional range of motion in patients with FAI leads to high impaction loads at terminal ranges, which can ultimately result in a number of compensatory disorders. Furthermore, some case series have found associations between FAI and other extra-articular hip conditions including athletic pubalgia and osteitis pubis [22,41]. One study found that 33 % of athletes with chronic groin pain had two or more separate pathologies causing their symptoms [28]. Therefore, physicians must consider the possibility that there exist multiple and often concomitant pathologies in a patient presenting with groin pain. Otherwise, a substantial risk exists that the patient will continue to be symptomatic even after treatment. Although some patients presenting with groin pain may successfully recover with nonsurgical treatment, patients do frequently require surgical intervention. The surgical management of FAI generally involves either femoroplasty or acetabuloplasty done through either arthroscopic, open, or mini-open methods. However, failure to simultaneously address other underlying extra-articular pathologies such as athletic pubalgia through surgical treatment results in high rates of persistent

U. Jorgensen (✉)
Department of Orthopaedic Surgery and Sports Traumatology, Odense University Hospital, Institute of Clinical Research, University of Southern Denmark, Sdr. Boulevard 29, Odense C DK-5000, Denmark
e-mail: Uffe.Joergensen@rsyd.dk

N.S. Horner • D. de SA • O.R. Ayeni
Division of Orthopaedic Surgery, Department of Surgery, McMaster University, Hamilton, ON, Canada

O.R. Ayeni et al. (eds.), *Diagnosis and Management of Femoroacetabular Impingement*,
DOI 10.1007/978-3-319-32000-7_15

symptoms and inability to return to sport [21, 37, 38, 41]. This chapter looks to address the history, physical examination, investigations, and management of some common extra-articular hip conditions frequently associated with FAI including (1) athletic pubalgia, (2) osteitis pubis, and (3) internal snapping hip syndrome. Table 15.1 presents a brief summary of the pathology, recommended investigations, and management for each of these three conditions.

15.2 Athletic Pubalgia

Athletic pubalgia is a syndrome that is most commonly seen in high-performance athletes. It consists of lower abdominal/inguinal pain upon activity and often progresses to include adductor pain. Athletes participating in sports requiring cutting or frequent acceleration and deceleration (e.g., soccer, ice hockey, and football) appear to be most susceptible to athletic pubalgia [18, 32]. Although the mechanism of athletic pubalgia has been debated in the literature, the majority of evidence appears to suggest that the syndrome is caused by a complex injury of the flexion/adduction apparatus of the lower abdomen and hip [43]. A number of alternative terms have been used to describe athletic pubalgia in the literature including "Gilmore's groin" [18], "sports hernia" [21], "sportsman's hernia" [51], and "pubic inguinal pain syndrome" [9].

Patients presenting with athletic pubalgia will most commonly complain of lower abdominal pain and proximal adductor pain. Although this pain is generally gradual in onset, it less commonly occurs as a result of an acute injury. These acute injuries are generally caused by hyperabduction of the hip and/or hyperextension of the trunk leading to a tear of the rectus abdominis [43, 57]. Athletic pubalgia appears to be much more common in males; however, an increasing proportion of females have been diagnosed in the last decade [44]. A number of physical examination maneuvers may be useful in the diagnosis of athletic pubalgia including painful resisted hip adduction in flexion and extension [36], reproduced symptoms with Valsalva maneuver [43], and reproduced symptoms with a resisted sit-up with simultaneous palpation of the inferolateral distal rectus abdominis [43]. Moreover, palpation of the proximal adductor muscles, abdominal obliques, transverse abdominis, and rectus abdominis is recommended [36].

If after a thorough history and physical examination athletic pubalgia is suspected, a plain radiograph and MRI are the recommended investigations [36]. Although there are no characteristic radiograph findings of athletic pubalgia, a plain radiograph is useful in ruling out other causes of groin pain. MRI has been shown to

Table 15.1 Summary of three pathologies known to be associated with FAI

Condition	Pathology	Recommended imaging/ investigations	Surgical treatment options
Athletic pubalgia	Complex injury of the flexion/adduction apparatus of the lower abdomen and hip	1. Plain radiograph 2. MRI 3. Ultrasound-guided diagnostic injection	1. External oblique repair 2. Transversalis fascia repair 3. Transversus abdominis repair
Osteitis pubis	Chronic overuse injury of the pubic symphysis and the parasymphyseal bone	1. Plain radiograph 2. MRI 3. Diagnostic injection	1. Wedge resection 2. Arthrodesis 3. Pubic symphysis curettage 4. Endoscopic pubic symphysectomy
Internal snapping hip syndrome	Iliopsoas tendon slides over the iliopectineal eminence of the femoral head resulting in a snapping sensation	1. Plain radiograph (including elongated neck lateral view) 2. Ultrasound 3. Possible MRI	1. Iliopsoas tendon release/lengthening

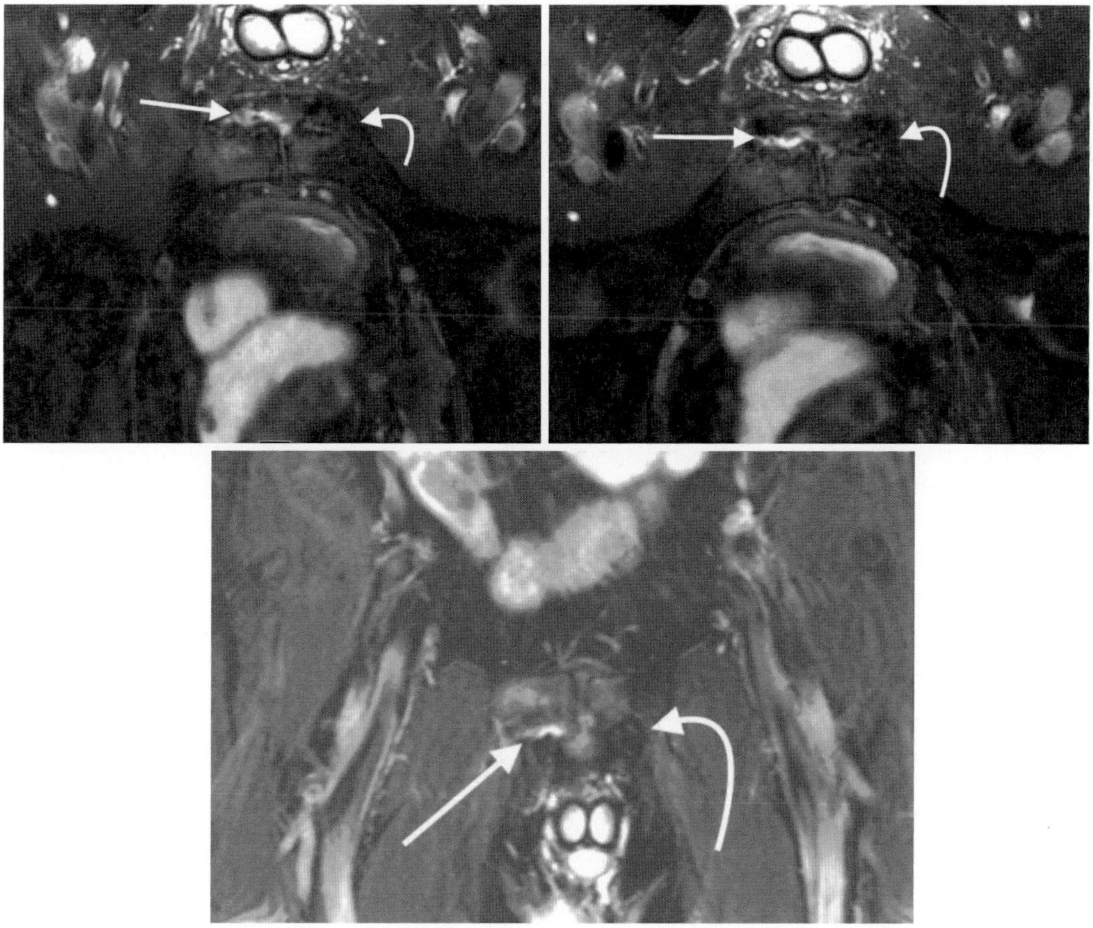

Fig. 15.1 (*Top left, top right*) Axial and (*bottom middle*) coronal T2-weighted fast spin echo fat-saturated MR images show disruption with hematoma/granulation tissue (*white arrows*) at the right rectus abdominis-adductor aponeurotic plate attachment at the anteroinferior pubis. Note the normal-appearing aponeurotic plate attachment on the asymptomatic left side (*curved white arrow*)

have high sensitivity and specificity for adductor and rectus abdominis pathology [57]. Figure 15.1 shows typical MRI findings in a patient with athletic pubalgia. It should be noted that Silvis et al. [52] found in one study that 36 % of asymptomatic professional hockey players had MRI findings consistent with athletic pubalgia. Additionally, a diagnostic ultrasound-guided intra-articular injection can be useful in ruling out intra-articular pathology as the source of the patients' symptoms [3].

Athletic pubalgia can be managed both nonsurgically and surgically. Nonsurgical treatment recommendations include a trial of physiotherapy and rest followed by gradual reintroduction to sport activity [4, 34]. However, the current literature suggests that nonsurgical management of athletic pubalgia may offer no benefit compared with placebo [53]. On the other hand, surgical outcomes in the literature are much more positive. There have been a number of different surgical procedures described. These procedures include, but are not limited to, external oblique, transversalis fascia, and transversus abdominis repairs either with or without mesh and through either open or laparoscopic methods [6, 17, 33, 43]. The various surgical treatment options report generally positive outcomes with anywhere between 80 and 100 % rates of return to sport.

Recently, there has been evidence appearing that suggests there is an association between athletic pubalgia and FAI [22, 37, 38]. Larson et al. [37, 38] showed in a case series of 37 patients with both symptomatic athletic pubalgia and FAI that patients only had a 25 % rate of return to sport if only athletic pubalgia surgery was performed. Similarly, patients who only had hip arthroscopy performed for FAI had a relatively low (50 %) rate of return to sport. However, those patients who had procedures to correct both the athletic pubalgia and the FAI had an almost 90 % rate of unrestricted return to sport. In this study, the surgical procedure for athletic pubalgia was unspecified, and in all cases, the FAI was treated arthroscopically. The only complications reported were two superficial wound infections.

Another 38 patient case series on individuals with both FAI and athletic pubalgia reported similar findings [22]. In this study, no patients who had only athletic pubalgia correction surgery were able to return to sport; however, 100 % of patients who had surgical treatment of their athletic pubalgia followed by surgical treatment of their FAI at a later date were able to return to sport. The mean duration prior to return to play was 5.9 months. In this study, the procedure performed to treat the athletic pubalgia was not specified. The FAI was treated arthroscopically, and it was reported that 65 % of patients underwent both femoroplasty and acetabuloplasty, 21 % had only femoroplasty, and the remaining 13 % had only acetabuloplasty.

Sansone et al. [48] found that more than 60 % of patients stated that they were unsatisfied after either adductor tenotomy or rectus tenotomy for athletic pubalgia had a positive hip impingement test at postoperative follow-up. These results imply that undiagnosed FAI may be a common reason for failure of athletic pubalgia surgery.

These studies highlight the importance of ensuring that physicians consider the possibility of concurrent athletic pubalgia in the patient with FAI. The evidence suggests that hip arthroscopy or correction of the athletic pubalgia alone is unlikely to completely alleviate a patient's symptoms with both conditions. However, the literature currently reports that in patients with both athletic pubalgia and FAI simultaneous correction of both conditions results in generally good outcomes with a high proportion of patients successfully being able to return to sport. Overall, the treatments both appear to be safe as only a very low rate of minor complications are reported after surgical treatment of patients with both FAI and athletic pubalgia.

15.3 Osteitis Pubis

Athletic osteitis pubis is a chronic overuse injury of the pubic symphysis and the parasymphyseal bone [27]. It should be noted that osteitis pubis can also be caused by etiologies other than mechanical sport injuries such as vaginal delivery, infection, and pelvic/perineal surgery [16]. However, for the purpose of this chapter, discussion will be limited to osteitis pubis in athletes. Patients presenting with osteitis pubis most commonly complain of central pubis pain and/or medial groin pain that is worsened with activity [27]. Patients may also have superior pubic rami, adductor, perineal, inguinal, or scrotal pain [16, 54]. Physical examination findings may include reduced external/internal rotation of the hip, adductor/abductor weakness, and a waddling, antalgic gait [40, 41].

Radiographs in patients with osteitis pubis are generally unremarkable in the acute setting, however, sclerotic or cystic changes may occur in patients with chronic osteitis pubis [48]. Bone marrow edema of the pubic symphysis on MRI is a common finding in patients with osteitis pubis [45]. That being said, one study found that 65 % of asymptomatic athletes also had bone marrow edema of the pubic symphysis on MRI [45]. Figure 15.2 shows the MRI findings in a patient with severe osteitis pubis. Steroid injections into the pubic symphysis have been recommended both as a nonsurgical treatment option and to aid in diagnosis [29]. A systematic review of treatment of osteitis pubis found that 58.6 % of patients were able to fully return to sport after management with steroid injections into the pubis symphysis [10].

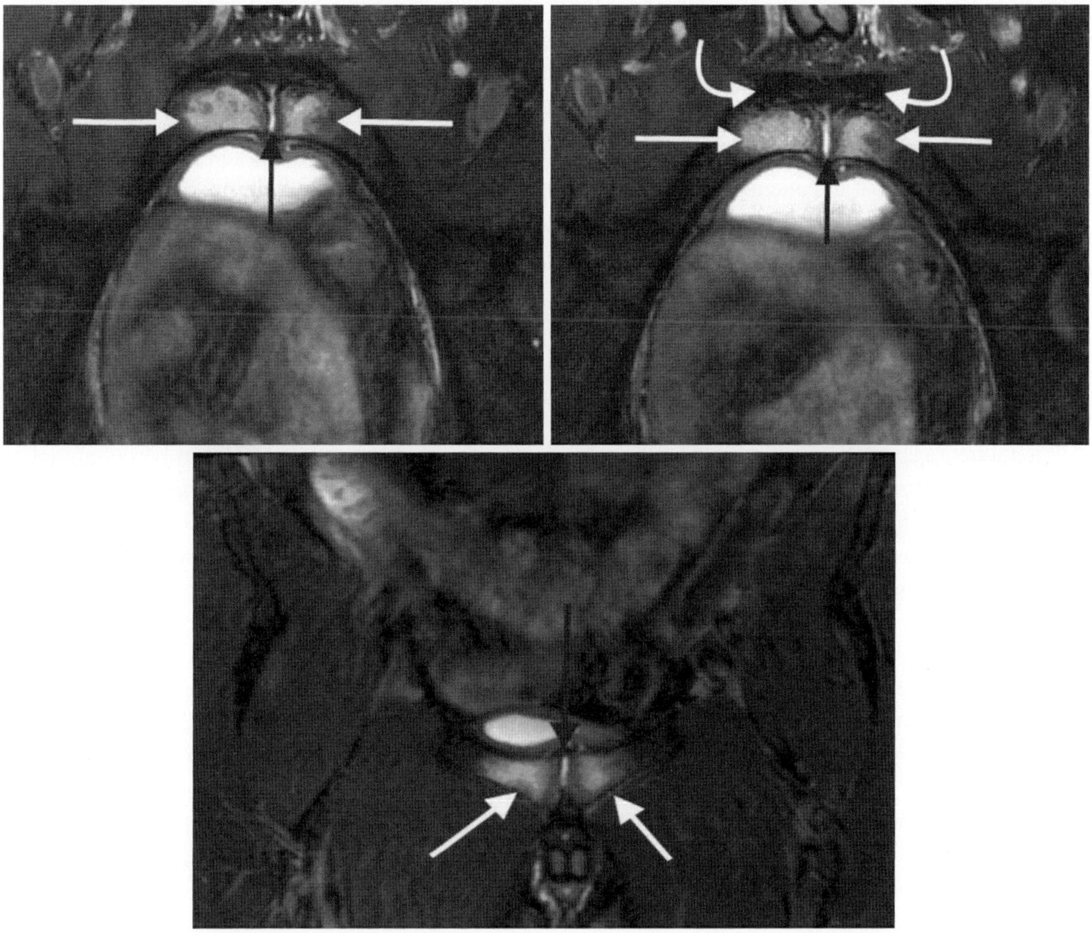

Fig. 15.2 (*Top left, top right*) Moderate bone marrow edema spanning the subchondral region of the pubic symphysis anterior to posterior on an axial fat-saturated T2-weighted image (*white arrows*) typical for severe osteitis pubis. There is fluid in the pubic symphyseal cleft (*black arrows*). The rectus abdominis-adductor aponeurosis is intact (*curved white arrows*). (*Bottom middle*) Coronal fat-saturated T2-weighted image shows osteitis pubis with bone marrow edema (*white arrows*) and symphyseal fluid (*black arrow*)

Nonsurgical treatment options in the management of osteitis pubis include rest, NSAIDs, physiotherapy, steroid injections, and cross training [29, 47]. Literature rates of return to sport after nonsurgical treatment (not including steroid injection) of osteitis pubis range from 81 to 100 % with time to return to sport varying from 3 days to 24 months [27]. Nevertheless, definitive treatment of osteitis pubis relies on surgical treatment. Surgical treatment options for osteitis pubis include wedge resection [19], arthrodesis [42], pubic symphysis curettage [48], and endoscopic pubic symphysectomy [41]. Radic and Annear [48] reported 16 of 24 patients undergoing pubic symphysis curettage were able to return to sport at 2.5–12 months. Similarly Matsuda et al. [41] reported positive outcomes treating osteitis pubis with an endoscopic pubic symphysectomy. Although surgical treatment does appear to provide benefit to patients, there is currently no evidence to strongly support one form of surgical treatment over the others [27]. In fact, some authors even suggest that surgical treatment should not be performed for osteitis pubis and that for the vast majority of patients, nonsurgical treatment options are sufficient [16].

It has been suggested that FAI may cause osteitis pubis as a result of a compensatory increase in range of motion at the pubic symphysis due to the reduced range of functional range of motion of the hip [55]. In a retrospective case series, Matsuda et al. [41] reported that in patients with both symptomatic FAI and osteitis pubis, simultaneous hip arthroscopy and endoscopic pubic symphysectomy resulted in significantly improved VAS and NAHS scores as well as a mean patient satisfaction rating of 8.3 (scale 0–10). The only complications reported were two patients who had postoperative scrotal swelling which resolved spontaneously. Although the literature appears to suggest that a relationship between FAI and osteitis pubis probably exists, very limited clinical information, specifically addressing the treatment and outcomes of patients with both conditions, is reported in the literature.

15.4 Internal Snapping Hip Syndrome

Internal snapping hip syndrome is a condition in which the iliopsoas tendon moves over the iliopectineal eminence or the femoral head resulting in a snapping sensation [1, 5]. Internal snapping hip syndrome has the potential to produce labral tears and even chondral damage [2,14]. Unlike labral tears secondary to FAI, which typically produce lesions at the 1–2 o'clock position, labral tears caused by internal snapping hip syndrome typically produce a characteristic labral tear at the 3 o'clock position [7].

In addition to the snapping sound and/or sensation, patients with internal snapping hip syndrome will frequently complain of pain with repetitive twisting or flexion of the hip. Physical examination findings for internal snapping hip syndrome include a positive flexion-adduction-internal rotation (FADIR) impingement test and tenderness over the iliopsoas at the level of the anterior joint line [14]. The snapping can often be reproduced on physical exam by slowly transitioning the hip from a flexed, abducted, externally rotated position to an extended, internally rotated position with the patient supine [8]. Figure 15.3 shows how this physical exam maneuver can be completed. Alternatively with the patient in the lateral position, transitioning the hip back and forth from extension to flexion will often recreate the snapping of the hip [8]. In the diagnosis of internal snapping hip syndrome, anteroposterior pelvis and elongated neck lateral radiographs are recommended in all patients [23]. A diagnostic ultrasound can also be useful in confirming the diagnosis of internal snapping hip syndrome. Real-time ultrasound or fluoroscopy with contrast injected into the iliopsoas bursa allows the examiner to observe for a jerk in the iliopsoas tendon at the same time as a snap in the hip is heard or felt [8, 56]. Although some studies suggest that an MRI can be beneficial in the diagnosis of tendinopathies [11], other authors suggest that a good history and physical examination are typically sufficient for the diagnosis of internal snapping hip syndrome [20].

Recommended nonsurgical treatment for internal snapping hip syndrome includes physiotherapy, intra-articular injections, and/or iliopsoas bursa injection [23]. Gruen et al. (2002) found in a case series that 37 % of patients failed nonsurgical management of internal snapping hip syndrome and required surgical treatment. Ilizaliturri et al. [31] stated that surgical treatment only be considered in patients who have failed nonsurgical treatment options. A number of surgical treatment options have been described in the literature for internal snapping hip syndrome including iliopsoas tendon release at the lesser trochanter [30], at the level of the joint [15], or at the level of the peripheral compartment [31]. Iliopsoas tendon releases can be done either through open approaches or through endoscopic techniques [13, 30]. One randomized control trial found no significant clinical difference between endoscopic iliopsoas tendon release at the level of the lesser trochanter compared with at the level of the peripheral compartment and that both procedures significantly improved WOMAC scores in 100 % of patients [31]. Another study reported 100 % of patients experienced no continued snapping after iliopsoas release and that 82 % of patients experienced excellent pain relief (Gruen et al. 2002). A systematic review of surgical management of internal snapping hip syndrome found that open treatment had a 21 % rate of complications, whereas arthroscopic treatment had only a 2.3 % complication rate [35]. This systematic review found the fol-

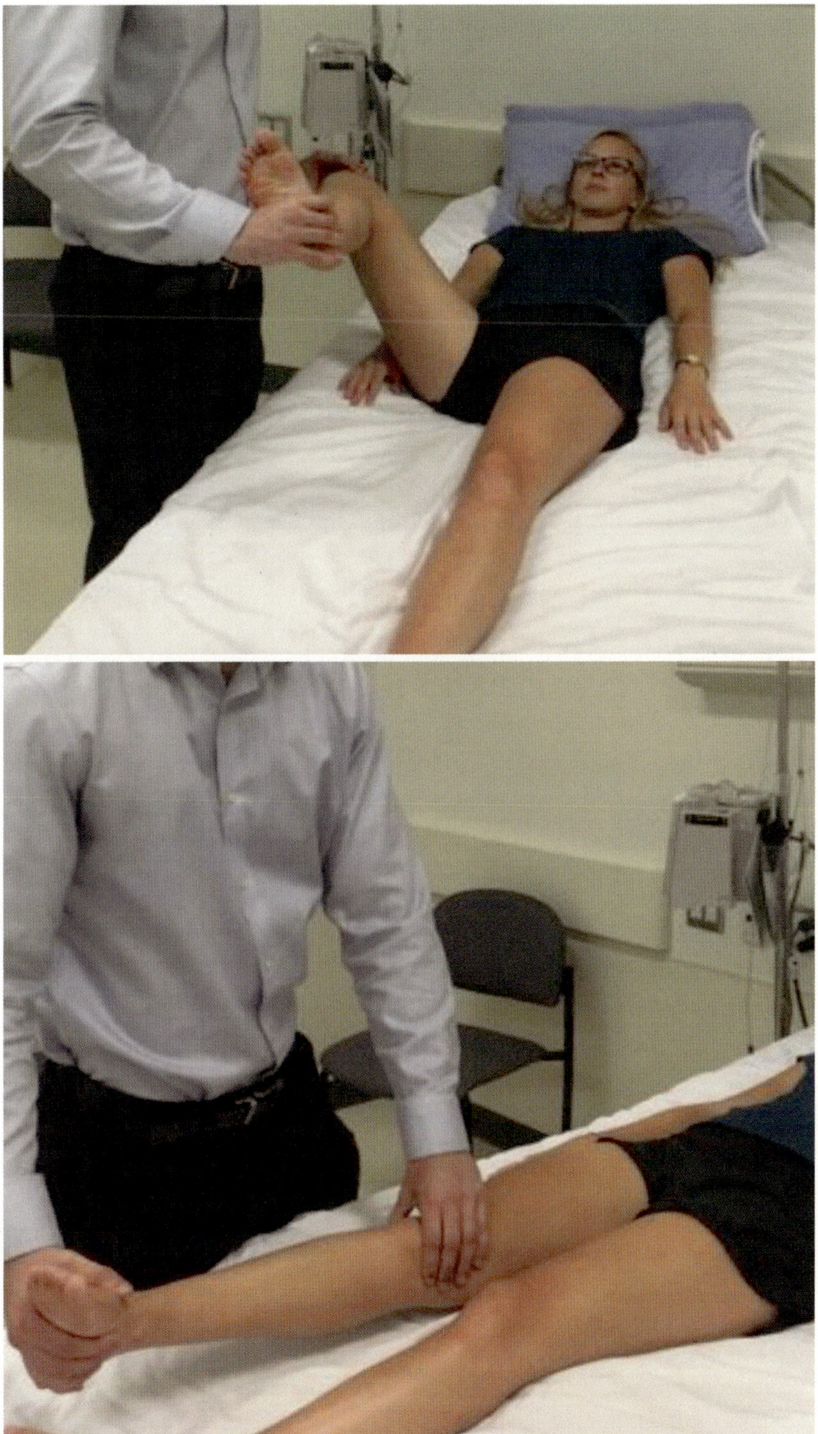

Fig. 15.3 By transitioning the hip from a flexed, abducted, and externally rotated position (*top*) to an extended and internally rotated position (*bottom*), snapping of the hip may be reproduced

lowing complications reported in the literature after surgical treatment of snapping hip syndrome: hip flexor weakness, anterior thigh paresthesia, anterolateral thigh numbness, greater trochanteric bursitis, ischial bursitis, superficial infections, and a hematoma. They also reported that among the 11 included studies, arthroscopic surgery had a 100 % success rate of resolution of snapping, whereas open procedures only had a 77 % success rate.

In one case study of 75 patients undergoing iliopsoas tendon lengthening for internal snapping hip, it was observed that 76.4 % of patients also required acetabuloplasty for pincer impingement and 52.7 % of patients required femoroplasty for CAM impingement [5]. Patients with FAI may have a higher propensity for developing internal snapping hip syndrome as a result of compensatory effects secondary to the reduced functional range of motion associated with FAI [23]. Heyworth et al. [26] found that failing to address a tight iliopsoas tendon during index hip arthroscopy is a frequent cause of patients requiring revision surgery. In this study, four of the nine patients who required revision surgery after index hip arthroscopy for FAI had a psoas tendon release performed during the revision surgery. One systematic review of revision hip arthroscopies found that a psoas release was performed in 15.3 % of revision hip arthroscopies [50]. It should be noted, however, that this study was looking at revision hip arthroscopies for all index indications, not exclusively for FAI.

Patients who have simultaneous iliopsoas tendon lengthening and FAI correction have been shown to have significant improvement across a variety of hip outcome scores and patient reported outcomes [5]. In this study, both the FAI and the internal snapping hip were treated arthroscopically. Iliopsoas fractional lengthening was performed through the central compartment at the level of the joint line where the iliopsoas is approximately 50 % muscle and 50 % tendon. The iliopsoas tendon was incised while avoiding the muscular portion in order to cause fractional lengthening of the tendon. The only complications reported were one patient with transient groin numbness, one patient with superficial infection, and one patient with heterotopic ossification. Revision surgery was required in 14.5 % of the patients, with re-rupture of the labrum being the most common indication for revision hip arthroscopy. No patients required revision surgery for continued snapping of the hip.

15.5 Other Extra-articular Conditions Associated with FAI

Although this chapter largely focuses on patients presenting with both FAI and either athletic pubalgia, osteitis pubis, or internal snapping hip syndrome, there is a number of other compensatory conditions that may occur as a result of underlying FAI. For example, hip flexor strains may be associated with FAI as a result of the hip flexor muscles eccentrically contracting when the hip is pushed past its reduced physiologic ROM as a result of the abnormal bony anatomy that occurs in FAI [23]. These types of injuries can almost always be treated conservatively. Proximal hamstring tendinopathy may occur secondary to FAI due to patients developing a compensatory pelvic tilt in order to reduce the occurrence of anterior impingement [23]. Although this is also often treated nonoperatively, up to 20 % of patients will fail conservative treatment, some of which will ultimately require surgical intervention [39]. There currently exists little to no evidence in the literature on the success of simultaneous management of these conditions in patients with FAI.

It should also be mentioned that in certain cases hip impingement may actually have an extra-articular etiology. The most notable cause of extra-articular hip impingement occurs when an abnormal prominence of the anterior inferior iliac spine (AIIS) at the acetabular rim results in decreased available space for soft tissue and ultimately causes impingement during flexion of the hip [25]. In addition to x-ray and/or MRI, an anesthetic injection into the AIIS area can be diagnostic for AIIS impingement. Currently there exists very limited evidence on the management of AIIS impingement. The largest case series to date on this topic is a 163 patient case series which used an arthroscopic method for decompression of the AIIS [24]. This case series showed significant improvement in postoperative MHHS, SF-12, and VAS; however, it is unclear how much of the improvement was attributable to the AIIS decompression as opposed to the simultaneous osteoplasties that were performed for

CAM and/or pincer impingement. Other smaller case series using either an open or arthroscopic method for AIIS decompression also showed positive outcomes across a variety of outcome scores [25, 37, 38, 46]. No complications associated with the AIIS decompression were reported in any of these case series. Although AIIS impingement appears to be the most frequently reported form of extra-articular impingement, there are case reports in the literature of other extra-articular sources of impingement including psoas impingement, ischiofemoral impingement, and greater trochanteric/pelvic impingement [12].

Take-Home Points

1. The literature supports that there exists an association between FAI and some extra-articular hip conditions including athletic pubalgia, osteitis pubis, and internal snapping hip syndrome. In fact the literature states that one in three athletes with chronic groin pain will have more than one pathologic process causing their symptoms.
2. In patients with FAI and an extra-articular pathology, surgically treating only the extra-articular or intra-articular pathology will result in a high likelihood of persistence of symptoms, inability to return to sport, and/or high rates of further surgery.
3. In patients with FAI and extra-articular pathology, treating both sources of pain simultaneously results in outcomes that are satisfactory without increased morbidity. Case series reporting outcomes on surgical outcomes in patients with both FAI and extra-articular pathology generally report low rates of minor complications, and therefore surgical treatment can be considered relatively safe.
4. Some researchers recommend a trial of nonsurgical treatment prior to surgical treatment of athletic pubalgia [4]. However, other studies have found that nonsurgical treatment provides no added benefit relative to placebo [53]. Nonsurgical management of osteitis pubis and internal snapping hip syndrome appears to have more promising outcomes than the results published for athletic pubalgia.
5. There is currently a lack of high-quality studies such as randomized control trials that have been done on patients with both FAI and extra-articular pathology, and therefore the conclusions made from the available literature should be interpreted with caution.

Key Evidence Related Sources

1. de Sa D, Alradwan H, Cargnelli S, Thawer Z, Simunovic N, Cadet E, Bonin N, Larson C, Ayeni OR. Extra-articular hip impingement: a systematic review examining operative treatment of psoas, subspine, ischiofemoral, and greater trochanteric/pelvic impingement. Arthroscopy. 2014;30(8):1026–41.
2. Hammoud S, Bedi A, Magennis E, Meyers WC, Kelly BT. High incidence of athletic pubalgia symptoms in professional athletes with symptomatic FAI. Arthroscopy. 2012;28:1388–95.
3. Hammoud S, Bedi A, Voos JE, Mauro CS, Kelly BT. The recognition and evaluation of patterns of compensatory injury in patients with mechanical hip pain. Sports Health. 2014;6(2):108–18.
4. Khan M, Adamich J, Simunovic N, Philippon MJ, Bhandari M, Ayeni OR. Surgical management of internal snapping hip syndrome: a systematic review evaluating open and arthroscopic approaches. Arthroscopy. 2013;29(5):942–8.
5. Larson CM. Sports hernia/athletic pubalgia: evaluation and management. Sports Health. 2014;6(2):139–44.
6. Matsuda DK, Ribas M, Mastuda NA, Domb BG. Multicenter outcomes of endoscopic pubic symphysectomy for osteitis pubis associated with femoroacetabular impingement. Arthroscopy. 2015;31(7):1255–60.

References

1. Allen WC, Cope R. Coxa saltans: the snapping hip revisited. J Am Acad Orthop Surg. 1995;3(5):303–8.
2. Alpert JM, Kozanek M, Li G, Kelly BT, Asnis PD. Cross-sectional analysis of the iliopsoas tendon and its relationship to the acetabular labrum: an anatomic study. Am J Sports Med. 2009;37(8):1594–8.
3. Ayeni OR, Farrokhyar F, Crouch S, Chan K, Sprague S, Bhandari M. Pre-operative intra-articular hip injection as a predictor of short-term outcome following arthroscopic management of femoroacetabular impingement. Knee Surg Sports Traumatol Arthrosc. 2014;22(4):801–5.
4. Becker LC, Kohlriesser DA. Conservative management of sports hernia in a professional golfer: a case report. Int J Sports Phys Ther. 2014;9(6):851–60.
5. Bitar YF, Stake CE, Dunne KF, Botser IB, Domb BG. Arthroscopic iliopsoas fractional lengthening for internal snapping of the hip: clinical outcomes with a minimum 2-year follow-up. Am J Sports Med. 2014;42(7):1696–703.
6. Brown RA, Mascia A, Kinnear DG, Lacroix V, Feldman L, Mulder DS. An 18-year review of sports groin injuries in the elite hockey player: clinical presentation, new diagnostic imaging, treatment, and results. Clin J Sport Med. 2008;18(3):221–6.
7. Byrd JW. Evaluation and management of the snapping iliopsoas tendon. Instr Course Lect. 2006;55:347–55.
8. Byrd JW. Evaluation of the hip: history and physical examination. N Am J Sports Phys Ther. 2007;2(4):231–40.
9. Cavalli M, Bombini G, Campanelli G. Pubic inguinal pain syndrome: the so-called sports hernia. Surg Technol Int. 2014;24:189–94.
10. Choi H, McCartney M, Best TM. Treatment of osteitis pubis and osteomyelitis of the pubic symphysis in athletes: a systematic review. Br J Sports Med. 2011;45(1):57–64.
11. De Paulis F, Cacchio A, Michelini O, Damiani A, Saggini R. Sports injuries in the pelvis and hip: diagnostic imaging. Eur J Radiol. 1998;27(S1):S49–59.
12. de Sa D, Alradwan H, Cargnelli S, Thawer Z, Simunovic N, Cadet E, Bonin N, Larson C, Ayeni OR. Extra-articular hip impingement: a systematic review examining operative treatment of psoas, subspine, ischiofemoral, and greater trochanteric/pelvic impingement. Arthroscopy. 2014;30(8):1026–41.
13. Dobbs MB, Gordon JE, Luhmann SJ, Syzmanski DA, Schoenecker PL. Surgical correction of the snapping iliopsoas tendon in adolescents. J Bone Joint Surg Am. 2002;84(3):420–4.
14. Domb BG, Shindle MK, McArthur B, Voos JE, Magennis EM, Kelly BT. Iliopsoas impingement: a newly identified cause of labral pathology in the hip. HSS J. 2011;7(2):145–50.
15. Fabricant PD, Bedi A, De La Torre K, Kelly BT. Clinical outcomes after arthroscopic psoas lengthening: the effect of femoral version. Arthroscopy. 2012;28(7):965–71.
16. Fricker PA, Taunton JE, Ammann W. Osteitis pubis in athletes: infection, inflammation or injury? Sports Med. 1991;12(4):266–79.
17. Gentisaris M, Goulimaris I, Sikas N. Laparoscopic repair of groin pain in athletes. Am J Sports Med. 2004;32(5):1238–42.
18. Gilmore J. Groin pain in the soccer athlete: fact, fiction and treatment. Clin Sports Med. 1998;17(4):787–93.
19. Grace JN, Sim FH, Shives TC, Coventry MB. Wedge resection of the symphysis pubis for the treatment of osteitis pubis. J Bone Joint Surg Am. 1989;71(3):358–64.
20. Gruen GS, Scioscia TN, Lowenstein JE. The Surgical Treatment of Internal Snapping Hip. Am J Sports Med. 2002;30(4):607–13.
21. Hackney RG. The sports hernia: a cause of chronic groin pain. Br J Sports Med. 1993;27(1):58–62.
22. Hammoud S, Bedi A, Magennis E, Meyers WC, Kelly BT. High incidence of athletic pubalgia symptoms in professional athletes with symptomatic FAI. Arthroscopy. 2012;28:1388–95.
23. Hammoud S, Bedi A, Voos JE, Mauro CS, Kelly BT. The recognition and evaluation of patterns of compensatory injury in patients with mechanical hip pain. Sports Health. 2014;6(2):108–18.
24. Hapa O, Bedi A, Gursan O, Akar MS, Guvencer M, Haviticioglu H, Larson CM. Anatomic footprint of the direct head of the rectus femoris origin: cadaveric study and clinical series of hips after arthroscopic anterior inferior iliac spine/subspine decompression. Arthroscopy. 2013;29(12):1932–40.
25. Hetsroni I, Poultsides L, Bedi A, Larson CM, Kelly BT. Anterior inferior iliac spine morphology correlates with hip range of motion: a classification system and dynamic model. Clin Orthop Relat Res. 2013;471(8):2497–503.
26. Heyworth BE, Shindle MK, Voos JE, Rudzki JR, Kelly BT. Radiologic and intraoperative findings in revision hip arthroscopy. Arthroscopy. 2007;23(12):1295–302.
27. Hiti C, Stevens K, Jamati M, Garza D, Matheson G. Athletic osteitis pubis. Sports Med. 2011;41(5):361–76.
28. Holmich P. Long-standing groin pain in sportspeople falls into three primary patterns, a "clinical entity" approach: a prospective study of 207 patients. Br J Sports Med. 2007;41(4):247–52.
29. Holt MA, Keene JS, Graf BK, Helwig DC. Treatment of osteitis pubis in athletes. Results of corticosteroid injections. Am J Sports Med. 1995;23(5):601–6.
30. Ilizaliturri Jr VM, Villalobos Jr FE, Chaidez PA, Valero FS, Aguilera JM. Internal snapping hip syndrome: treatment by endoscopic release of the iliopsoas tendon. Arthroscopy. 2005;21(11):1375–80.
31. Ilizaliturri Jr VM, Chaidez C, Vilegas P, Briseno A, Camacho-Galindo J. Prospective randomized study of

2 different techniques for endoscopic iliopsoas tendon release in the treatment of internal snapping hip syndrome. Arthroscopy. 2009;25(2):159–63.
32. Irshad K, Feldman LS, Lavoie C, Lacroix VJ, Mulder DS, Brown RA. Operative management of "hockey groin syndrome": 12 years experience in National Hockey League players. Surgery. 2001;130(4):759–64.
33. Jakoi A, O'Neill C, Damsgaard C, Fehring K, Tom J. Sports hernia in National Hockey League players: does surgery affect performance? Am J Sports Med. 2013;41(1):107–10.
34. Kachingwe AF, Grech S. Proposed algorithm for the management of athletes with athletic pubalgia (sports hernia): a case series. J Ortho Sports Phys Ther. 2008;38(12):768–81.
35. Khan M, Adamich J, Simunovic N, Philippon MJ, Bhandari M, Ayeni OR. Surgical management of internal snapping hip syndrome: a systematic review evaluating open and arthroscopic approaches. Arthroscopy. 2013;29(5):942–8.
36. Larson CM. Sports hernia/athletic pubalgia: evaluation and management. Sports Health. 2014;6(2):139–44.
37. Larson CM, Kelly BT, Stone RM. Making a case for anterior inferior iliac spine/subspine hip impingement: three representative case reports and proposed concept. Arthroscopy. 2011;27(12):1732–7.
38. Larson CM, Pierce BR, Giveans MR. Treatment of athletes with symptomatic intra-articular hip pathology and athletic pubalgia/sports hernia: a case series. Arthroscopy. 2011;27:768–75.
39. Lempainen L, Johansson K, Banke IJ, Ranne J, Makela K, Sarimo J, Niemi P, Orava S. Expert opinion: diagnosis and treatment of proximal hamstring tendinopathy. Muscles Ligaments Tendons J. 2015;5(1):23–8.
40. Macintyre J, Johson C, Schroeder EL. Groin pain in athletes. Curr Sports Med Rep. 2006;5(6):293–9.
41. Matsuda DK, Ribas M, Mastuda NA, Domb BG. Multicenter outcomes of endoscopic pubic symphysectomy for osteitis pubis associated with femoroacetabular impingement. Arthroscopy. 2015;31(7):1255–60.
42. Mehin R, Meek R, O'Brien P, Blachut P. Surgery for osteitis pubis. Can J Surg. 2006;49(3):170–6.
43. Meyers WC, Foley DP, Garret WE, Lohnes JH, Mandlebaum BR. Management of severe lower abdominal or inguinal pain in high-performance athletes. Am J Sports Med. 2000;28(1):2–8.
44. Meyers WC, McKechnie A, Philippon MJ, Horner MA, Zoga AC, Devon O. Experience with "sports hernia" spanning two decades. Ann Surg. 2008;248(4):656–65.
45. Paajanen H, Hermunen H, Karonen J. Pubic magnetic resonance imaging findings in surgically and conservatively treated athletes with osteitis pubis compared to asymptomatic athletes during heavy training. Am J Sports Med. 2008;36(1):117–21.
46. Pan HL, Kawanabe K, Akiyama H, Goto K, Onishi E, Nakamura T. Operative treatment of hip impingement caused by hypertrophy of the anterior inferior iliac spine. J Bone Joint Surg Br. 2008;90-B(5):677–9.
47. Pizzari T, Coburn PT, Crow JF. Prevention and management of osteitis pubis in the Australian Football League: a qualitative analysis. Phys Ther Sport. 2008;9(3):117–25.
48. Radic R, Annear P. Use of pubic symphysis curettage for treatment-resistant osteitis pubis in athletes. Am J Sports Med. 2008;36(1):122–8.
49. Sansone M, Ahlden M, Jonasson P, Thomee R, Falk A, Sward L, Karlsson J. Can hip impingement be mistaken for tendon pain in the groin? A long-term follow-up of tenotomy for groin pain in athletes. Knee Surg Sports Traumatol Arthrosc. 2014;22(4):786–92.
50. Sardana V, Philippon MJ, de Sa D, Bedi A, Ye L, Simunovic N, Ayeni OR. Revision hip arthroscopy indications and outcomes: a systematic review. Arthroscopy. 2015. doi:10.1016/j.arthro.2015.03.039.
51. Sheen AJ, Paajanen H. The next step towards rational treatment for 'The sportsman's groin'. Br J Sports Med. 2015;49(12):764–5.
52. Silvis MI, Mosher TJ, Smetana BS, Chinchilli VM, Flemming DJ, Walker EA, Black KP. High prevalence of pelvic and hip magnetic resonance imaging findings in asymptomatic collegiate and professional hockey players. Am J Sports Med. 2011;39(4):715–21.
53. Swan KG, Wolcott M. The athletic hernia: a systematic review. Clin Orthop Relat Res. 2007;455:78–87.
54. Verrall GM, Slavotinek JP, Fon GT. Incidence of pubic bone marrow edema in Australian rules football players: relation to groin pain. Br J Sports Med. 2011;35(1):28–33.
55. Voos JE, Mauro CS, Kelly BT. Femoroacetabular impingement in the athlete: compensatory injury patterns. Oper Tech Orthop. 2010;20(4):231–6.
56. Winston P, Awan R, Cassidy JD, Bleakney RK. Clinical examination and ultrasound of self-reported snapping hip syndrome in elite ballet dancers. Am J Sports Med. 2007;35(1):118–26.
57. Zoga AC, Kavanagh EC, Omar IM, Morrison WB, Koulouris G, Lopez H, Chaabra A, Domesek J, Meyers WC. Athletic pubalgia and the "sports hernia": MR imaging findings. Radiology. 2008;247(3):797–807.

The Evidence for Rehabilitation After Femoroacetabular Impingement (FAI) Surgery: A Guide to Postsurgical Rehabilitation and Supporting Evidence

16

Darryl Yardley

Contents

D. Yardley, MSc PT (Canada), MClSc, FCAMPT
Clinical Operations and Development, DSD Management, Hamilton, ON, Canada

Hip Preservation Program,
The West End Physiotherapy Clinic,
Hamilton, ON, Canada

Department of Physical Therapy, Faculty of Health Sciences, Western University, London, ON, Canada

Private Practice Division, Canadian Physiotherapy Association, Ottawa, ON, Canada
e-mail: darryl.yardley@gmail.com

16.1 Introduction

The global interest in hip arthroscopy cases and related scientific literature continues to evolve [1–4]. Recent advancements in the understanding of hip biomechanics have led to the development of techniques to correct femoroacetabular impingement (FAI) and repair and/or preserve the labrum during hip arthroscopy. Although considerable attention in the literature is devoted to diagnosis and operative treatment, the information about postoperative rehabilitation and outcomes has been slower to emerge. Thus, the purpose of this chapter is to

O.R. Ayeni et al. (eds.), *Diagnosis and Management of Femoroacetabular Impingement*,
DOI 10.1007/978-3-319-32000-7_16

identify a rehabilitation framework following arthroscopic intervention for FAI. Presently, the rehabilitation protocols available in the literature have minimal support from clinical outcome data [4]. The utilization of validated, patient-reported outcome (PRO) measures should be a key component to guide postoperative management.

16.2 Postoperative Rehabilitation Framework

The framework is developed from the critical appraisal of the available evidence in order to guide clinical practice. Current evidence supports a postoperative period of restricted weight-bearing and mobility restrictions; however, the specific interventions within the postoperative phases are variable with no comparative trials published to date [5]. Understanding the complex relationship among the bony architecture of the acetabulum and femur, the labrum, as well as the proximate soft tissues (i.e., ligaments and muscles) is important to optimize postoperative rehabilitation. Case reports and case series designs (level IV evidence [6]) identify the need to balance the healing properties of tissues, with restoration of hip motion, stabilization of the lumbo-pelvic-hip complex, and reestablishing muscular coordination and balance in the lower extremity and lower kinetic chain. However, existing reports are descriptive in nature; hence the superiority of a particular program cannot be determined. Clinicians require more than "general guidelines" and/or orthopedic surgeon recommendations to augment postoperative clinical outcomes.

Available studies describe successful postoperative outcomes utilizing a four- or five-phase rehabilitation program [4, 5, 7–9, 23, 34]. In order to bridge the gap between clinical practice consensus and evidence, this chapter will outline a five-phase framework for hip arthroscopy rehabilitation based on:

- Healing milestones based on tissue properties and integrity at specific postoperative timelines of recovery [9, 34]
- Recognizing the patient's preoperative health status and activity level, as well as postoperative physical demands and participation levels
- Current best evidence – case reports and case series designs, as well as clinician's expert opinion, and level IV and V evidence, respectively [6] – to identify interventions to address impairments of body function and structure, activity limitations, and participation restrictions associated with the postoperative rehabilitation [10]

16.3 Prehabilitation

Prehabilitation typically refers to improving the functional capacity of a patient to be able to withstand the stressors of pain and inflammation, functional limitations, and participation restrictions associated with a hip arthroscopic procedure. If a patient maintains a higher level of functional ability before a surgery, they may recover more quickly through the rehabilitation process postoperatively [95]. To optimize postoperative timelines to achieve maximal recovery and functional outcomes, it is important to identify and manage pain and any predisposing factors that may contribute to a patient's hip pathology [11].

Griffen et al. [12] described the value and importance of preoperative management for patients preparing for hip arthroscopy. Establishing preoperative baseline functional and PRO measures can aid in a patient's predicted postoperative outcome. The emphasis generally revolves around patient education and pain management. Managing perioperative pain is crucial for the success of hip arthroscopy. There are many pain management strategies, some of the common ones include:

- Education and counseling around activity modification and controlling aggravating factors and avoiding positions (e.g., sitting in low, soft chairs) that create impingement on the joint and lead to intra- and extra-articular pain.
- The utilization of superficial thermal agents (i.e., cryotherapy, heat) and electrical physical agents (i.e., electrical stimulation – transcutaneous

electrical nerve stimulation (TENS)) to aid in pain mitigation. *The contraindications/precautions for electrophysical agents*, Special Issue (62:5) of Physiotherapy Canada by Houghton, Nussbaum, and Hoens, provide further details regarding the appropriate use and application of these electrophysical agents (EPAs) [16].

- Improving gait mechanics with/without assistive devices to reduce compensatory movement strategies that may lead to muscle weakness and inhibition resulting in other pathologies (i.e., tendinopathies, bursitis). Gait training with assistive devices, when used correctly, can reduce the amount of force through the hip joint and reduce intra-articular pain and inflammation.

Patient education related to the arthroscopic procedure, postoperative care and expectations, as well as predicted outcomes, is an important element for the surgical pathway of care. Knowledge around expectations for postoperative restrictions and common pitfalls is necessary to promote postoperative compliance. Understanding the potential benefits of assistive devices can also facilitate postoperative recovery. Collaborating with an occupational therapist (OT) to ensure adaptive equipment is available and in place in the patient's home and/or workplace (i.e., raised toilet seat, grab bars, shower bench, seat cushions, sock aid) can help protect healing tissue and uphold postoperative restrictions.

As the growing body of research on pain science continues to evolve it needs to be acknowledged as an appropriate patient education intervention for those undergoing an arthroscopic procedure. Given the average timeline to diagnosis of FAI has been shown to be up to 3.1 years [96], it would be rational to expect changes in central pain processing and central sensitization. Additionally, psychological and behavioral factors, such as depression, fear-avoidance beliefs, and pain catastrophizing, often require intervention. A patient's familiarity with pain expectations and strategies to best control postoperative pain and inflammation has the potential to reduce the anxiety and threat of those symptoms. Mitigating the threat of pain may allow damaged tissues to heal to the best extent possible in a few weeks or months without any prolongation or chronicity. Thus, evaluation from a modern pain science perspective and patient education from a therapeutic neuroscience approach may lead to superior rehabilitation outcomes [98]. Another probable fear-provoking postoperative symptom that requires education is nerve dysfunction or neuropraxia. Dippmann (2014) demonstrated that 46 % of patients reported symptoms of nerve dysfunction within the first 6 weeks following hip arthroscopy [99]. It is important for patients to understand the nerve injury may be caused from external compression (related to surgical table setup and perineal post) causing ischemia to the nerve and/or the traction time applied during the arthroscopic procedure. Patients need to be aware that this is often a temporary issue; once nerve conduction is restored, recovery is spontaneous within a period of days up to 3 months [3, 17]. In the Dippmann (2014) study, 18 % of patients reported nerve dysfunction at 1 year postoperatively. There are a small proportion of documented cases that do not fully recover. The nerves most commonly affected are the pudendal and sciatic. Pudendal neuralgia is one of the most commonly reported complications following hip arthroscopy [100]. The diagnosis of pudendal neuralgia tends to get overlooked despite patients presenting with perineal hypesthesia and dysesthesia. Pailhé (2013) demonstrated that the incidence of pudendal neuralgia is two percent, which was previously underestimated in the literature [100].

To improve a patient's functional capacity preoperatively, it is advised that clinicians assess movement patterns to reduce compensatory strategies that lead to joint pain [18]. Interventions to address altered motor control strategies in the lumbo-pelvic-hip region, hip-muscle weakness and inhibition, imbalances in the lower kinetic chain, and postural malalignment must be addressed cautiously [11]. Preoperative teaching of correct gait mechanics using assisted devices (i.e., crutches) within the prescribed postoperative weight-bearing restrictions can help eliminate persistent pain-avoidance strategies. Also, teaching appropriateness and correct execution of postoperative exercises may help improve neuromuscular efficiency to induce compensatory changes in muscle activation patterns and facilitate early functional stability [19]. It is essential that a patient be aware of the timely commencement for postoperative rehabilitation to maximize his/her recovery.

One of the most beneficial components of prehabilitation is the formation of a patient's support network. In addition to family and friends, establishing a rehabilitation team is of critical importance. In particular, research on the therapeutic alliance acknowledges the importance of a positive interpersonal relationship between a clinician and patient and recognizes this to be an essential component of patient-centered care [13, 14]. Building trust and establishing an emotional bond with a patient are critical dimensions of the therapeutic alliance that lead to therapeutic progress [15]. Recent evidence supports the theory that biopsychosocial factors, especially the therapeutic alliance, may account for up to 60 % of a clinical outcome [14]. The findings of this study suggest that the alliance between patient and clinician positively correlates with clinical outcomes for individuals in physical rehabilitation settings, including treatment adherence and treatment satisfaction [14]. Failing to acknowledge the importance of the therapeutic alliance and the need to understand the patient's goals can interfere with clinical outcomes.

16.4 Phase I: Maximum Protection (Day 1–3 Weeks)

Phase I overview: the primary rehabilitation goals are (1) to reduce postoperative pain and inflammation, (2) limit the stress to the femoral neck and labrum (if repaired/reconstructed), and (3) protect the integrity of the soft tissues, in particular the capsule. The secondary focus is to commence restoration of uniplanar range of motion (ROM) and normalization of gait with an assistive device.

Systematic review of the literature states hip arthroscopy has an overall complication rate around four percent. There is a very low rate of major complications such as dislocation, fracture, infection, and avascular necrosis [24]. Nevertheless, a hip arthroscopic procedure requires that clinicians take into consideration the excision of the anterior capsule (capsulotomy), osteochondroplasty to remove the bony abnormality, and the location of the labral tear (if present and repaired/reconstructed). Appropriate healing of a labral repair/reconstruction can restore multiple aspects of hip mechanics, including regulation of synovial fluid flow, maintenance of a suction seal and joint stability, proprioception, and force transmission to the articular cartilage [8, 26–29]. The hip fluid seal, in addition to regulating intra-articular fluid pressurization, contributes to hip stability. Evidence supports that labral repair and reconstruction improves distractive stability at small displacements and reduces micro-instability within the hip joint. Additionally, the capsule contributes to the suction effect by providing distractive stability at larger displacement forces [97]. As a clinician, being aware of capsular and/or labral alterations during FAI surgery is imperative to know which interventions to apply versus avoid early into the rehabilitation process to enable the restoration of stability and function. This phase also requires significant patient education to uphold postoperative restrictions in weight bearing, ROM, and muscle activation to avoid the many possible pitfalls.

The utilization of weight-bearing restrictions is critical to reduce the risk of fracture [3, 25] and to optimize healing of the labral repair/reconstruction (if applicable) [20]. Osteochondroplasty (resection of the bone) of the femoral head-neck junction for a CAM impingement and/or acetabular rim for pincer FAI warrants protection to prevent a femoral neck fracture or stress fracture. Commonly, a labral repair accompanies FAI surgery and also requires load protection [4]. The most common documented area of labral tears occurs in the anterior-superior region, which bears the most loads and experiences the greatest shear forces [8]. Without appropriate load restrictions, inflammation will linger and delay tissue healing, which may negatively impact later phases of the rehabilitation process. The majority of patients are prescribed protected weight bearing with underarm crutches postoperatively [4, 5, 7–9, 21–23, 34]. The percentage of protected weight bearing is variable throughout the literature. Weight-bearing status tends to be dependent on the surgeon's orders and, if additional considerations occur at the time of surgery, related to the extent of the procedure and the healing timelines for the involved tissues (i.e., bone, cartilage, labrum). Patients and clinicians need to adhere to the suggested weight-bearing guidelines and be instructed to progress gradually, in collaboration with the treating surgeon. Typically, patients will be instructed to apply 10 kg (approximately 22 lb) of load onto the surgical extremity during phase I [9, 22, 34]. Additionally, throughout gait retraining it is important that the patient initiates flat-foot contact with the surgical limb. Avoiding toe-touch weight bearing may decrease iliopsoas irritation by reducing sustained hip flexion [8]. Clinicians must ensure gait training with the appropriate assistive device on level surfaces, as well as stairs are addressed with the patient.

The capsulotomy is used to improve visualization and instrument maneuverability [3] during hip arthroscopy by many surgeons, and its integrity should be protected throughout early postoperative rehabilitation. Pushing a patient through painful ROM and/or end-range stretching can result in capsular laxity and hypermobility [5]. Focal laxity most commonly occurs as anterior capsular laxity secondary to repetitive movements involving hip external rotation and/or extension, possibly resulting in iliofemoral ligament insufficiency [30]. Thus, ROM restrictions have been implemented to allow the capsule appropriate healing. Additionally, adhering to these ROM restrictions reduces stresses (i.e., compressive and shear) to the labrum, which can reduce the likelihood of failure of the labral repair and/or reconstruction [31, 101]. Hip ROM is addressed in all three planes of motion within the following limitations: anecdotally extension within 0–10°, external rotation under 10° [4], abduction under 25° [31], and flexion less than 90°. Clinicians must avoid combined movements at this stage, especially *extension-abduction-external rotation* due to the associated risk of dislocation. With regard to flexion, Sink et al. (2010) demonstrated that the anterior-superior cartilage damage coincided with the area of FAI when the hip was positioned into flexion and internal rotation [32], hence another reason to avoid combined movements of the hip during this phase. Upholding these ROM restrictions will help reestablish the passive structures [33] and avoid hypermobility/instability later on in the recovery process. Panjabi (1992) presented the conceptual basis of a stabilizing system in the spine through three subsystems: (1) passive, (2) active, and (3) neural. The passive subsystem he affirmed can be extrapolated to the bones, capsules, and ligaments of the hip joint. Restoration of passive stability is important, as there are documented cases of over-resection of the bone from the acetabular rim for pincer FAI that may also predispose the hip to structural instability [25].

Other factors that may influence the protection phase of the rehabilitation protocol include whether a capsular repair occurred, microfracture procedure was performed, psoas tendon was released, or biological solutions [3] were introduced into the joint. Some surgeons advocate for the utilization of a rigid, postoperative hip brace that is combined with crutches for ambulation. When prescribed, it is often used for additional protection of the repair and to preserve ROM restrictions [23]. Communication with the surgeon and the rehabilitation team becomes of utmost importance to ensure that the appropriate restrictions are applied in each individual case [4]. Poor verbal or nonverbal communication between the primary clinician and the surgeon is a major link to postoperative pitfalls and likely suboptimal patient clinical outcomes.

16.4.1 Recommended Interventions

16.4.1.1 Manual Therapy

The clinician, within the patient's pain tolerance, can commence a series of passive ROM immediately postoperatively. These physiological movements must not bring the range to a point beyond the above noted restrictions. Restoring internal rotation before external rotation [22] due to ROM limitations can reduce the incidence of intra-articular adhesions [32]. Additionally, the utilization of gentle circumduction [7, 23, 34] ROM for the hip joint in this early phase of the rehabilitation process has evidence to support favorable outcomes [7, 8, 23, 34, 35]. Both strategies, especially circumduction [37], are integral to reduce postoperative adhesions (fibrosis). These adhesions, if formed, can result in ongoing pain and dysfunction, which has a negative impact on recovery and may be an associated cause of revision surgery [36, 37].

16.4.1.2 Therapeutic Exercise

Early controlled mobility can begin through the use of a stationary bike. Gentle motion through the joint can facilitate joint lubrication [38]. The patient should be limited to an upright frame with an adjustable seat that prevents the hip from flexing beyond 90°. If any stress (soreness) is experienced in the hip flexors, adjust the pedaling to a pendular motion and ensure the contralateral side is being used to assist [34]. There should be no resistance during this phase, and the patient may progress as tolerated for 20 minutes up to two sessions per day [34, 39].

The patient, within his/her pain tolerance, can commence a series of active assisted exercises. There is caution not to push the range of motion to a point of discomfort either with exercise or in daily activities. Some case series and surgeon protocols recommended the use of a continuous passive motion (CPM™) unit immediately postoperatively to facilitate a gradual restoration of hip flexion and to limit intra-articular adhesions. There are no strict guidelines for its use; commonly documented surgeon preferences are 4–8 hours per day, for up to 6 weeks postoperatively. Performing a hip pendulum within a small arc of motion of the hip joint may be a suitable exercise to endure the benefits of hip circumduction at home. In order to prevent a flexion contracture, and begin to restore hip extension, the patient is encouraged to lie prone (on the stomach) for at least 2 hours per day [23, 31]. This can be progressed to include a gentle lengthening of rectus femoris via adding knee flexion (heel to bum); subsequently a modified Thomas position over the side of the bed can be utilized.

Patients must participate in therapeutic exercises to reestablish postural awareness for a neutral lumbar spine. Once established, retraining the motor control of the lumbo-pelvic stabilizers is important in this first phase. Lumbo-pelvic stabilization refers to the inner unit, which is comprised of the pelvic floor muscles, transversus abdominis, multifidi, and the diaphragm [40]. An increasingly common approach used within the management of low back pain has been low-load, high-repetition training of the abdominal and trunk muscles (stabilizers), to improve the control and activation of the back and abdominal muscles [49].

Clinicians must consider the degree of neuropraxia that results from irritation of the neurovascular structures within the lumbo-pelvic-hip complex from the sustained traction of the procedure or from the external compression from the surgical setup [3]. A neuropraxia results in decreased motor unit recruitment [45]. The effect of dysfunction must be taken into account when considering strengthening exercises due to the altered connection between the neurological system (in particular the brain) and targeted muscles [45]. Albeit some case studies initiate isometric exercises for the quadriceps and gluteal muscles during this phase, strengthening is generally delayed until neuropraxia subsides [4, 34].

16.4.1.3 Electrophysical Agents (EPAs)

It is important to manage the pain *and* inflammatory consequences of a hip arthroscopy procedure. The most commonly applied intervention to address both impairments is cryotherapy. While the research continues to evolve, there is good evidence for the utilization of cryotherapy in situations of inflammation and pain [41]. Another (*preferred*) option is the combination of cold *and* compression units, such as the Cryo/Cuff or Game Ready™ [42]. This type of unit provides both cold and compression simultaneously and has been shown to be both safe and effective [43, 44]. Anytime clinicians integrate EPAs into a treatment plan, clinical judgment must be used to determine how to "titrate the dose" specific to the depth of the tissue and clear any contraindications and precautions [16] for patient safety.

16.4.1.4 Patient Education

A patient's overall health behaviors and recovery can be significantly improved depending on the process by which a clinician imparts information to patients and their support network (i.e., family members). Comprehension of the arthroscopic procedure and compliance with postoperative restrictions are crucial to avoiding known pitfalls in recovery. Restrictions such as avoiding prolonged sitting on low soft surfaces, not pivoting on or actively lifting the surgical limb, avoiding sit-ups, crossing the legs, and walking for exercise must be understood. As well, maintaining appropriate bed mobility, safe positioning, and hygiene of incisions can greatly impact postoperative recovery [34]. Patients must be mindful that rehabilitation programs should not reproduce pain and exacerbate their symptoms. It is critical that clinicians emphasize the importance of not irritating the hip flexors (i.e., psoas major and rectus femoris) during activities of daily living (ADLs) and prescribed exercises to reduce the risk of developing tendinopathy [30].

16.5 Phase II: Mobility and Neuromuscular Retraining (3–6 Weeks)

Phase II overview: the primary rehabilitation goals are to (1) restore uniplanar ROM, (2) restore lumbo-pelvic core stability, (3) reestablish neuromuscular control, and (4) normalize gait with an assistive device. The clinician should continue to focus on (1) limiting the stress to the femoral neck, (2) reducing postoperative pain and inflammation, and (3) protecting the integrity of the soft tissues, in particular, the capsule and labrum (if repaired).

Phase II is centered on restoring mobility of the hip joint with a moderate focus on protection given that the majority of restrictions are supported throughout this phase. With the understanding that each phase in the rehabilitation process builds upon the previous, clinicians must continue to respect the ROM restrictions associated with the capsulotomy and labral repair (if applicable). The aim is to progressively regain 80 % of full ROM by the end of this phase [34]. Gaining mobility too slowly may result in residual stiffness and intra-articular adhesions, which can result in unnecessary load and shear forces applied within the joint and delay recovery. Conversely, pushing a patient through painful ROM and/or aggressive end-range stretching of the hip capsule (especially anterior) may result in hypermobility or micro-instability [5]. Simultaneously, the need to reduce muscle inhibition through isolated muscle activation in order to regain correct neuromuscular control is a fundamental element [23]. Normalization of gait with the appropriate assistive device, while respecting the healing process, is critical at this phase to restore movement patterns and load transfer. Lastly, patient compliance with restrictions and activity modifications remains important throughout this phase.

Following a hip arthroscopic procedure, simply restoring mechanical restraints is not enough for a functional recovery of the hip. Neuromuscular training enhances unconscious motor responses by stimulating both afferent signals and central mechanisms responsible for static and dynamic joint stability [46]. A lag in the neuromuscular reaction time can result in dynamic joint instability with recurrent episodes of joint deterioration and possible subluxation. Information about the position and movement of the hip comes from the mechanoreceptors located in and around the articular tissues. Disruption to the mechanoreceptors creates an inhibitory effect on the normal neuromuscular system. The objectives of neuromuscular retraining following FAI surgery are to improve the central nervous system's (CNS) ability to generate and relearn optimal muscle-firing patterns, diminish movement coordination impairments, and achieve a state of readiness in the muscles to manage joint forces that results in enhanced motor control and dynamic joint stability [46, 47, 50, 55]. Another goal is to obtain equilibrium of loaded segments in static and dynamic situations and acquire postural control in situations resembling conditions of daily life and more strenuous activities [19]. It is important to appreciate the focus in this phase on neuromuscular training versus strength training, which focuses on increasing motor output. Neuromuscular training aims principally at improving quality and efficiency of movements [19]. Meaningful repetition of the retraining movements over time is necessary to cause lasting change [48]. Hence, neuromuscular control will prime the system for strengthening in phase III. Placing emphasis on strengthening before restoration of mobility and neuromuscular control often leads to compensatory movement patterns that precipitate soft tissue irritation (i.e., tendinopathy, bursitis).

16.5.1 Recommended Interventions

16.5.1.1 Manual Therapy

Passive physiological movements must not bring the ROM into pain reproduction, or to a degree beyond the prescribed restrictions. Hip ROM continues to be addressed in all three planes of motion within altered limitations: extension to 15°, external rotation under 20° [4], and no combined extension-abduction-external rotation until the end of phase II. Hip flexion can be increased to 120 degrees (at discretion of surgeon) and internal rotation can be fully restored throughout the sagittal plane.

Clinicians can select from multiple techniques to restore the mobility of the hip joint: passive physiological ROM, joint mobilizations, Mobilizations with Movement (MWM), and Muscle Energy Techniques (METs). Passive techniques need to remain within R2 (range into mild resistance) [60], pain-free, and isolated to the hip joint to avoid excessive strain on the lumbar spine and sacroiliac joints. It is important to note that mobilization of the joint capsule without definitive clinical findings (i.e., early capsular end-feel) and reasoning may be detrimental to the patient's recovery [34]. The preferred methods of manual techniques that build upon passive ROM are MWM and METs. Through biomechanical and neurophysiological effects, MWM can attain hip centeredness/centration [53] to improve and maintain pain-free hip mobility. Joint centration may enable the neurological system to normalize muscle tone around the hip complex and optimize movement efficiency and reduce the likelihood of soft tissue impingement. Gains in hip mobility using METs may be attributed to the nature of proprioceptive neuromuscular facilitation (PNF) exercises, which are primarily designed to maximize improvements in mobility. These techniques utilize the neuromuscular system's inhibitory reflexes to improve muscular relaxation and greater stretch magnitude [51]. Regardless of chosen manual technique, the common pitfall is inappropriate dosing and aggressiveness applied to the healing (soft) tissues.

Myofascial (*aka* soft tissue) mobilization is commonly integrated into this phase to manage and alter the increased postoperative muscle tone that develops. The primary areas of focus are the adductor group, tensor fascia lata, and rectus femoris. Clinically, it appears while other pelvic and hip stabilizers are inhibited due to pain and/or neuromuscular dysfunction, the adductors are often the first muscle group to compensate. Research has demonstrated that the adductor longus acts as a hip flexor and the adductor magnus acts as a hip extensor [52]. Following hip arthroscopy, the psoas muscle is often inhibited. Clinically, the tensor fascia lata and rectus femoris are superficial hip flexors, which tend to compensate for the lack of function of the psoas and become overused and irritated throughout the postoperative rehabilitation process [34]. These muscles in addition to the gluteus medius and minimus, piriformis, quadratus lumborum, and paraspinals all benefit from myofascial mobilization to reduce tone throughout the rehabilitation process. Scar tissue at the portal sites requires special attention to restore full hip mobility. The degree of myofascial mobilization that has been identified to aid in a patient's postoperative recovery can benefit from concurrent treatment in an interprofessional model of care (i.e., registered massage therapist).

There is limited evidence to looking specifically at rhythmic stabilization in the hip. However, there is strong evidence to support its benefit in the shoulder and lower back pain literature [50, 51, 54]. An adjunct to the implementation of specific interventions that restore neuromuscular control during this phase of rehabilitation can be rhythmic stabilization and reciprocal submaximal isometric muscle contractions of the deep internal and external rotators of the hips [54, 61]. Additionally, PNF is used with rhythmic stabilization and slow reversal holds to reestablish proprioception and dynamic stabilization of the hip joint. The main objective is to enable the unconscious process of interpreting and integrating the peripheral sensations received by the CNS into appropriate motor responses [50]. These drills are to facilitate appropriate agonist/antagonist muscle cocontractions. Efficient coactivation assists in restoring muscle balance around the hip, thus enhancing joint congruency and joint compression [54]. Research indicates a significant increase in joint ROM, as well as dynamic and static muscle endurance following concentrated rhythmic stabilization training [51]. Rhythmic stabilization exercises in the open-chain position can encourage cocontraction of the musculature about the hip, providing a foundation for dynamic neuromuscular stabilization. Initially, these drills should focus on all three anatomical planes of motion of the hip joint, although avoiding the sagittal plane (due to hip flexor irritation) until the end of the phase, as long as the technique is pain-free [30].

16.5.1.2 Therapeutic Exercise

Continued use of a stationary bike to facilitate lubrication and nutrients via the synovial fluid is recommended [38]. The patient remains limited to an upright frame with an adjustable seat that prevents the hip from flexing beyond 90°. Progressing to mild resistance toward the end of this phase can occur as long as no stress is experienced in the hip flexors. The duration may progress as tolerated for 30 min up to two sessions per day [34, 39]. For those patients who are prescribed a CPM and continue to use it into phase II, generally have their daily usage reduced as the duration on the bike increases.

The patient will progress the series of active assisted exercises into stretching/self-mobilization to restore the ROM of the hip joint. It is important that these stretches address capsular and soft tissue end-feels [47] within the prescribed restrictions. The emphasis is placed on hip flexor and adductor stretching to avoid myotendinous inflammation and intra-articular adhesions [8]. There is caution not to push the stretches to a point of pain and to target thc hip joint specifically. At this phase, introducing strategies to perform ROM exercises of pelvis-on-femur rotation (pelvic dissociation) needs to accompany femur-in-pelvis rotation in all three planes of motion [31]. Common exercises are performed in supine, prone, half-kneel, and quadruped positions to address the ROM goals. Implementation of a foam roller regimen for self-myofascial mobilization to improve tissue extensibility and reduce muscle tone is often introduced in the later portion of this phase to augment ROM exercises. There is also level V evidence that a foam roller can increase muscle activation, which may have a positive impact on normalizing movement patterns and motor control around the hip joint [56].

Neuromuscular retraining exercises prescribed will have emphasis put on the efficiency and quality of each movement [19]. The emphasis needs to be placed on the ability of the CNS to properly recruit the correct muscles to produce and reduce force, as well as dynamically stabilize the body's structure in all three planes of motion. The introduction of active ROM exercises at the hip joint (single plane) and in movement synergies of all joints in the surgical limb is to be performed within the correct movement pattern and with acceptable muscle coordination [47]. These exercises may begin gravity-eliminated and progress to against-gravity providing they do not exacerbate symptoms. Again, hip flexion is to be avoided until later in this phase due to the low threshold for irritation [30, 34]. In a small percentage of patients, active external rotation may be avoided up to 6 weeks to avoid tone and spasm of the obturator internus muscle in cases of exacerbation of pelvic girdle pain [57]. Additionally, optimization of neuromuscular control, based on biomechanical and neuromuscular principles, aims to improve sensorimotor control and achieve compensatory functional stability. Using sensorimotor exercises for balance and proprioception to drive muscle activation patterns can be initiated at this stage as long as weight-bearing restrictions are maintained. Improving load transfer onto the surgical limb through weight shifting with assisted devices (e.g., side-side, front-back, diagonal patterns) is a critical step for normalizing gait.

With the introduction of neuromuscular training, the clinician must be monitoring the kinesthetic input and quality of the movement patterns and not simply counting the number of sets and repetitions [50]. Clinicians too often feel compelled to progress patients by giving them "new" exercises at each therapy session. It cannot be stressed enough that it is not beneficial to prescribe exercises that patients do not have the proprioceptive ability to perform. It is important to observe the quality of an exercise or movement. Proprioceptive deficits, fatigue, and/or weaknesses in specific muscles can lead to compensatory and faulty movement patterns. Faulty patterns are then integrated into unconscious motor programs that perpetuate preoperative dysfunction. More specifically, a faulty firing pattern of the gluteal muscles reduces their stabilization capabilities at the hip joint and potentially allows for excessive anterior translation and levering of the femoral head during hip extension. If these patterns are not corrected early, any joint and tissue structures along the lower kinetic chain [63] become susceptible to injury or irritation (i.e., tendinopathies, bursitis, micro-instability). Therefore, clinical reasoning and judgment must be applied to reeducate firing patterns prior to initiating any strengthening and/or dynamic and loaded activity.

Emphasizing lumbo-pelvic stabilization continues simultaneously with the addition of neuromuscular retraining. Once the sequencing and timing of the inner unit have been achieved, progressive exercises to strengthen the core can begin. Furthermore, incorporating progressive loading exercises (i.e., quadruped positions, bridging) to challenge rotational stability (transverse motion plane) is endorsed [4, 34]. A thorough assessment of the lumbo-pelvic region is necessary and will need to be continually monitored throughout phase III as the rehabilitation is concentrated around the twenty-seven muscles acting upon the hip joint [64]. A stable core is required for the primary movers and stabilizers of the hip and lower extremity to function optimally [59]. Anecdotally, inadequate stability and faulty movement patterns contribute to hip flexor dysfunction and persistent tendinopathy. If a patient continues to demonstrate clinical signs and symptoms of a dysfunctional core by the end of phase II, collaboration with a pelvic health physical therapist (PT) can be effective in preparing the patient for phase III success. Pelvic health PTs are trained to perform intravaginal and intrarectal digital assessments with patients of all genders in order to determine the relative strength and tone of the different pelvic floor muscles. Patients with inadequate core function would benefit from confirmation of proper performance of Kegel exercises through digital internal examination or biofeedback [77]. This way of assessment and treatment makes it possible to assign specific interventions and protocols to address individual muscle imbalances.

Normalization of gait is an essential focus in this phase. Patients and clinicians need to adhere to the suggested weight-bearing guidelines that typically get increased to 50 % load onto the surgical limb by 4 weeks postoperatively, anecdotally. It is important that clinicians ensure gait training occurs with the appropriate assistive device on level surfaces with correct mechanics at foot contact, weight acceptance (load transfer), functional extension, and a progressive swing phase. Inappropriate use of assistive devices and amplified weight-bearing status increases the patient's risk for complication (i.e., tendinitis, fracture, failed repair/reconstruction). The use of hydrotherapy in retraining gait and weight acceptance is very effective once the incisions are healed [31, 34]. Additionally, the AlterG™ (antigravity treadmill) can be introduced by approximately week four postoperatively to restore gait mechanics through controlled loading that preserves the weight-bearing restrictions. There is level V evidence that the AlterG is an effective modality for achieving earlier functional recovery in level overground gait and may supplement cardiovascular training [58].

Orthopedic surgeons tend to remove weight-bearing restrictions by 6 weeks postoperatively and prescribe weight bearing as tolerated. Thus, by the end of this phase, the requirements for a normalized gait are to have no notable Trendelenburg or modified Trendelenburg sign, full hip extension from mid-stance to toe off, and normal progression of the extremity through swing phase such that the lumbo-pelvic complex is not rotating in the transverse plane to facilitate lower extremity advancement [34].

16.5.1.3 Electrophysical Agents (EPAs)

It is important to continue managing the pain *and* inflammatory consequences from the arthroscopic procedure through the application of cryotherapy or Cryo/Cuff. At this stage some clinicians support the use of electrical stimulation (*e*-stim) for pain relief (TENS) and/or muscle reeducation (neuromuscular electrical stimulation (NMES)). With the inclusion of *e*-stim, clinicians once again must use their skills in clinical reasoning to determine how to "titrate the dose," apply the current for maximal therapeutic benefit, and clear any contraindications and precautions [16] for patient safety.

16.5.1.4 Patient Education

It is important to continue to educate patients on the arthroscopic procedure, postoperative care and restrictions, healing expectations, activity modifications, and positioning [34]. Comprehension and compliance of postoperative restrictions are crucial to facilitate the recovery process and avoid common pitfalls, especially when patients often feel ahead of the recovery process and the current status of their healing tissues in phase II. Patients need to be reminded that their rehabilitation program should not reproduce pain and exacerbate their symptoms. Early excessive activity and rapid progressions of rehabilitation intensity can delay the recovery process.

16.6 Phase III: Muscle Balance and Strengthening (6–12 Weeks)

Phase III overview: the primary rehabilitation goals are to (1) restore full hip ROM, (2) reestablish muscle balance through neuromuscular control and muscle strengthening, (3) optimize proprioception, (4) demonstrate dynamic lumbo-pelvic stability during low-demand exercises, and (5) normalize gait without an assistive device. The clinician should continue to monitor (1) pain and inflammation; (2) the integrity of soft tissues, in particular, the hip flexors, capsule, and labrum (if repaired/reconstructed); and (3) patient adherence to activity modification guidelines.

This phase is based on minimal protection of the surgical procedure. In the majority of cases, patients have their restrictions removed by the beginning of phase III following their postoperative appointment with the surgeon. Endorsement to restore full return of ROM hrough the inclusion of combined hip movements, plus the appropriate weaning of assistive devices to restore loading forces and normalize gait. Thus, it is important in this phase to monitor the pain score of the patient during ADLs. Patients should regain function and independence in ADLs without discomfort by the completion of this phase [34].

Following a hip arthroscopic procedure, restoring muscle balance requires three components: (1) adequate muscle length-tension relationships, (2) appropriate muscle recruitment via subconscious neuromotor pathways, and (3) optimal muscle power and endurance. Adequate stability and motor control of the lumbo-pelvic girdle in low-demand weight-bearing activities are important to restore surgical limb loading and normalize gait cycle early within this phase. Additionally, clinical expertise suggests that Manual Muscle Test (MMT) grading of greater than or equal to 4/5 should be achieved for all hip girdle musculature by the end of this phase. Strength impairments of the trunk, hip, and lower extremity identified through clinical reasoning should be addressed by the commencement of this phase. It is recommended that any asymmetrical muscle weakness be addressed with a strengthening program for the specific weakened individual muscle and/or muscle group. Strength and endurance exercises should build upon the activation improvements of the deep glutei and hip rotators from phase II. However, clinicians must ensure that the patient can actively perform the correct movement pattern within an adequate arc of motion, as well as demonstrate correct firing patterns and timing prior to adding resistance exercises. Following an osteochondroplasty, patients likely have an increase in physiological internal/external arc of motion (particularly in flexion), as well as an increase in abduction range. Clinically, these increases in range of motion seem to be dependent on patient age. Thus, it is important to enhance the activation and strength of the deep hip rotators to control the greater ROM.

16.6.1 Recommended Interventions

16.6.1.1 Manual Therapy

As in phase II, clinicians can select from multiple techniques to restore the mobility of the hip joint: passive physiological ROM, joint mobilizations, MWM, and METs. Even though the goal in this phase is to restore full combined (tri-planar) ROM, the passive techniques must still be within R2 [60], remain pain-free, and isolated to the hip joint to avoid excessive strain on the joints above and below the hip. The principle of joint centration is still encouraged to optimize joint congruency and establish normalized muscle tone around the joint to avoid any soft tissue impingement. Progressive myofascial mobilization techniques are utilized in this phase to address hypertonicity and/or shortening of the myofascial system, as well as adverse tension in the neural system. Addressing muscle groups and fascial planes that are limiting tri-planar movement patterns requires attention and appropriate dosing to restore full hip mobility. It is important to address myofascial restrictions right at the end ranges of motion. Common interventions in the rehabilitation environment include clinician applied hands-on techniques (i.e., ART®, Soft Tissue Release) and/or instrument-assisted tissue release techniques. Furthermore, interprofessional collaboration with other rehabilitation providers (i.e., registered massage therapist, chiropractors) remains important during this phase to address myofascial limitations. Anecdotally, addressing the myofascial limitations prior to any residual capsular tightness tends to facilitate recovery. It is important to repeat that mobilizing the joint capsule without conclusive clinical (arthrokinematic and/or capsular) findings and reasoning may be detrimental to a patient's recovery [34].

16.6.1.2 Therapeutic Exercise

Patients often continue the use of a stationary bike and progress the resistance and duration as able, but need to continue to monitor overload of the hip flexors. Patients are deconditioned secondary to preoperative activity modifications, the arthroscopic procedure, and decreased activity levels due to surgical restrictions and pain. Cardiorespiratory/aerobic conditioning is required to promote optimal health and wellness [47]. Other activities that enable aerobic conditioning with limited stress to the hip joint postoperatively include swimming, AlterG®, and elliptical trainer. It is recommended that the treadmill be reserved due to the change in gait mechanics (e.g., stride length) often associated with the dismissal of an assistive device. Premature integration of treadmill walking can intensify loads on the hip musculature and cause uneven force distribution across the joint surface. Uneven force distribution over the articular cartilage surfaces and labrum may lead to the advancement of articular cartilage degeneration and/or a failed labral repair/reconstruction [8, 31].

The patient will progress their series of stretching/self-mobilization exercises to address the tri-planar movements of the hip, but must avoid causing (soft tissue) impingement and pain. End-range stretching/self-mobilization is emphasized in both flexion and extension quadrants of the hip. Continuing to incorporate strategies to perform ROM exercises of pelvis-on-femur and femur-in-pelvis is important to address intra-articular/capsular adhesions and myofascial limitations [31]. However, at this stage it is important for the clinician to reason through passive ROM and corresponding end-feels (soft tissue versus capsular) [47] and length-tension relationships to determine appropriate mobility exercises. When analyzing the length-tension relationship of muscles, truly shortened presentations require direct stretching, as compared to a hypertonic status that requires modulation through muscle balancing efforts via strength and endurance retraining. At this stage, it is common to see a muscular imbalance around the pelvic girdle among the hip flexors, adductors, glutei, erector spinae, and abdominals [31]. A systematic foam roller (pre-exercise) regimen or other myofascial release equipment can improve extensibility and alter muscle tone to enhance the effectiveness of ROM exercises. Educating and teaching patients to apply *self*-myofascial release and mobilization exercises at home is fundamental for sustaining the manual therapy treatments clinicians apply.

Progressive exercises emphasizing dynamic lumbo-pelvic stabilization and motor control continue concurrently. The addition of full weight-bearing and functional (i.e., sit-to-stand, ¼ squat) exercises to challenge core stability is endorsed now that weight-bearing restrictions are removed [4, 34]. Concentrating on optimizing the neuromuscular control of the lumbo-pelvic-hip complex can improve sensorimotor control. Using sensorimotor exercises for balance and proprioception to drive muscle activation patterns can now be performed in full weight-bearing positions. Proprioceptive exercises (*without assisted devices*) in bilateral stance are initiated and typically progressed from closed kinetic chain (CKC) supported to unsupported (e.g., balance mats, wobble board, trampoline) with minimal capsular stress [34, 37]. A common pitfall during this phase is a rapid progression of weight-bearing exercise volume and intensity. Patients must be able to effectively "load transfer" onto their surgical extremity before any unilateral stance exercises can be prescribed and practiced.

Neuromuscular retraining exercises are continued and advanced to focus on the timing and coordination of active movements throughout (*full*) available ROM [47]. The timing of gluteal muscle function must repeatedly be reassessed and addressed throughout the rehabilitation process. Although 6 weeks postoperatively seems quite long to commence resisted exercises, clinicians must remember that patients cannot strengthen a muscle that their brain (CNS) cannot effectively activate. Hence, training muscle "activation" must come before strengthening, which is why phase III is designed to build upon the primary goals of phase II. Furthermore, enhancing the timing of cocontraction of the core muscles can aid in restoring optimal function of the primary movers and stabilizers of the hip. Anecdotally, having core musculature that fires automatically and efficiently leads to faster gains in hip strength [59]. Monitoring the quality of isokinetic strengthening exercises is once again critical to ensure fatigue and/or weaknesses in specific muscles do not lead to faulty movement patterns and subsequent injury or irritation in the lumbo-pelvic-hip complex and lower extremity (particularly around the knee).

Low-level evidence exists for rehabilitation programs focusing on *hip rotation* to address the weakness and/or inhibition of the deep glutei (gluteus medius and gluteus minimus) and short external rotators [61, 62]. It is necessary to dedicate time to the deep glutei, as their primary role is to assist with stabilizing the femoral head in the acetabulum and abduction on the weight-bearing side during gait [65]. Open kinetic chain (OKC) strength training of the deep internal and external rotators should concentrate on low resistance and high repetitions [4, 62]. More specifically, moderate electromyographic (EMG) activity of 21–40 % maximal voluntary isometric contraction (MVIC) is best used to facilitate neuromuscular reeducation and endurance, compared to a higher activation of 41–60^{+} percentage MVIC used to facilitate strength gains [102, 103]. Technique is critical for gaining maximum benefit from this rotational program. For instance, maximal-effort hip internal rotation torque increases when the hip is flexed more than 60° as compared to a neutral position [61]. Clinically, it is recommended that the rotational exercise be performed daily until the end of phase III [62]. In cases where a labral repair accompanies an FAI procedure, evidence supports the need for the stabilization capability of the hip internal and external rotators to compensate for the loss of passive rotational stability and impaired hip fluid seal [18]. As neuromuscular improvements and endurance are gained in the OKC, the clinician may challenge the patient with stronger resistance bands/weights, transition from slow to faster speeds, simple to complex coordination of tasks, and gradual to sudden challenges with perturbations. Once the timing and coordination of the deep glutei have improved and OKC internal rotation and external rotation MMTs are adequate bilaterally, additional hip stabilization and gluteal strengthening exercises can be integrated. Additional strengthening exercises include progressions into weight-bearing/CKC. Electromyographic studies have demonstrated effective CKC exercises to promote deep glutei and gluteus maximus activity [62, 66, 104–107].

It is recommended that reeducation of the psoas muscle be initiated during this phase. There is much debate over the primary function of the psoas as a hip flexor or a lumbar stabilizer. Evidence also suggests that the psoas may have a role in stabilizing the femoral head anteriorly, given its location across the anterior hip joint [3, 47]. Anecdotally, many patients often present with inhibition of the psoas muscle following hip arthroscopy [34]. Hence, the need exists to be resourceful when retraining psoas, not just prescribe basic concentric hip flexion exercises. Clinical experience has demonstrated effectiveness in addressing psoas *eccentrically* from the trunk down compared to concentrically from the surgical limb up. The patient is instructed to isolate a "lean back" from the hip joint while maintaining a stable lumbar spine [34]. It is important to note that clinicians should not eliminate the concentric portion of an exercise, but rather clinicians should have an increased awareness for designing exercises to have a greater eccentric emphasis. Also consider how eccentric exercise should be a part of a systematic and progressive approach to training after a hip scope. On another note, it is common for patients to have difficulty performing concentric hip flexion exercises due to postoperative muscle imbalance and/or intra-articular adhesions, which often develops into tendinitis of the psoas or the secondary (i.e., tensor fascia lata, rectus femoris, sartorius) hip flexors. Thus, it is important for the clinician to use their decision-making skills to appropriately manipulate training variables (i.e., load, volume, intensity, frequency) to provide a progressive stimulus to retrain the psoas major in preparation for the functional training of phase IV.

Gait retraining is an essential focus in this phase as well, given that clinicians must wean patients from any assistive device. Assistive devices should only be abandoned when gait is pain-free and does not demonstrate any compensatory limp, which can amplify weight-bearing loads on the hip and increase the risk for tendinopathy. A symmetrical gait pattern is necessary to prevent concomitant stress throughout the lower extremity and spine. Again, the use of hydrotherapy or the AlterG™ can be effective modalities to aid in quicker normalization of gait and functional recovery. Similar to phase II, the requirements for a normalized gait without assistive devices are to have no observable Trendelenburg sign, full hip extension from midstance to toe off, and normal progression of the extremity through swing phase without any compensatory lumbo-pelvic girdle rotation to facilitate lower limb progression [34].

16.6.1.3 Electrophysical Agents (EPAs)

Typically, the pain *and* inflammatory consequences of hip arthroscopy are resolved. At this stage some clinicians continue to use NMES to aid in muscle reeducation during the strengthening program. However, if pain continues to be a factor, phase II EPAs are carried through.

The addition of moist heat has the capability to improve circulation, enhance tissue repair, and increase tissue elasticity. The primary application principle in phase III is to reduce tonicity through the effect of heating the sensory receptors in the skin, which reduces reflex muscle tone [16, 67]. This effect prepares the state of the muscle for ROM exercises, myofascial release, and/or joint mobilizations. With the inclusion of heat, clinicians once again must use their skills in clinical reasoning to determine how to "titrate the dose," maximize the therapeutic effect, and clear any contraindications and precautions [16] for patient safety.

16.6.1.4 Patient Education

It is important to continue to educate patients on their compliance with activity modifications [34], how to appropriately wean from their assistive device, abide by quality versus quantity of exercises, as well as how to manage symptom provocation during/with ADLs. Patients need to be reminded that their rehabilitation program should not reproduce pain and exacerbate their symptoms, and early excessive activity as well as rapid progressions of rehabilitation intensity can result in incorrect movement patterns and muscle imbalance, which may delay their functional recovery.

16.6.1.5 Return to Work

The transition from phases II to III or III to IV is based on postoperative follow-up with the orthopedic surgeon. At these time periods, it is common for the surgeon to address a patient's return-to-work plan. Reintegration into the workplace is dependent on the individual patient, the physical demands of the workload, and their recovery status. It is common for graduated hours and/or modified duties to be assigned and carried over into phase IV until better functional strength and endurance can be attained. In more complex cases, the collaboration with an OT can be effective in preparing a patient for a safe return to the work environment. An OT has the knowledge and skills to provide quality and comprehensive return-to-work services. Return-to-work services enable the reintegration of patients into the workplace following interruption due to physical and/or mental health issues [68]. OTs collaborate with injured workers, health professionals, work teams, managers, unions, and health and safety committees to facilitate return-to-work services [68]. The expertise to assess how the influences of work environments, occupational performance (via functional ability evaluations or job demand analyses), and health conditions (i.e., recovery from a hip arthroscopy) can positively impact return-to-work options and success.

16.7 Phase IV: Functional Training of the Hip and Lower Extremity (12–18 Weeks)

Phase IV overview: the primary rehabilitation goals are to (1) build both strength and endurance – it is very important that the trunk, hip, and thigh muscle strength is adequately achieved by the end of phase III (MMT grading of ≥4/5) to avoid alterations of lower extremity alignment during functional activities, (2) normalize gait mechanics with adequate lateral hip stability (i.e., no Trendelenburg sign) before lower kinetic chain *strengthening is advanced* [4, 31, 70], *and (3) demonstrate suitable dynamic balance and proprioception. The clinician needs to gauge if a patient can (1) demonstrate non-compensated activities and higher-demand work functions* [34], *(2) be independent with home and gym programs and remain asymptomatic following these workouts* [34], *and (3) maintain adherence to activity modification guidelines.*

The focus of functional training within the rehabilitation program is to improve *quality* movement, which is grounded on a balance between mobility and stability. Functional training for the lower extremity to move optimally is through the use of specific exercises with the premise that improvements are noted in areas that are specifically trained. Proficient execution of an activity with a multi-joint structure requires balancing the biomechanical relationships between the joints and body segments over a base of support [63]. Movements involved in ADLs, sports, and work environments require an integration of various muscles for multi-joint movements, rather than isolated muscle function or joint movement. Functional training exercises are intended to reproduce everyday demands, developing muscles as a system so that sport- and work-related activities can be performed effectively and efficiently and accelerate postoperative recovery. Functional exercises can activate the entire kinetic chain from the shoulder girdle and trunk stabilizers of the upper body, to the hip, knee, and ankle stabilizers of the lower extremity. The effectiveness of functional training requires that exercises be performed in a way that reinforces the neuromuscular activation patterns in optimal postural alignment and movement execution. This is a proprioceptive/kinesthetic awareness concept that builds upon the neuromuscular retraining that was introduced in phase II and early stages of the postoperative recovery.

The natural progression of exercises should focus on the continuum of difficulty from phase III. The literature on exercises for the trunk (core), hip, and thigh muscles is vast and suitable to guide clinicians when selecting specific exercises [4, 40, 61, 66, 70–74, 104–106]. Clinicians need to appreciate the unique ability of the hip musculature to control movement in all planes of motion about the hip joint, which makes it key for optimal movement execution in the lower kinetic chain [63, 69]. Clinical reasoning skills must be applied to determine the appropriateness of a prescribed exercise, how to adequately dose each exercise, optimize the "intensity" to "movement quality" ratio, and the interaction of the environment to appropriately challenge an *individual* patient's system. Clinicians should be encouraged to select exercises designed to enhance how well a patient moves and performs an activity. The goal should be to enhance a patient's baseline and raise their capacity for recovery. Attempting to identify a progressive list of exercises for *all* postoperative patients would be contradictory to evidence-based, clinical decision-making around exercise prescription and patient-centered care. Moreover, a recipe-based list of exercises may prevent a patient from achieving their individual maximal recovery.

Understandably, a functional rehabilitation approach can be complex due to the nature of a multi-joint system and the ease of movement dysfunction subsequent to proprioceptive/kinesthetic impairments associated with the arthroscopic procedure and resulting trauma. Thus, the skilled clinician must be able to analyze the functional drills prescribed and identify correct versus compensatory movement patterns. If an optimal posture is not maintained or compensations are allowed, then practicing a compensatory movement pattern may lead to recurrent pathology (i.e., tendinitis, bursitis), a delay in recovery, and/or limit the benefits of functional training. Drills must involve multi-planar and weight-bearing exercises that are specific to a patient's occupational and/or sport/recreational demands [4]. Furthermore, drills should progress from double limb to single limb, from slow speed to fast speed, from stable surfaces to unstable surfaces, from gradual challenges to sudden challenges (e.g., external perturbation), and from simple coordination to complex coordination when concentrating on the sequencing of functional movement patterns in the lower kinetic chain.

Compression garments (shorts or pants) with directional/zoned compression are often recommended during this phase. The anecdotal rationale in phase IV is to encourage mechanical support to facilitate the functional rehabilitation program and aid in the successful reintegration to work and/or recreational activities. There are some cases where a compression garment may be prescribed earlier in phase III. Compression products are becoming more popular among athletes and nonathletes alike and have evolved into a multimillion dollar industry [109]. Many companies claim to offer compression through various garment styles, although the recommended pressure intensity is 15–20 mmHg and is considered the lower end to be of medical grade [110]. Current evidence in the subject area is low and inconclusive and typically performed on healthy subjects. At this time, clinical decision-making for this patient population should be based on comparative objective analysis with versus without a garment, as well as patient-reported improvements in functional tests and ADLs (i.e., single-leg stance, stairs, etc.). Commonly reported mechanisms behind the use of medical grade compression are (1) improved postural control and balance [108], (2) proprioceptive enhancement [108, 111], (3) improved dynamic support and motion control of the hips and legs (especially with frontal and/or transverse plane movement) [109, 111], (4) decreased ipsilateral hip adductor activity during single limb tasks (a commonly overactive muscle group in the postoperative hip arthroscopy population [34]) [109], (5) improved blood circulation [109], and (6) reduced fatigue of exercising muscles during submaximal activities [110]. Future studies to evaluate the influence of compression are necessary in order to determine the scientific mechanisms specifically on neural input, such as muscle recruitment or activation, and normalization of muscle tone, during movement and activities. Learning more about the role of medical grade compression to accelerate recovery and prevent (re-) injury is of significant value.

Once the patient has achieved adequate dynamic core stability and hip [69] and thigh strength (MMT grading of ≥4/5), low-level plyometric drills can be added to the rehabilitation program [4]. Without an adequate baseline of strength, there is the potential for injury to occur if the intensity and volume of plyometric training exceed the capacity of the patient [78]. Plyometric training can condition the body through dynamic and resistance exercises, such as hops and jumps. This type of exercise advances a group of muscles to restore maximal strength. These exercises exploit the muscles' lengthening and shortening cycle to increase power output. Plyometric exercises begin with a rapid stretch of a muscle (eccentric phase) and are followed by a rapid shortening of the same muscle (concentric phase), which help bridge the gap between speed and strength training. Thus, this form of training conditions the nervous system to react more rapidly to the stretch-shortening cycle that can increase speed of movement and improve power production [78]. In the literature, attention has been given to eccentric hip-muscle function to improve performance, both in sport and occupational settings. Addressing the eccentric actions of the hip musculature should be considered in comprehensive postoperative programs to enhance functional recovery and performance [79].

In cases where hip mobility is not symmetric and pain-free, ROM exercises are encouraged to continue as previously outlined. Interventions should concentrate on end-range loading. Myofascial mobilization is continued to restore ROM, but is also aimed at restoring muscle timing, coordination, and sequencing to enhance movement quality. Clinical experience supports that there is soft tissue accommodation periods that occur following hip arthroscopy. As previously mentioned, myofascial release techniques are effective when there is a need to discriminate between tissue tightness (decreased ROM) and increased muscle tone (hypertonicity). Additionally, *Intramuscular Stimulation* (IMS™) or Contemporary Medical Acupuncture can be considered at this stage to increase local blood flow, address chronic muscle shortening and/or to desensitize supersensitive structures [75, 76, 113]. The intention is to restore ROM through contracture release [75], reduce myofascial pain and possibly induce a healing response, or neuromuscular reset to targeted tissues [76, 113]. The underlying mechanisms of these techniques are beyond the scope of this chapter, but the body of evidence is advancing for clinicians to seek further knowledge and practical training. Like any intervention it is important to use clinical reasoning skills to determine its appropriateness, the most suitable application regimen based on examination (e.g., needling of the myofascial structures crossing the hip joint and the associated spinal segments), and to understand safety measures, precautions, and contraindications. It is strongly endorsed that trained clinicians wait 12 weeks to *introduce acupuncture needles* in the region of a surgical site or any tissue that communicates with the involved hip joint to avoid increasing infection risk.

16.8 Phase V: Advanced Training – Specificity for Return to Sport and/or Work (18–24 Weeks)

Phase V overview: the primary rehabilitation goals are to (1) achieve the trunk, hip, and thigh muscle strength equivalent to 5/5 using MMT grading, (2) dynamic lumbo-pelvic stability during high-demand single-limb exercises, and (3) optimize functional strength, endurance, and power within the lower kinetic chain. The clinician needs to monitor that a patient is (1) independent with an advanced home and gym program and remains asymptomatic following these workouts [34] *and (2) safe and effective in their return to sporting or work activities at their pre-injury level. By the end of this phase, patients should return to a pain-free competitive state without any type of acute inflammatory response during that process. Thus, this phase must be closely monitored, since the patient will be the most active as they have been in months, possibly years.*

Later stage exercise prescription builds upon the functional retraining that transpired in phase IV and progresses to dynamic performance drills in this final phase of the postoperative program. It is important to note here that ROM should be checked periodically to ensure that loading the hip with advanced exercises does not alter neuromuscular responses and joint mechanics. Maintaining a balance between mobility and stability is essential for a patient to function optimally. Using a systematic approach to functional training allows for continual feedback where progressions are based on movement appraisal. When fundamental improvements are observed, increases in volume, intensity, and complexity can be utilized. A similar approach can be used to challenge core stability when a patient performs high-demand single-limb drills and impact exercises that require adequate control within the transverse plane. Advanced balance activities need to challenge the sensory inputs through the manipulation of three systems: the visual, the vestibular, and the somatosensory (proprioceptors). Maintaining a state of equilibrium and quality movement patterns throughout drills that advance unstable surfaces and incorporate preplanned and unanticipated perturbations is a key component to optimal performance. Depending on a patient's goals and pre-injury activity levels, higher-level plyometric drills can be incorporated into the rehabilitation program with the strength gains attained in phase IV. Three additional types of advanced training should be incorporated into phase V.

16.8.1 Resistance Training

Resistance training is one of the more powerful tools available to clinicians and, when applied appropriately, plays a significant role in the postoperative rehabilitation process. Key areas of focus for resistance training include increasing muscle size (hypertrophy), strength, power, speed, endurance, coordination, general health, and maximal postoperative recovery [80]. A program should aim to collectively improve these components in an integrative approach. It is important to note the sole act of resistance training does not ensure optimal gains in muscle strength and recovery. Rather, it is the magnitude of the individual effort and systematic structuring of the stimulus that determine the outcomes affiliated with resistance-type training [80].

For improvements to occur, patients need to be forced to adapt to changing training stimuli. Thus, incorporating resistance training postoperatively, clinicians must use their clinical reasoning skills to integrate three training principles: overload, variation, and specificity.

Overload is described as "a stimulus of sufficient strength, duration, and frequency (such) that it forces a patient to adapt" [81]. The adaptive process of the body only responds if a patient is continually required to exert a greater magnitude of force to meet higher physiological demands [80, 81]. This principle is necessary for maximal muscle fiber recruitment and subsequently muscle fiber hypertrophy and strength increases [80]. This is commonly tracked by volume load (repetitions x intensity), but can be impractical in a clinic setting. Thus, the Rating of Perceived Exertion (RPE) has been demonstrated as a reliable measure of exercise intensity and a practical method for clinicians to use [82]. If a patient can understand how to use the RPE scale appropriately, a patient who exercises at a level of "fairly light" to "somewhat hard" or "hard" is usually exercising at an appropriate heart rate, VO_2 reserve, or metabolic equivalents [87]. Unless the patient has participated in a maximum-effort-graded exercise test, any prescription using the other measures is only an estimate in a clinical setting.

Variation describes the manipulation of training variables for the stimulus to remain optimal. It has been shown that systematically varying volume and intensity are most effective for long-term progression and benefit.

Specificity refers to the physiological changes the body makes in response to the training stimulus applied. The physiological adaptations to training are specific to the muscle actions, contraction types, dynamics of the effort, rate of force development, range of motion, muscle groups trained, energy systems (anaerobic versus aerobic power), and intensity and volume of training.

The manipulation of variables in exercise prescription covers more than just sets and repetitions following hip arthroscopy. Exercise prescription requires continual clinical decision-making through the many conflicting demands patients experience outside of the clinical environment. The program should incorporate all planes of motion, integrate working proximal to distal and distal to proximal, and be applied to both a controlled and uncontrolled environment. At this stage, the program must include all components of training that improve explosive power. Training variables such as repetitions, velocity, intermuscular coordination, rate of force development [83], positional holds, and technique must be incorporated to any late-phase program. One common problem when prescribing resistance exercise is determining the appropriate combination of training variables. Anecdotally, manipulating one variable per session may offer the greatest chance of avoiding a setback or system breakdown. Excessive manipulation in volume and/or intensity may produce less than optimal results and may actually create a situation of symptom exacerbation or impaired recovery.

16.8.2 Aerobic Training

Treatment recommendations for this phase are to increase both volume and intensity of aerobic activity, regardless of the equipment choice. Commonly, cross-training occurs between elliptical trainer, bicycling, Stairmaster™, swimming (*no whip kick*), and treadmill walking. Based on clinical experience, 30–40 min of continuous exercise at moderate intensity is a benchmark of this phase. Some programs will strive for 60 min if a patient's capacity allows for it, and it replicates their specific energy demands for sport or work. For activities that are more anaerobic in nature, doing some interval work after a couple of weeks of endurance exercise would help enhance both the aerobic and anaerobic energy systems.

There are numerous case series and cohort studies that support an earlier timeline than phase V to initiate a running program. However, a running program should not be initiated until patients can demonstrate good repetitive single-leg landing control, adequate control of frontal and transverse plane mechanics of the hip and knee, dynamic stability during high-demand single-limb exercises, sufficient eccentric hip-muscle function, and a symmetric and proficient gait pattern. Appropriate gait retraining early in the rehabilitation program is integral for a successful return to running to prevent abnormal joint and tissue loading in the hip and lower kinetic chain. Without optimal mechanics, gait modifications redistribute and alter forces during running. Furthermore, the patient needs to be able to demonstrate appropriate muscular endurance and ability to generate power [31]. A patient's hip must not present with pain during or after any resistance training drills or cardiovascular exercises. Resistance training, in particular, can be used to justify the initiation of running by way of increasing a tissues tolerance and response to loading. Clinically, it takes time for the above-mentioned factors to be suitably trained to foster safe return to running. Typically, it is recommended that a program commence with interval running prior to reinstating a pre-injury regimen. Periodization is key for a successful return to running to allow the soft tissues to have the chance to adapt and avoid tissue failure *(failure is caused when demands on the body exceed its ability to adapt)*. If patients understand the importance of system adaptability, then they will more likely understand the importance of a graded return to running to foster the adaptation of different stresses on the joint and surrounding soft tissues. However, when initiated too early, or progressed too rapidly, running tends to result in symptom exacerbation and setback due to the impact and abnormal forces transmitted to the hip. Tissue failure results in pain and the need to desensitize the nervous system and unload the affected tissues to modify the application of stress, which ultimately delays the recovery process and timeline for return to pre-injury level of function.

16.8.3 Agility Training

Agility is the ability to move and change the body's direction and position quickly and effectively with control in response to a stimulus [88]. Agility drills typically commence by introducing proper footwork, timing, and speed, as well as cognitive components [88] such as anticipation and pattern recognition. In most sports, an athlete must be able to accelerate, decelerate, and change directions rapidly with good body control in order to perform well and reduce the risk of injury. Similar drills can be incorporated into training programs for the general population and nonathletes to improve performance in recreational and daily activities. Drills that assist in the development of generalized motor programs can boost a patient's proprioceptive capabilities [86]. Retraining a patient's nervous system can have a positive impact on their movement efficiency and skill. For instance, the same movements being produced by an athlete in a game setting compared to a nonathlete playing with their children or crossing a busy street may require similar intensity and movement demands. Thus, agility drills used in conjunction with resistance training in a comprehensive postoperative program can better prepare patients for the demands of their daily lives.

An ideal implementation strategy is to select a fundamental movement skill associated with the patient's goals and then maintain the clinician's instruction and focus on that specific skill. It is important to provide the patient with a setting in which the skill would be performed in. These drills should commence by introducing large angles and low speeds (i.e., large figure 8s) and progress to more advanced drills with sharper angles and increasing speeds [85]. Once a patient is able to successfully and appropriately run in a straight line, without difficulty and pain, nonlinear activities may be initiated, such as cutting and pivoting. Clinicians must ensure patients focus 100 % of their energy on the skill, and each rep is focused on *quality* to signal correct movement patterns before advancing or combining skills. Be sure to stop the exercise if the execution is poor. If clinicians are teaching too many different skills and are not emphasizing technique, intensity of effort, and speed, the meaning of the skill(s) is lost and retraining will be negatively impacted even in this later postoperative phase. Once the targeted movement of the skill has been mastered, the patient can increase the intensity or speed of the drill. Remember the brain is programming these movement patterns. If they are poor that is how they will be reprogrammed in the CNS. Clinicians must demand top-notch movement quality and execution. It is important that clinicians build a foundation of movement in which greater skills can be built upon. There are many examples of agility drills in the literature. Nevertheless, clinicians must use their clinical reasoning to select the appropriate drills based on a patient's skills and functional demands when integrating agility into an individualized postoperative training program.

16.9 Return to Pre-injury Activity Levels

Studies support that the majority of improvements in pain and function (self-reported using the *modified Harris hip score*) occur between 0 and 3 months and again between 3 and 6 months postoperatively. Thus, a gradual recommencement of pain-free activities over a 6-month period can be anticipated [9, 89]. Patients may experience continued improvement in symptoms and functional outcomes throughout the first year postoperatively [11, 84]. Based on current evidence and study populations, no *clinically significant* improvements are noted in the literature from 6 to

12 months that would support delaying return to sport and/or work [9]. While 6 months seems to be an appropriate benchmark, progress may be faster or slower depending on the individual patient. Thus, determination of safe and appropriate timelines for a return-to-work and/or sport activities should be assessed on a case-by-case basis in consultation with the orthopedic surgeon. Variations in timelines may be related to:

- Preoperative level of activity and pre-diagnosed duration of symptom involvement. A cautionary consideration when returning a patient to sport is the use of the uninjured lower extremity as it has been demonstrated in the literature that a significant detraining effect can occur [94].
- The extent of the surgical procedure performed and the healing properties of the resected impinging lesion and associated soft tissues repaired (labral tears, chondral damage, and so on).
- The type and performance level (recreational versus professional) of sport, as well as the demands and competition environment.
- The type of occupational environment, demands, and performance and support from the patient's manager(s) with regard to compliance with any recommendations for graduated hours and/or modified duties.
- The complexities associated with patients who sustain their injury in a work-related incident or motor vehicle collision, as compared to the athletic and pre-arthritic population. There is a much smaller proportion of evidence assessing outcomes and disability status in these populations. A recent study showed postoperative functional outcomes in workers' compensation groups to be lower compared to those in the nonworkers' compensation group [112]. Furthermore, the effect of litigation and financial compensation on outcomes following hip arthroscopy requires further exploration.

A systematic review identified and summarized the available evidence pertaining to the rate of return to sport following surgical intervention for FAI in athletes. Of the total athletes, 90.7 % returned to sport and 88 % returned to pre-injury activity levels at a minimum of 6 months [89]. In the review, assessment of the subgroups showed that among the recreational athletes, the return-to-sport rate was 87 % and the return to pre-activity levels was 84 %. For the subgroup of professional athletes, the rate of return to sport was 95 % and the rate of return to pre-injury activity levels was 92 %. On the other hand, there are case series (level IV evidence) that suggest a return to sport can occur anywhere between 4 and 6 months [84]. Two particular case series suggested a return to full competitive activity at an average of 3.4 months in professional athletes [30, 90]. There is evidence suggesting that reported clinical outcomes found in athletic populations may be applicable to the nonathletic/general population [89]. However, clinicians must be cognizant of the differences in body systems between professional athletes, recreational athletes, and the general population with regard to healing timelines and recovery. It is important to note that the patients included in these studies participated in a wide range of sports with correspondingly wide range of skill levels. Thus, successful return to sport based on the type of sport or level of participation still requires further evaluation. It is recognized that activities with higher degrees of rotational stresses, hyperextension, and hyperflexion may be more difficult to return to because of the stresses placed on the labrum and chondral surfaces (when repaired) [47]. Some common activities that fall into this category are distance running, ballet, golf, ice hockey, soccer, and mixed martial arts, which are common recreational activities seen among the general population.

16.10 Outcome Measurement

Postoperative rehabilitation following hip arthroscopy is not linear. It requires a good understanding of the underlying pathology, awareness of the patient's goals, clinical experience and skilled clinical reasoning, patience, as well as continual communication with the orthopedic surgeon. In current practice, the timeline provided with each *phase* should serve as a guideline, rather than an absolute, as progressions are criterion based. Timelines will vary considerably based on the individual patient, general health history, the osseous and soft tissue structures impacted during the arthroscopic procedure, and compliance with activity modification education. Evidence would suggest that progressions through the different phases of this *five-phase rehabilitation program* should be based on a validated hip outcome tool that is patient reported, not just postoperative timelines and clinician experience [92, 93]. With the integration of an appropriate measurement tool, more explicit phases and interventions of this postoperative rehabilitation program and more accurate outcomes of hip arthroscopy can be ascertained. Large-scale prospective studies need to be conducted to determine the *scores* of a validated outcome tool that will identify mastery of each rehabilitation phase after FAI arthroscopic surgery.

Patient-reported outcomes (PROs) are becoming an integral part of measuring treatment effectiveness with the advancement of hip preservation surgery. It is important for a tool to address the before and after impact of interventions on impairments of body function and structure, activity limitations, and participation restrictions in a patient who has undergone hip arthroscopy [47]. Traditionally the modified Harris hip score (*1969*) has been used as the standard outcome measure for the evaluation of hip arthroscopy outcomes in the FAI literature. More recently, new PRO tools in the field have been developed [91]. In a 2015 systematic review, six PRO tools were identified with description or comparison of their measurement properties. Critical appraisal of the development, measurement properties, and head-to-head comparison studies verified that the International Hip Outcome Tool (iHOT33) scored the best of the most recently developed PRO tools [91]. The iHOT33 is a 33-item tool that uses a visual analog scale response format to measure health-related quality of life in young, active patients with hip disorders [92]. A shorter version of the 33-item tool was developed for easier implementation in the routine clinical practice. The 12-item tool (iHOT12) has demonstrated very similar characteristics to the original, losing very little information despite being only one-third of its length. It is valid, reliable, and responsive to change. Thus, the iHOT12 or iHOT33 is recommended as a primary tool to capture PROs for FAI surgery. The iHOT12 is more likely for routine clinical practice and the iHOT33 most likely to be used in the research setting for prospective clinical trials [92, 93].

To take this one step further, future study needs to be conducted with the intention of developing functional testing guidelines specific to FAI and hip arthroscopic surgery. As no single instrument or functional/objective test is currently capable of measuring all the myriad of factors believed to relate to outcome, it is reasonable to accept that a range of tests should be administered to facilitate a comprehensive evaluation of postoperative outcome. A series of tests will be required to measure *both* the quantitative and qualitative aspects of functional performance after hip arthroscopy. In short, the addition of PRO tools and functional testing criteria to postoperative timelines and clinical experience would provide the best accuracy of postoperative rehabilitation program advancement, appropriate rate and level of return to activities after FAI surgery in all patient populations, and a method for evaluating a successful outcome after hip arthroscopy for FAI.

Conclusion

This chapter is intended to provide clinicians with evidence-based rehabilitation guidelines, instruction, and functional goals for the postoperative management of a patient who has undergone an arthroscopic hip procedure for FAI (with or without labral repair/reconstruction). This five-phase rehabilitation program is not a substitute for a clinician's clinical reasoning during a patient's postoperative recovery. Clinical reasoning should be based on individual symptoms, physical signs, progress, and/or the presence of operative modifications and/or complications. If a clinician requires assistance or guidance at any stage of recovery, they should consult with the patient's orthopedic surgeon. Verbal or nonverbal communication with the surgeon is imperative before any adjustments are made to their *current* postoperative protocol. Modifications often are prescribed following an arthroscopic procedure and require strict implementation. Each surgeon is unique, as are their surgical techniques, and thus slight variations will exist within all protocols.

As clinicians, we must continue to evaluate advances in scientific research and assess new rehabilitation perspectives. Future research is required to focus on comparative trials to determine the effect of specific postoperative rehabilitation guidelines and begin to determine superiority of particular approaches and interventions at different timelines postoperatively. At this time, it is through collaboration with medical and clinical colleagues, peer review, and PRO tools that we aim to deliver the highest outcomes following FAI surgery.

Take-Home Points

1. At this time, the evidence-based literature surrounding postoperative rehabilitation after FAI surgery is in its infancy. What we do know is that the rehabilitation is not linear and thus requires a good understanding of the underlying pathology, awareness of the patient's goals, clinical experience and skilled clinical reasoning, patience, and frequent communication with the orthopedic surgeon.
2. Communication between the clinician and orthopedic surgeon is critical to ensure the appropriate protocol and any necessary modifiers are applied for each individual patient case. Communication with the surgeon and among the rehabilitation team is of utmost importance to ensure that the appropriate restrictions are applied. Poor verbal or nonverbal communication is a major link to postoperative pitfalls and poor outcomes.
3. The five-phase postoperative rehabilitation program provides evidence-based guidelines, instruction, and functional objectives for the management of a patient who has undergone an arthroscopic procedure. Based on this guideline, it is necessary for a clinician to understand that each phase builds upon the previous. However, clinical experience has demonstrated that some patients will go through the phases faster or slower than others depending on variations in preoperative condition, general health status, complexity of the FAI procedure with or without labral involvement, and the presence of postoperative complications.
4. Patients can experience continued improvement in pain and function throughout the course of 1 year postoperative. However, studies support that the majority of improvements occur within the first 6 months postoperative. Improvements seen from 0 to 6 weeks are associated with protecting the surgical site through compliance with weight-bearing and ROM restrictions. From 6 to 12 weeks, emphasis is placed on restoration of mobility and neuromuscular control, muscle balance, and strength of the hip and trunk. The improvements recognized from 3 to 6 months are linked to functional and resistance training of the hip, trunk, and lower kinetic chain. The emphasis is on movement quality and optimization to enhance performance and successfully reintegrate patient's return-to-work and/or recreational activities.
5. The addition of patient-reported outcome tools and functional testing criteria to postoperative timelines and clinical experience can enhance the accuracy of postoperative rehabilitation advancement and appropriate rate and level of return to activities after FAI surgery in all patient populations and be a method for evaluating a successful outcome after hip arthroscopy.

Key Evidence Related Sources

1. Spencer-Gardner L, Eischen JJ, Levy BA, et al. A comprehensive five-phase rehabilitation programme after hip arthroscopy for femoroacetabular impingement. Knee Surg Sports Traumatol Arthrosc. 2014;22:848–59.
2. Stalzer S, Wahoff M, Scanlan M. Rehabilitation following hip arthroscopy. Clin Sports Med. 2006;25(2): 337–57.
3. Edelstein J, Ranawat A, Enseki K, et al. Post-operative guidelines following hip arthroscopy. Curr Rev Musculoskelet Med. 2012;5(1):15–23.
4. Beck M. Groin pain after open FAI surgery: the role of intraarticular adhesions. Clin Orthop Relat Res. 2009;467(3): 769–74.
5. Selkowitz DM, Powers CM. Which exercises target the gluteal muscles while minimizing activation of the tensor fascia lata? Electromyographic assessment using fine-wire electrodes. J Orthop Sports Phys Ther. 2013;43(2): 54–65.

References

1. Colvin AC, Harrast J, Harner C. Trends in hip arthroscopy. J Bone Joint Surg Am. 2012;94(4):e23, 1–5.
2. Montgomery SR, Ngo SS, Hobson T, et al. Trends and demographics in hip arthroscopy in the United States. Arthroscopy. 2013;29(4):661–5.
3. Glick JM, Valone F, Safran M. Hip arthroscopy: from the beginning to the future – an innovator's perspective. Knee Surg Sports Traumatol Arthrosc. 2014;22:714–21.
4. Spencer-Gardner L, Eischen JJ, Levy BA, et al. A comprehensive five-phase rehabilitation programme after hip arthroscopy for femoroacetabular impingement. Knee Surg Sports Traumatol Arthrosc. 2014;22:848–59.
5. Cheatham S, Eneki KR, Kolber MJ. Post-operative rehabilitation after hip arthroscopy: a search for the evidence. J Sports Rehabil. 2015;24(4):413–8.
6. Phillips B, Ball C, Sackett D, et al. Oxforce centre for evidence-based medicine – levels of evidence. 2009. Available at: http://www.cebm.net/index.aspx?o=1025. Accessed 21 Nov 2014.
7. Stalzer S, Wahoff M, Scanlan M. Rehabilitation following hip arthroscopy. Clin Sports Med. 2006;25(2):337–57.
8. Cheatham SW, Kolber MJ. Rehabilitation after hip arthroscopy and labral repair in a high school football athlete. Int J Sports Phys Ther. 2012;3(1):70–2.
9. Dippman C, Thorborg K, Kraemer O, et al. Hip arthroscopy with labral repair for femoracetabular impingement: short-term outcomes. Knee Surg Sports Traumatol Arthosc. 2014;22:744–9.
10. World Health Organization. International classification of functioning, disability and health: ICF. Geneva: World Health Organization; 2009.
11. Shindle M, et al. Arthroscopic management of labral tears in the hip. J Bone Joint Surg Am. 2008;90:2–19.
12. Griffin KM, Henry CO, Byrd JWT. Rehabilitation after hip arthroscopy. J Sport Rehabil. 2000;9:77–88.
13. Potter M, Gordon S, Hamer P. The physiotherapy experience in private practice: the patient's perspective. Aust J Physiother. 2003;49:195–202.
14. Hall A, Ferreira P, Maher C, et al. The influence of the therapist-patient relationship on treatment outcome in physical rehabilitation: a systematic review. Phys Ther. 2010;90(8):1099–108.
15. Bordin ES. The generalizability of the psychoanalytic concept of the working alliance. Psychotherapy. 1979;16:252–60.
16. Houghton PE, Nussbaum EL, Hoens AM. Electrophysical agents: contraindications and precautions. Physiother Can. 2010 Special Issue; 62(5):5–80.
17. Wojciech K, Mydlarz MD, Encyclopedia of Otolaryngology. Neuropraxia. Head Neck Surg. 2013:1855. http://link.springer.com/referenceworkentry/10.1007%2F978-3-642-23499-6_200122
18. Lewis CL, Sahrmann SA. Acetabular labral tears. Phys Ther. 2006;86:110–21.
19. Ageberg E, Nilsdotter A, Kosek E, Roos E. Effects of neuromuscular training (NEMEX-TJR) on patient-reported outcomes and physical functioning in severe primary hip or knee osteoarthritis: a controlled before and after study. BMC Musculoskelet Disord. 2013;14:232.
20. Dorfmann H, Boyer T. Arthroscopy of the hip: 12 years of experience. Arthroscopy. 1999;15:67–72.
21. Larsen CM, Giveans MR. Arthroscopic debridement versus refixation of the acetabular labrum associated with femoracetabular impingement. Arthroscopy. 2009;25(4):369–76.
22. Philippon MJ, Briggs KK, Yen YM, et al. Outcomes following hip arthroscopy for femoracetabular impingement with associated chondrolabral dysfunction: minimum two-year follow-up. J Bone Joint Surg Br. 2009;91(1):16–23.
23. Wahoff M, Ryan M. Rehab after hip femoracetabular impingement arthroscopy. Clin Sports Med. 2011; 30(2):463–82.
24. Kowalczuk M, Bhandari M, Farrokhyar F, et al. Complications following hip arthroscopy: a systematic review and meta-analysis. Knee Surg Sports Traumatol Arthrosc. 2013;21(7):1669–75.

25. Zingg PO, Buehler TC, Poutawera VR, Alireza A, Dora C. Femoral neck fractures after arthroscopic femoral neck osteochondroplasty for femoroacetabular impingement. Knee Surg Sports Traumatol Arthrosc. 2014;22(4):926–31.
26. Fry R, Domb B. Labral base refixation in the hip: rationale and technique for an anatomic approach to labral repair. Arthroscopy. 2010;26:S81–9.
27. Takechi H, Nagashima H, Ito S. Intra-articular pressure of the hip joint outside and inside the limbus. Nihon Seikeigeka Gakkai Zasshi. 1982;56:529–36.
28. Kim YT, Azuma H. The nerve endings of the acetabular labrum. Clin Orthop Relat Res. 1995;320:176–81.
29. Ferguson SJ, Bryant JT, Ganz R, Ito K. An in vitro investigation of the acetabular labral seal in hip joint mechanics. J Biomech. 2003;36:171–8.
30. Philippon MJ, Schenker M, Briggs K, Kuppersmith D. Femoroacetabular impingement in 45 professional athletes: associated pathologies and return to sport following arthroscopic decompression. Knee Surg Sports Traumatol Arthrosc. 2007;15:908–14.
31. Garrison JC, Osler MT, Singleton SB. Rehab after arthroscopy of an acetabular labral tear. N Am J Sports Phys Ther. 2007;2(4):241–50.
32. Sink EL, Zaltz I, Heare T, Dayton M. Acetabular cartilage and labral damage observed during surgical hip dislocation for stable slipped femoral epiphysis. J Pediatr Orthop. 2010;30:26–30.
33. Panjabi M. The stabilizing system of the spine. Part I. Function, dysfunction, adaptation, and enhancement. J Spinal Disord. 1992;5(4):383–9.
34. Edelstein J, Ranawat A, Enseki K, et al. Post-operative guidelines following hip arthroscopy. Curr Rev Musculoskelet Med. 2012;5(1):15–23.
35. Philippon MJ, Christensesn JC, Wahoff MS. Rehab after arthroscopic repair of intra-articular disorders of the hip in a professional football athlete. J Sport Rehabil. 2009;18(1):118–34.
36. Beck M. Groin pain after open FAI surgery: the role of intraarticular adhesions. Clin Orthop Relat Res. 2009;467(3):769–74.
37. Willimon SC, Briggs KK, Philippon MJ. Intra-articular adhesions following hip arthroscopy: a risk factor analysis. Knee Surg Sports Traumatol Arthrosc. 2014;22:822–5.
38. Nugent-Derfus GE, Takara T, O'Neill JK, et al. Continuous passive motion applied to whole joints stimulates chondrocyte biosynthesis of PRG4. Osteoarthritis Cartilage. 2007;15:566–74.
39. Enseki KR, Martin RL, Draovitch P, et al. The hip joint: arthroscopic procedures and postoperative rehab. J Orthop Sports Phys Ther. 2006;36:516–25.
40. Richardson C, Hodges P, Hides J. Therapeutic exercise for lumbo-pelvic stabilization: a motor control approach for the treatment and prevention of low back pain. 2nd ed. London: Churchill Livingstone; 2004.
41. Bleakley C, McDonough S, MacAuley D. The use of ice in the treatment of acute soft-tissue injury: a systematic review of randomized controlled trials. Am J Sport Med. 2004;32:251–61.
42. Rennie S. ELECTROPHYSICAL AGENTS – Contraindications and precautions: an evidence-based approach to clinical decision making in physical therapy. Physiother Can. 2010;62(5):1–80.
43. Kullenberg B, Ylipaa S, Soderlund K, Resch S. Postoperative cryotherapy after total knee arthroplasty. J Arthroplasty. 2006;21:1175–9.
44. Holmstrom A, Hardin B. Cryo/Cuff compared to epidural anesthesia after knee unicompartmental arthroplasty. J Arthroplasty. 2005;20:316–21.
45. Visser C, Coene L, Brand R, Tavy D. The incidence of nerve injury in anterior dislocation of the shoulder and its influence on functional recovery a prospective clinical and emg study. J Bone Joint Surg Br. 1999;81-B(4):679–85.
46. Risberg MA, Mork M, Krogstad Jenssen H, Holm I. Design and implementation of a neuromuscular training program for anterior cruciate ligament reconstruction. J Orthop Sports Phys Ther. 2001;31(11):620–31.
47. Enseki K, Harris-Hayes M, White DM, et al. Nonarthritic hip joint pain: clinical practice guidelines linked to the International Classification of Functioning, Disability and Health from the Orthopaedic Section of the American Physical Therapy Association. J Orthop Sports Phys Ther. 2014;44(6):A1–32.
48. Dorion J. Facial neuromuscular retraining. Article in Perspectives on Swallowing and Swallowing Disorders (Dysphagia). 2005;14(2):18–23.
49. Cairns MC, Foster NE, Wright C. Randomized controlled trial of specific spinal stabilization exercises and conventional physiotherapy for recurrent low back pain. Spine. 2006;19:670–81.
50. Guido JA, Stemm J. Reactive neuromuscular training: a multi-level approach to rehabilitation of the unstable shoulder. N Am J Sports Phys Ther. 2007;2(2):97–103.
51. Kofotolis ND, Vlachopoulos SP, Kellis E. Sequentially allocated clinical trial of rhythmic stabilization exercises and TENS in women with chronic low back pain. Clin Rehabil. 2008;22:99.
52. Green DL, Morris JM. Role of the adductor magnus and adductor longus in postural movements and in ambulation. Am J Phys Med. 1970;49:223–40.
53. Vicenzino B, Hing W, Rivett D, Hall T. Mobilisation with movement: the art and the science. Edinburgh: Churchill Livingstone; 2011.
54. Wilk KE, Meister K, Andrews JR. Current concepts in the rehabilitation of the overhead throwing athlete. Sports Med. 2002;30(1):136–51.
55. Denegar CR, Saliba E, Saliba S. Impact of injury and pain on neuromuscular control. In: Therapeutic modalities for musculoskeletal injuries. 2nd ed. Champaign: Human Kinetics; 2006.
56. TMG Case Study. Self-myofascial release protocols assessment: application notes. Ljubljana: Tensiomyography; 2011.
57. Prather H, Dugan S, Fitzgerald C, et al. Review of anatomy, evaluation, and treatment of musculoskeletal pelvic floor pain in women. PM R. 2009;1:346–58.
58. AlterG. http://www.alterg.com/. Accessed 14 Dec 2014.

59. Flack NA, Nicholson HD, Woodley SJ. A review of the anatomy of the hip abductor muscles, gluteus medius, gluteus minimus, and tensor fascia lata. Clin Anat. 2012;25:697–708.
60. Maheu E. Choice of grades of passive movement in treatment. Orthopaedic Division Syllabus. Canadian Physiotherapy Association; 2007.
61. Lindsay DM, Maitland ME, Lowe RC, Kane TI. Comparison of isokinetic internal and external hip rotation torque using different testing positions. J Orthop Sports Phys Ther. 1992;16(1):43–50.
62. Johnson CAM, Lindsay DM, Wiley JP. Treatment of iliopsoas syndrome with a hip rotation strengthening program: a retrospective case series. J Orthop Sports Phys Ther. 1999;29(4):218–24.
63. Werstine M, Werstine R. LE dysfunction and management. Orthop Div Rev. 2006;18–23.
64. Neuman DA. Kinesiology of the musculoskeletal system: foundations for physical rehabilitation. St. Louis: Mosby Inc.; 2002.
65. Gottschalk F, Kourosh S, Leveau B. The functional anatomy of tensor fascia latae and gluteus medius and minimus. J Anat. 1989;166:179–89.
66. Distefano LJ, Blackburn JT, Marshall SW, et al. Gluteal muscle activation during common therapeutic exercises. J Orthop Sports Phys Ther. 2009;39: 532–40.
67. Belanger AY. Evidence-based guide to therapeutic physical agents. Philadelphia: Lippincott Williams & Wilkins; 2003.
68. Canadian Association of Occupational Therapists of Ontario. Position State: return-to-work and occupational therapy. 2009. http://www.caot.ca/default.asp?pageid=3883. Accessed 25 Jan 2015.
69. Grimaldi A. Assessing lateral stability of the hip and pelvis. Man Ther. 2011;16:26–32.
70. Ekstrom RA, Donatelli RA, Carp KC. Electromyographic analysis of core trunk, hip and thigh muscles during 9 rehabilitation exercises. J Orthop Sports Phys Ther. 2007;37(12):754–62.
71. Ayotte NW, et al. Electromyographical analysis of selected LE muscles during 5 unilateral weight-bearing exercises. J Orthop Sports Phys Ther. 2007;37(2):48–55.
72. Boudreau SN, et al. Hip-muscle activation during the lunge, single-leg squat, and step-up-and-over exercises. J Sport Rehabil. 2009;18:91–103.
73. Bolga LA, Uhl TL. Electromyographic analysis of hip rehabilitation exercises in a group of healthy subjects. J Orthop Sports Phys Ther. 2005;35(8):487–94.
74. O'Sullivan K, et al. Electromyographic analysis of the three subdivisions of gluteus medius during weight-bearing exercises. Sports Med Arthrosc Rehabil Ther Technol. 2010;2:17–25.
75. Gunn CC. Review Article: Intramuscular Stimulation (IMS) – the Technique. Institute for the Study and Treatment of Pain. 2002. Based *on material from The Gunn Approach to the Treatment of Chronic Pain Intramuscular Stimulation (IMS) for Myofascial Pain of Radiculopathic Origin, by C. Chan Gunn, 1996 Churchill Livingstone. Figures and Table are used with permission. © iSTOP.*
76. Zylstra ED. Functional dry needling – applications for management of movement impairment, pain and sports injuries. Kinetacore Physical Therapy Education. Course notes – Jan 2013.
77. Magali Robert M, Ross S, et al. Conservative management of urinary incontinence. SOGC Clin Pract Guidel. 2006;186:1113–8.
78. Faigenbaum AD, Chu DA. Plyometric training for children and adolescents. Am Coll Sports Med. http://www.acsm.org/access-public-information/brochures-fact-sheets/fact-sheets. Accessed 9 Jan 2015.
79. Baldon RM, Lobato DFM, Carvalho LP, et al. Relationship between eccentric hip isokinetic torque and functional performance. J Sport Rehabil. 2012;21(1):26–33.
80. Kraemer WJ, Ratamess NA. Fundamentals of resistance training progression and exercise prescription. Med Sci Sports Exerc. 2004;36(4):674–88.
81. Carinale M, Newton R, Nosaka K. Strength and conditioning: Biological Principles and Practical Applications. John Wiley & Sons Ltd, The Atrium, Southern Gate, Chichester, West Sussex, PO19 8SQ, UK.
82. Day ML, McGuigan MR, Brice G, Foster C. Monitoring exercise intensity during resistance training using the session RPE scale. J Strength Cond Res. 2004;18(2):353–8.
83. Newton RU, Kraemer WJ. Developing explosive muscular power: implications for a mixed methods training strategy. Strength Cond J. 1994;16:20–31.
84. Byrd JW, Jones KS. Arthroscopic femoroplasty in the management of cam-type femoroacetabular impingement. Clin Orthop Relat Res. 2009;467:739–46.
85. Hewett TE, Paterno MV, Myer GD. Strategies for enhancing proprioception and neuromuscular control of the knee. Clin Orthop Relat Res. 2002;402:76–94.
86. Schmidt RA, Lee TD. Motor control and learning: a behavioral emphasis. 4th ed. Champaign: Human Kinetics; 2005. p. 91–101. 280–5, 401–31.
87. Thompson WR, Gordon NF, Pescatello LS, editors; American College of Sports Medicine. ACSM's guidelines for exercise testing and prescription. 8th ed. Baltimore: Lippincott Williams & Wilkins; 2009.
88. Sheppard JM, Young WB. Agility literature review: classifications, training and testing. J Sports Sci. 2006;25(9):919–32.
89. Alradwan H, Philippon MJ, Farrokhyar F, et al. Return to preinjury activity levels after surgical management of femoroacetabular impingement in athletes. Arthroscopy. 2012;28(10):1567–76.
90. Philippon MJ, Weiss DR, Kuppersmith D, et al. Arthroscopic labral repair and treatment of femoroacetabular impingement in professional hockey players. Am J Sports Med. 2010;38:99–104.
91. Ramisetty N, Kwon Y, Mohtadi N. Patient-reported outcome measures for hip preservation surgery – a

systematic review of the literature. J Hip Preserv Surg. 2015;2(1):15–27. doi: 10.1093/jhps/hnv002. eCollection 2015.

92. Mohtadi NGH, Griffin DR, Pedersen ME, et al. The development and validation of a self-administered quality-of-life outcome measure for young, active patients with symptomatic hip disease: the international hip outcome tool (iHOT33). Arthroscopy. 2012;28(5):595–610.
93. Griffin DR, Parsaons N, Mohtadi NGH, et al. A short version of the international hip outcome tool (iHOT12) for use in routine clinical practice. Arthroscopy. 2012;28(5):611–8.
94. Hiemstra LA, Webber S, MacDonald PB, Kriellaars DJ. Contralateral limb strength deficits after anterior cruciate ligament reconstruction using a hamstring tendon graft. Clin Biomech (Bristol, Avon). 2007;22:543–50.
95. Nielsen PR, Jorgensen LD, Dahl B, et al. Prehab and early rehabilitation after spinal surgery: randomized clinical trial. Clin Rehabil. 2010;24:137–48.
96. Clohisy JC, Knaus ER, Hunt DM, et al. Clinical presentation of patients with symptomatic anterior hip impingement. Clin Orthop Relat Res. 2009;467(3): 638–44.
97. Nepple JJ, Philippon MJ, Campbell KJ, et al. The hip fluid seal-part II: the effect of an acetabular tear, repair, resection and reconstruction on hip stability to distraction. Knee Surg Sports Traumatol Arthrosc. 2014;22:730–6.
98. Louw A, Puentedura E. Therapeutic neuroscience education, pain, physiotherapy and the pain matrix. Int J Health Sci. 2014;2(3):33–45.
99. Dippmann C, Thorborg K, Kraemer O, et al. Symptoms of nerve dysfunction after hip arthroscopy: an under-reported complication. Arthroscopy. 2014;30(2):202–7.
100. Pailhé R, Chiron P, Reina N, Cavaignac E, Lafontan V, Laffosse JM. Pudendal nerve neuralgia after hip arthroscopy: retrospective study and literature review. Orthop Traumatol Surg Res. 2013;99(7): 785–90.
101. Safran MR, Giordano G, Lindsey DP, Gold GE, Rosenberg J, Zaffagnini S, Giori NJ. The biomechanical behaviour of the acetabular labrum. Am J Sports Med. 2011;39(1):92S–102.
102. Reiman MP, Bolgla LA, Loudon JK. A literature review of studies evaluating gluteus maximus and gluteus medius activation during rehabilitation exercises. Physiother Theory Pract. 2012;28(4): 257–68.
103. Escamilla RF, Fleisig GS, Yamashiro K, Mikla T, Dunning R, Paulos L, Andrews JR. Effects of a 4-week youth baseball conditioning program on throwing velocity. J Strength Cond Res. 2010;24(12): 3247–54.
104. Boren K. Electromyographic analysis of gluteus medius and gluteus maximus during rehabilitation exercises. Int J Sports Phys Ther. 2011;6(3): 206–23.
105. Stastny P, Lehnert M, Zaatar Zaki AM, Svoboda Z, Xaverova Z. Does the dumbbell carrying position change the muscle activity during split squats and walking lunges? J Strength Cond Res. 2015; 29(11):3177–87.
106. Krause D. Electromyographic analysis of the gluteus medius in five weight-bearing exercises. J Strength Cond Res. 2009;23(9):2689–94.
107. Selkowitz DM, Powers CM. Which exercises target the gluteal muscles while minimizing activation of the tensor fascia lata? Electromyographic assessment using fine-wire electrodes. J Orthop Sports Phys Ther. 2013;43(2):54–65.
108. Michael JS, Dogramaci SN, Steel KA, Graham KS. What is the effect of compression garments on a balance task in female athletes? Gait Posture. 2014; 39(2):804–9.
109. Chaudari AMW, Jamison ST, McNally MP, et al. Hip adductor activations during run-to-cut maneuvers in compression shorts: implications for return to sport after groin injury. J Sports Sci. 2014; 32(14):1333–40.
110. Miyamoto N, Kawakami Y. Effect of pressure intensity of compression short-tight on fatigue of thigh muscles. Med Sci Sports Exerc. 2014;46(11): 2168–74.
111. Bernhardt T, Anderson GS. Influence of moderate prophylactic compression on sport performance. J Strength Cond Res. 2005;19(2):292–7.
112. Salvo JP, Hammoud S, Flato R, Sgromolo N, Mendelsohn ES. Outcomes after hip arthroscopy in patients with worker's compensation claims. Orthopedics. 2015;38(2):e94–8.
113. Shah JP, Gilliams EA. Uncovering the biochemical milieu of myofascial trigger points using in-vivo microdialysis: An application of muscle pain concepts to myofascial pain syndrome. Journal of Bodywork and Movement Therapies. 2008;12(4): 371–84.

Complications of FAI Surgery: A Highlight of Common Complications in Published Literature

17

Cécile Batailler, Elliot Sappey-Marinier, and Nicolas Bonin

Contents

C. Batailler, MD • E. Sappey-Marinier, MD
N. Bonin, MD (✉)
Hip and Sports Medicine Department, Lyon Ortho Clinic, Clinique de la Sauvegarde,
29 B avenue des Sources, Lyon 69009, France
e-mail: n.bonin@gmail.com

A complication is an event that results in prolonged operation time, or prolonged recovery from surgery, or requires a specific medical treatment, a secondary procedure, or a revision of the index procedure. Major complications are defined as those that have life-threatening sequelae or endanger the viability of the limb involved [1]. In FAI surgery, major complications are represented by deep infection, pulmonary embolism, intra-abdominal fluid extravasation, large-vessel vascular injury, definitive nerve injury, avascular necrosis, femoral neck fracture, trochanteric nonunion, dislocation, and death. Minor complications are iatrogenic chondrolabral damage, skin damage, temporary nerve palsy, capsular adhesion, deep vein thrombosis, broken instrumentation, heterotopic ossification, and microinstability [2].

This chapter will give an overview of the general complications that can occur during hip preservation surgery, management of specific complications related to FAI surgery in general, and according to the surgical technique in particular. The failures of FAI surgery (incomplete reshaping, recurrence of FAI, evolution toward osteoarthritis, etc.) will not be discussed in this chapter.

For each complication, we will review its incidence in published literature, with its risk factors, before exposing how to make its diagnosis and how to prevent it.

O.R. Ayeni et al. (eds.), *Diagnosis and Management of Femoroacetabular Impingement*,
DOI 10.1007/978-3-319-32000-7_17

17.1 General Complications

17.1.1 Infection

FAI surgery has a low rate of septic complications and the majority are superficial infections. Three cases of septic arthritis have been described in the literature [2–4]. The reported incidence is approximately 1/1000 in hip arthroscopy, but it can reach 2 % in FAI open surgery.

There are no current recommendations of prophylactic antibiotic treatment. However, routine preoperative administration of broad-spectrum antibiotics is advised if osseous procedures are anticipated (osteoplasty or anchor placement).

17.1.2 Deep Venous Thrombosis and Pulmonary Embolism

The incidence of deep venous thrombosis varies between 0.1 and 3.7 % according to the studies. The incidence of pulmonary embolism is less than 1/1000 [1, 2, 4–7]. Risk factors are the usual risk factors to venous thromboembolism. In hip arthroscopy, lower limb traction against the padded bolster can also produce endothelial injuries and/or compression of pelvic and femoral veins. The American College of Chest Physicians guidelines do not recommend systematic thromboprophylaxis, but only for high-risk individuals, extrapolating from knee arthroscopy experience [8].

In hip surgical dislocation, low-molecular-weight heparin is prescribed until the resumption of full weight bearing.

17.2 Specific Complications

17.2.1 Hip Instability

Hip dislocation is a feared complication, although it remains exceptional. In the literature, only few cases of dislocation have been accurately described after hip arthroscopy [9–15] and no case after open surgery.

An excessive acetabular rim resection, to treat a pincer effect, seems to be the most logical risk factor, transforming an acetabulum with good or borderline coverage into an acetabulum with insufficient anterior coverage, equivalent of acetabular dysplasia. But in the dislocation case reports after hip arthroscopy, only two had an acetabular rim resection [9, 14]. Three hip dislocations had CAM resection associated to iliopsoas tenotomy [10, 11] and one, an isolated CAM resection [15]. The anterior hip joint capsule and the labrum have a major stabilizing role, especially for hips with low coverage of the acetabulum. Iliopsoas muscle plays an important role of anterior dynamic stability. A large capsulotomy without repair, an iliopsoas release, and the absence or inadequate labral repair increase the risk of anterior hip instability especially if present concurrently.

Hip microinstability corresponds to minor form of instability, with the same risk factors. It is probably more frequent, but hardly diagnosed, thus remaining underestimated. The diagnosis can be challenging, only suspected by the patient's history and clinical exam, without another possible diagnosis. Microinstabilities can be manifested by recurrent groin pain, with or without trigger movements. Provocative maneuvers are not reliable, but hyperlaxity needs to be evaluated. AP pelvic radiograph usually reveals low acetabular center-edge angle (CEA). MRI or arthro-MRI often does not demonstrate specific or direct signs of these microinstabilities, though occasionally capsular defects will be identified and frequently anterior chondrolabral lesions will be seen.

Identifying patients at risk of postoperative instability is crucial to adapt arthroscopic procedures in particular for patients with CEA <25°, general or isolated hip hyperlaxity, or for patients prone to extreme range of motion (ballet, dancers, gymnasts). The capsulotomy must be as limited as possible and should be repaired prior to closure for these patients. Acetabuloplasty should be avoided and is absolutely contraindicated in patients with CEA <20°. An iliopsoas tenotomy must be performed only in symptomatic patients and avoided in patients with a significant anteversion of the femoral neck. Capsular repair is strongly recommended when psoas release is performed [10, 11].

17.2.2 Femoral Neck Fracture

Femoral neck fracture remains exceptional after FAI surgical treatment, lower than 1/1000 according to the literature. In two recent systematic reviews, one case was described out of 6962 hip arthroscopic procedures for the first one [1] and three cases out of 6334 for the second one [2]. All fractures occurred after femoral CAM resection.

In a cadaveric model, Mardones et al. found that up to 30 % of the femoral neck diameter could be resected at the anterolateral aspect of the head-neck junction, without substantially affecting its load-bearing capacity [16]. However, a 30 % resection did decrease the amount of energy required to produce a fracture. The same conclusion was found after simulation with CT scan and 3D Finite Element model [17].

Additional risk factors for femoral neck fracture, in addition to excessive resection of the femoral neck, are patient's age and bone quality, level of postoperative weight bearing, and postoperative trauma [18].

In the open surgical dislocation procedure, the volume of resection can be directly estimated by complete exposure of the femoral head-neck junction. In the arthroscopic procedure, the field of view of the arthroscope prevents complete visualization of the femoral head-neck junction. A total examination with the arthroscope in different positions is necessary to understand the shape and size of CAM deformities, in order to avoid an excessive resection. A large capsulotomy or capsulectomy may be needed to expose the deformity [19]. If any doubt, intraoperative fluoroscopy can be helpful.

17.2.3 Avascular Necrosis of the Femoral Head

Avascular necrosis of the femoral head (AVN) is the most feared complication in hip surgical dislocation. Nevertheless, it remains exceptional with no reported cases when the hip surgical anterior dislocation technique, described by Ganz [20], is performed to treat an isolated femoroacetabular impingement. A few cases of AVN are only reported when another osteotomy is associated to FAI treatment, such as a reduction of a slipped capital femoral epiphysis or intertrochanteric osteotomy [4]. After hip arthroscopy, two case reports of AVN were published in the literature [21, 22]. Surprisingly, the two recent systematic reviews give quite different results about AVN's incidence after hip arthroscopy, one reporting one case out of 6962 procedures [1] and the other one reporting ten cases out of 6334 [2]. However, the methodology of these two studies is quite similar.

If AVN occurs when the medial femoral circumflex artery is injured during surgical dislocation, its etiology has not been clearly identified during hip arthroscopic procedures. AVN could be attributed to the vascular compromise caused by traction combined with high fluid pressure in the joint tamponading local intraosseous blood flow [23]. AVN could also result to an injury of the lateral femoral circumflex artery, during portal placement and capsulotomy [21], or to an injury of the lateral epiphyseal branches of the medial femoral circumflex artery, occurring either by a wide T capsulotomy or by a femoral CAM resection performed too far posterolaterally [21, 22].

Persistent mechanical or inflammatory groin pain, with sometimes a remission period after the arthroscopy, can suggest the osteonecrosis. The range of motion is often limited. The MRI is the best exam to confirm an early diagnosis.

To prevent AVN-related complications, extremely elevated traction and intra-articular fluid pressure must be applied with caution. The capsulotomy must be limited in the posterior part of the femoral neck, and the CAM resection must be carefully pursued laterally in the peripheral compartment.

17.2.4 Heterotopic Ossification

The incidence of heterotopic ossification (HO) after hip arthroscopy varies from 1 to 12 % according to the literature [8, 24–26]. It is lower than in series of open surgical dislocation of the hip, where HO can reach 20–30 % [25]. Arthroscopic surgery is typically muscle preserving and may benefit from continuous joint and periarticular tissue irrigation that evacuates hematoma and bone debris, both widely known to be precursors to HO [25].

Diagnosis is made on X-rays, with visible ossifications within the soft tissues of the hip joint (Fig. 17.1), described by the Brooker classification [27]. Brooker grades I and II can give minimal symptoms, without significant loss of range of motions. The HO grade III and IV can be revealed by stiffness and a discomfort with latero-trochanteric pains that differs from preoperative groin-based pain.

To prevent HO, instrument exchange should always be performed with a cannula left in place during hip arthroscopy; this reduces muscle injuries by instrument passage. Also, the literature suggests that the joint should be washed out at the end of the procedure to evacuate the generated bone debris [18]. Because even small ossifications might affect the patients' performance or function [28], HO prophylaxis with oral nonsteroidal anti-inflammatory drug (NSAID) is recommended. NSAID administered for 3–4 weeks postoperatively reduces significantly the rate of HO, after hip arthroscopy [25, 29]. However, the exact dosing and duration of treatment is still debated.

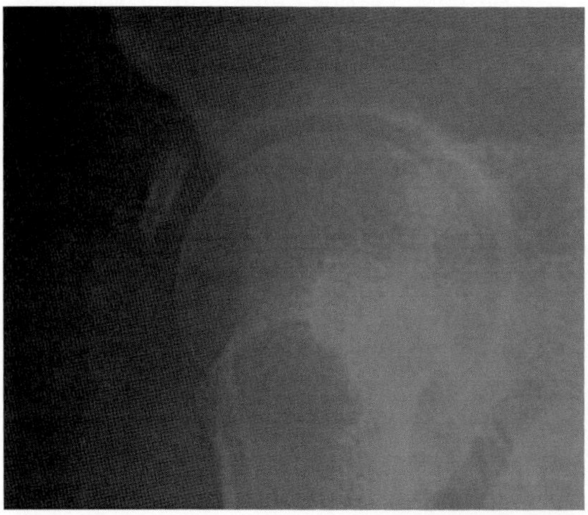

Fig. 17.1 Post operative heterotopic ossification on plain films

17.2.5 Suture Cut-Through During Labral Repair

Repairs of labral tears of the hip using suture anchors are now common. The suture can be positioned around the labrum as a cinch stitch or can pierce through the labral substance in a vertical mattress configuration. During passage of the suture through the labrum or in cases of excessive tightening, it is possible to cut the labrum, the stitch acting as a "butter slicer." It leads to sectioning off of some or all of the circumferential fibers of the labrum, disrupting the associated hoop stresses, with negative biomechanical consequences.

A cut-through is more likely with the vertical mattress technique as the suture is looped around hypoplastic labral tissue, leading some authors to recommend the cinch stitch technique. On the other hand, cinch stitch technique has been criticized for potentially everting the labrum and not restoring its normal triangular cross-section and labral seal function.

Therefore, our recommendations to prevent suture cut-through during labral repair are:

- To avoid overtightening sutures
- To favor cinch stitch technique when the labrum appears thin, hypoplastic, or fragile [18]

17.2.6 Adhesions

After surgical dislocation, 6.2 % arthroscopic adhesiolysis has been reported in 97 hips [30]. After hip arthroscopy, adhesions tend to develop between the labrum and the capsule (Fig. 17.2) and between the femoral neck and the capsule. Hypothetically, they would occur more frequently after acetabular and/or femoral osteoplasty with large capsular dissection.

Adhesions manifest by persistent postoperative pain, associated with a restricted flexion and rotation, by impairing the sealing function of the labrum or impinging against it. The diagnosis can be confirmed with MR arthrography.

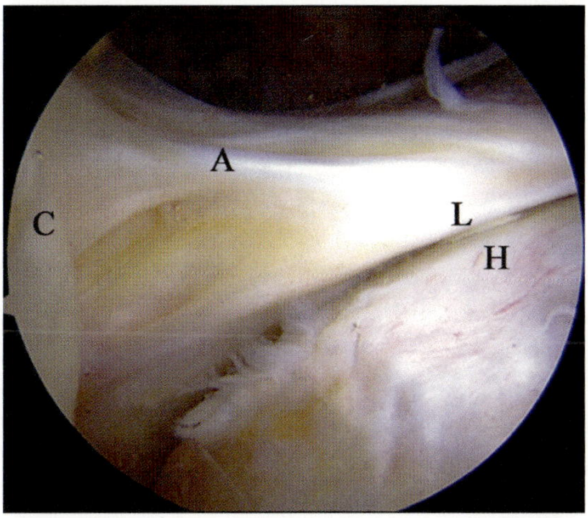

Fig. 17.2 Arthroscopic view of post operative adhesions

Early postoperative mobilization, particularly circumduction, is considered as the best prevention [18].

17.2.7 Pediatric Complications

The treatment of femoroacetabular impingement, either by arthroscopy or by open surgical dislocation, in the skeletally immature population, appears as safe as in the adult population without any case of slipped upper femoral epiphysis, osteonecrosis, triradiate cartilage injury, or growth disturbance [31, 32]. But the short-term follow-up and the low rate of hip osteoplasty in the literature can explain the absence of specific pediatric complications. Larger studies with longer follow-up on this unique population will enhance our understanding of the unique complications in pediatric patients.

17.3 Complications According to Surgical Technique

17.3.1 Specific Complications of Hip Arthroscopy

The complication rate, after arthroscopic treatment of femoroacetabular impingement, varies according to the studies from 1.3 to 15 %, with 0.3–1.7 % major complications [1, 2, 26, 33–36].

17.3.1.1 Complications Secondary to Traction

As hip is a congruent joint with a thick capsule and a large muscular envelope, important traction must be applied on the leg, to distract the joint and to allow safe access to the central compartment.

This strong traction can cause cutaneous and nerve related injuries.

Nerve Injury

The incidence of nerve injuries varies greatly according to the studies. It can reach up to 20 %, when authors consider temporary neuropraxia, with pudendal nerve palsy being the most frequent [2].

Pudendal neuropraxia is secondary to the nerve compression between the perineal support and the pubic ramus. It appears prematurely after arthroscopy, often by perineal hypoesthesia or dysesthesia [37].

Sciatic and peroneal nerve injuries remain unusual. They are secondary to stretching forces on the nerves, during the traction. Telleria [38] has monitored the sciatic nerve during hip arthroscopy and found sciatic nerve dysfunctions increasing after 32 min of traction, with traction force superior to 22.7 kg. The patient complains of dysesthesia on the lateral aspect of the leg and dorsum of the foot, with weakness of ankle dorsiflexion.

These injuries generally solve spontaneously in few days to 6 months. Long-term sequelae are exceptional.

Skin Perineal Damage

The overall rate of perineal skin damage is approximately 2/1000 [2]. It is secondary to a prolonged and important compression of the skin between the pubis ramus and the perineal support.

The injuries can be ranging from edema or hematoma to skin necrosis and pressure sore (Fig. 17.3). It can affect the perineum (scrotum and labia), the skin of the groin, and the inner part of the thigh.

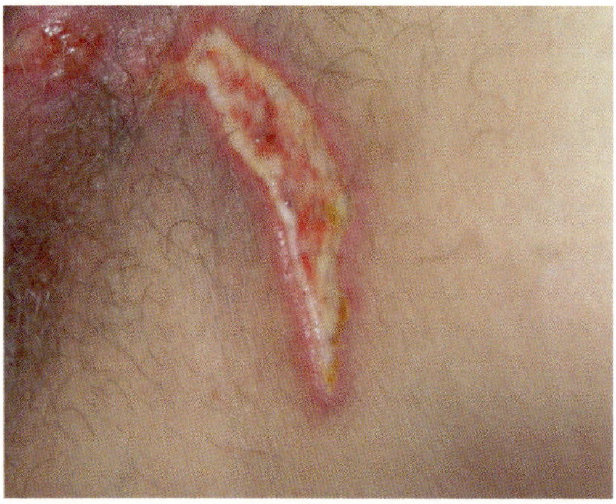

Fig. 17.3 Post operative skin necrosis

It is the same process as for the formation of bedsores, in accelerated procedures. This complication delays the hip rehabilitation, but again the long-term sequelae remain very rare.

To limit complications secondary to traction, two points are essential:

- *Traction force*: The general consensus is to distract the joint of approximately 10 mm (with a mean distraction force between 200 and 400 N). For a better distribution of compression forces, the well-padded bolster, in contact with the perineum, must be large (>10 cm in diameter) [39]. Initial abduction of the hip decreases the traction force on the perineum [40], as well as placing the patient in Trendelenburg position [41]. A peripheral compartment starting point allows to perform the capsulotomy without traction, decreasing the traction force necessary to distract hip during central compartment access, by a disruption of the hip joint suction-seal mechanism [42].
- *Traction time:* Traction time must be as short as possible. The surgeon's experience remains the best method to decrease it significantly. Peripheral compartment starting point allows one to perform capsulotomy and capsulolabral exposure without traction, decreasing also the traction time [42]. In situations where long traction periods are required (>2 h), traction should be released for a period of 15 min and then reapplied [43].

To overcome the traction-related complications, Sadri has described satisfying results with a hip distractor, an equivalent of external fixator, fixed on the acetabulum and femoral diaphysis [44]. Nevertheless, other specific complications to this technique are described.

17.3.1.2 Complications Secondary to Portals

Aberrant Portal Placement

Direct trauma of neurovascular structures can occur during portal placement, since every entry point is near neurovascular structures, in particular when the leg is under traction. The anterior portal is close to the lateral femoral cutaneous nerve (average distance, 5 mm), to the femoral nerve (average distance, 24 mm), and to the femoral artery (average distance, 39 mm) [45, 46]. The posterolateral portal is near the sciatic nerve at the level of capsule (average distance, 29 mm); and the anterolateral portal can come close to the superior gluteal nerve.

The lateral femoral cutaneous nerve, the nearest structure to the anterior portal, is at greatest risk of injury. Its incidence can reach 1 %, according to studies [45, 47]. It manifests by a numbness sensation in the anterolateral part of the thigh.

Knowledge of the anatomy around the hip joint is the best preventive measure of these complications. Neutral positioning of the leg is important during portal placement to ensure that the anatomy is not distorted.

Chondral and Labral Injury

Iatrogenic labral or chondral injuries are the most common complication of hip arthroscopy. The rate of this complication is very approximate and probably underreported by surgeons [2, 48, 49], varying from 0.67 to 20 % for labral injuries and from 0.3 to 39 % for chondral injuries, according to published studies.

The labral penetration is generally realized during establishment of the initial anterolateral portal, when performing central compartment first approach. It is localized in the superior or anterosuperior part of the labrum. The spinal needle can go through the labrum when it is placed too close to the acetabulum. The guidewire, and then the cannula, will follow the same track. The tear of the labrum will then have the same size as the diameter of the cannula (Fig. 17.4). On the other hand, positioning the needle too close to the femoral head can lead to direct chondral damage by the needle or the cannula. The second portal is typically safe since the needle penetrates in the joint under direct visualization by arthroscope.

Some indications of hip arthroscopy are more at risk to cause chondrolabral injuries, such as labral detachment, where the labrum occupies a large part of the joint space, or stiff hips, when sufficient distraction of 10 mm is not possible.

Once the surgeon has penetrated into the joint, there is less danger of labral damage, but chondral lesions can still occur. The repetitive exchange of instruments, in particular without the use of a cannula, and bad portal placement are risk factors of femoral head cartilage injuries. Acetabular cartilage injuries can also occur by intra-articular penetration of anchors, during labral repair.

These damages are immediately visualized during the arthroscopy. Badylak and Keene have shown that iatrogenic labral punctures do not affect the clinical results at short term, with a follow-up of 2 years or more [48]. However, their long-term consequences on the cartilage wear patterns have not been studied.

Peripheral compartment first approach allows reducing the risk of chondrolabral lesions, comparing to central compartment first approach [42]. Indeed, during peripheral approach, the instrumentation is introduced along the anterior femoral neck, at a safe distance to the labrum and cartilage. The capsulotomy is performed safely until the capsulolabral junction, which is easily visualized. Then, central compartment access can be performed under direct vision.

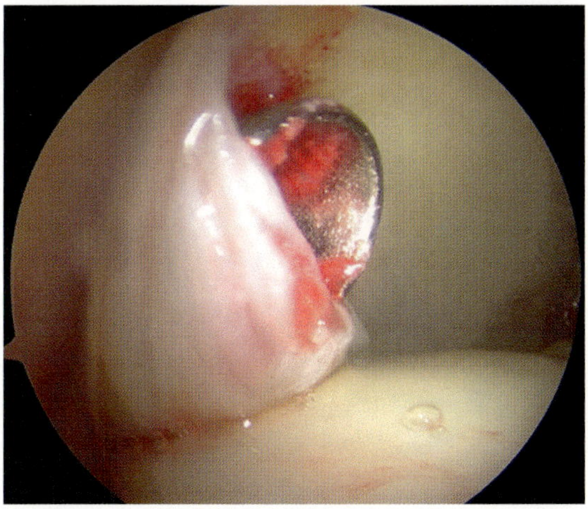

Fig. 17.4 Penetration of the labrum by metal cannula

To diminish risk of chondrolabral lesions when performing central compartment first approach, the needle and cannula should be inserted into the joint under fluoroscopic guidance, in order to obtain the best position level to penetrate the hip. Byrd has described a fluoroscopic sign to control if the needle has punctured the labrum during the portal placement [50]. After the needle has penetrated into the joint, a saline solution is injected. The needle should move distally with the femoral head, checked under fluoroscopy. If the needle stays proximal, a labral perforation is probable. The position of the needle should then be changed.

In order not to force the passage inside the hip with the hazard to create iatrogenic chondral lesions, instrument exchange should always be performed with a cannula. Also, to avoid intra-articular penetration of anchors, the position and direction of the drill should be carefully controlled before drilling. Hernandez [51] and then Lertwanich [52] have described the safe position for suture anchor insertion. The ideal starting point for anchor insertion is located on the capsular side of labral insertion, which is between 2.3 and 2.6 mm from the edge of the acetabular rim. The angle formed by the long axis of the drill and a perpendicular to the acetabular face is considered safe when it is between −7.2° and 20.4°, according to acetabular rim location and anchor size less than 3 mm. Nevertheless, drilling should always be supervised under arthroscopic vision of the acetabular articular surface

17.3.1.3 Complications Due to Arthroscopic Tools

Extra-articular Fluid Extravasation

A survey of the MAHORN group has identified 40 cases of intra-abdominal fluid extravasation on 25,648 hip arthroscopies, with an incidence of

0.16% [53]. According to other studies, the rate of this complication can reach 3/1000 [2]. This complication is probably due to the irrigation fluid diffusion along the iliopsoas sheath. The extravasation is generally retroperitoneal, sometimes intraperitoneal.

Possible risk factors can be a prolonged operative time (2 h or more), a high pressure of the irrigation fluid, an iliopsoas tenotomy at the beginning of the procedure, an extended capsulotomy, and the presence of an acetabular fracture [53].

Symptoms vary depending on the amount of extravasation volume. Verma et al. described five warning signs that must alert the surgeon and anesthetist during the surgery: inability to distend the joint, increased fluid requirement to maintain distension, frequent cutoff of pump irrigation systems, abdominal and thigh distension, and acute hypothermia [54]. In the recovery room, the patient can present with abdominal pain and distension, dyspnea, hypothermia, hemodynamic instability, and/or decreased venous return circulation from the lower extremities. Ultrasound or CT scan can confirm the diagnosis.

The preventive measures are to reduce the operative time, to limit the capsulotomy, to delay iliopsoas tenotomy to the end of surgery, to limit pump pressure 40–50 mmHg, to be cautious during hip arthroscopy for acute acetabular fractures, and to evaluate frequently the abdomen and the patient's hemodynamic status.

Mechanical Failure of Instrumentation

The risk of mechanical failure is high, compared to other joints, with an incidence varying between 0.2 and 3.5% according to the studies [2, 33, 34].

The most frequent is instrument breakage (Fig. 17.5) due to the need to use long instruments, often fragile, subjected to high stresses in this deep joint. Suture anchor failure is also described, due to the narrowness of the anterior acetabular rim [51].

To limit the risk, the needle, the Nitinol guidewire, the shaver, and the burr are usually disposable. Also, a sufficient capsulotomy increases instruments mobility, reducing stresses on the devices. Anchor placement should be controlled and resistance to manual traction should be tested before suture deployment.

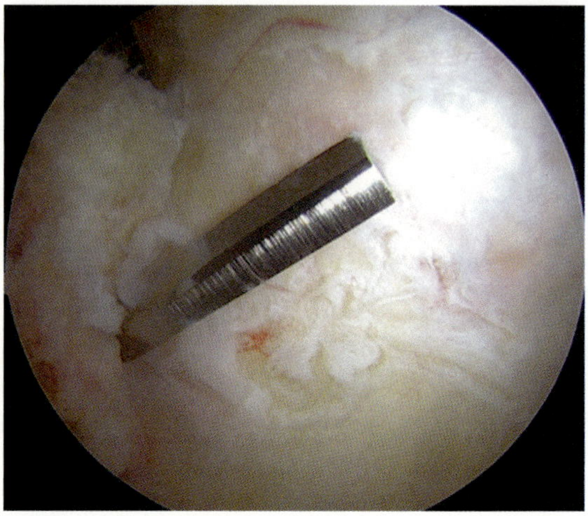

Fig. 17.5 Arthroscopic instrumentation breakage into the joint

In case of instrument breakage or anchor failure, the latter need to be removed, sometimes by arthrotomy, since they can cause serious chondral injuries.

17.3.1.4 Other Reported Complications

Other complications have been reported: hypothermia, inferior gluteal artery pseudoaneurysm, second-degree burn by fluid extravasation, snapping sounds, bleeding, and portal hematoma. These all are exceptional.

17.3.2 Specific Complications of Mini-open Approach Arthroscopically Assisted

The complication rate of mini-open approach surgery varies between 0 and 26% depending on the studies [3, 55–58].

17.3.2.1 Lateral Femoral Cutaneous Nerve (LFCN) Injury

Since mini-open approach incision for FAI treatment is just below and outside the passage of this nerve, LFCN injury is the most common specific complication of this surgery, reaching 22% in some studies.

The symptoms are dysesthesia in the anterolateral part of the thigh, which appears immediately after the surgery. It generally disappears spontaneously within weeks or months, without any sequelae.

Performing the incision 1.5 cm laterally to the classic incision described by Hueter reduces the risk of LFCN injury [3].

17.3.2.2 Other Complications

Few cases of femoral nerve injury have been noted [57]. The other complications are nonspecific to this mini-open approach and are described in the previous chapters. They remain rare and are secondary to open surgery, to hip arthroscopy with traction, and to FAI treatment.

17.3.3 Specific Complications of Hip Surgical Dislocation

The incidence of complications after hip surgical dislocation varies between 2 and 37 % according the studies, with a major complication rate up to 6 % [4, 20, 30, 59–61].

17.3.3.1 Trochanteric Nonunion or Migration

Nonunion of the trochanter is the most common major complication of this surgical technique, up to 6 % in some studies. During this approach, the trochanteric osteotomy is performed behind the posterior insertion of gluteus medius, leading the gluteus medius and vastus lateralis inserted on the trochanteric fragment. Therefore, high anterior forces are applied on the trochanter that can lead to nonunion and/or migration of the fragment. This complication occurs most often in the case of a flat trochanteric osteotomy [62], an inadequate fixation technique, an insufficient period of protection, or if the vastus lateralis muscle is released of the fragment [20].

The trochanteric nonunion can produce trochanteric mechanical pain, without a pain-free interval since surgery. Sometimes there is a residual abductor weakness or, at worst, a Trendelenburg gait. The diagnosis is confirmed on imaging: AP radiography or CT scan.

To reduce the risk of this complication, accurate surgical technique and cautious rehabilitation should be observed:

- A "digastric" osteotomy is better, the vastus lateralis muscle remaining inserted to counteract the gluteal muscle.
- A stepped osteotomy is better able to resist tensile and rotational forces [62].
- Strong fixation of the trochanteric osteotomy is required, with at least two or three cortical screws and sometimes other fixation materials [4, 7].
- Progressive rehabilitation with active abduction, passive adduction, and full weight bearing is allowed only after 6–8 weeks [20, 62].

17.3.3.2 Trochanteric Irritation, Bursitis, or Pain

This is the most common complication of the surgical dislocation technique, up to 26 % in some studies [30, 61, 63]. These trochanteric pains are secondary to bursitis or to metallosis, generally caused by the trochanteric hardware. Removal of fixation hardware usually gives a complete relief of this pain in the majority of cases.

17.3.3.3 Other Complications

Other complications of open surgery are described after hip surgical dislocation; but some are specific like sciatic nerve palsy or residual "saddlebag" deformities.

Take-Home Points

1. Be aware of rim resection, labral resection, capsulotomy, and iliopsoas tenotomy in patients at risk of postoperative instability (CEA <25°, hyperlaxity, patients prone to extreme range of motion).
2. Be precise when performing femoral CAM resection, in order to achieve enough but not over resection. Adequate capsulotomy and total CAM examination,

with the arthroscope in different positions, is required. Use fluoroscopy if there is any doubt.
3. Take care of traction force and traction time, to limit skin perineal damage and nerve injuries secondary to traction.
4. Use switching cannula during instrument exchange, to limit the risk of chondral damage or neurovascular lesions and to reduce muscular lesions, leading factor of heterotopic ossifications.
5. Pay special attention when performing trochanteric osteotomy, in order to avoid trochanteric nonunion. Digastric and stepped osteotomy with a strong fixation should be achieved.

Key Evidence Related Sources

1. Kowalczuk M, et al. Complications following hip arthroscopy: a systematic review and meta-analysis. Knee Surg Sports Traumatol Arthrosc. 2013;21(7): 1669–75.
2. Harris JD, et al. Complications and reoperations during and after hip arthroscopy: a systematic review of 92 studies and more than 6,000 patients. Arthroscopy. 2013;29(3):589–95.
3. Ilizaliturri Jr VM. Complications of arthroscopic femoroacetabular impingement treatment: a review. Clin Orthop Relat Res. 2009;467(3):760–8.
4. Pailhe R, et al. Pudendal nerve neuralgia after hip arthroscopy: retrospective study and literature review. Orthop Traumatol Surg Res. 2013;99(7): 785–90.
5. Griffin DR, Villar RN. Complications of arthroscopy of the hip. J Bone Joint Surg Br. 1999;81(4):604–6.
6. Kocher MS, et al. Intra-abdominal fluid extravasation during hip arthroscopy: a survey of the MAHORN group. Arthroscopy. 2012;28(11):1654–60.e2.

Bibliography

1. Kowalczuk M, et al. Complications following hip arthroscopy: a systematic review and meta-analysis. Knee Surg Sports Traumatol Arthrosc. 2013; 21(7):1669–75.
2. Harris JD, et al. Complications and reoperations during and after hip arthroscopy: a systematic review of 92 studies and more than 6,000 patients. Arthroscopy. 2013;29(3):589–95.
3. Laude F, Sariali E, Nogier A. Femoroacetabular impingement treatment using arthroscopy and anterior approach. Clin Orthop Relat Res. 2009;467(3):747–52.
4. Sink EL, et al. Multicenter study of complications following surgical dislocation of the hip. J Bone Joint Surg Am. 2011;93(12):1132–6.
5. Matsuda DK, et al. Comparative systematic review of the open dislocation, mini-open, and arthroscopic surgeries for femoroacetabular impingement. Arthroscopy. 2011;27(2):252–69.
6. Papalia R, et al. Femoroacetabular impingement syndrome management: arthroscopy or open surgery? Int Orthop. 2012;36(5):903–14.
7. Naal FD, et al. Midterm results of surgical hip dislocation for the treatment of femoroacetabular impingement. Am J Sports Med. 2012;40(7): 1501–10.
8. Chan K, et al. Complications following hip arthroscopy: a retrospective review of the McMaster experience (2009–2012). Can J Surg. 2013;56(6):422–6.
9. Matsuda DK. Acute iatrogenic dislocation following hip impingement arthroscopic surgery. Arthroscopy. 2009;25(4):400–4.
10. Austin DC, Horneff 3rd JG, Kelly 4th JD. Anterior hip dislocation 5 months after hip arthroscopy. Arthroscopy. 2014;30:1380–2.
11. Sansone M, et al. Total dislocation of the hip joint after arthroscopy and ileopsoas tenotomy. Knee Surg Sports Traumatol Arthrosc. 2013;21(2):420–3.
12. Mei-Dan O, McConkey MO, Brick M. Catastrophic failure of hip arthroscopy due to iatrogenic instability: can partial division of the ligamentum teres and iliofemoral ligament cause subluxation? Arthroscopy. 2012;28(3):440–5.
13. Ranawat AS, McClincy M, Sekiya JK. Anterior dislocation of the hip after arthroscopy in a patient with capsular laxity of the hip. A case report. J Bone Joint Surg Am. 2009;91(1):192–7.
14. Rosenbaum A, et al. Posterior dislocation of the hip following arthroscopy - a case report and discussion. Bull Hosp Jt Dis (2013). 2014;72(2):181–4.
15. Dierckman BD, Guanche CA. Anterior hip capsuloligamentous reconstruction for recurrent instability after hip arthroscopy. Am J Orthop (Belle Mead NJ). 2014;43(12):E319–23.
16. Mardones RM, et al. Surgical treatment of femoroacetabular impingement: evaluation of the effect of the size of the resection. J Bone Joint Surg Am. 2005;87(2):273–9.

17. Alonso-Rasgado T, et al. Changes in the stress in the femoral head neck junction after osteochondroplasty for hip impingement: a finite element study. J Orthop Res. 2012;30(12):1999–2006.
18. Papavasiliou AV, Bardakos NV. Complications of arthroscopic surgery of the hip. Bone Joint Res. 2012;1(7):131–44.
19. Ilizaliturri Jr VM. Complications of arthroscopic femoroacetabular impingement treatment: a review. Clin Orthop Relat Res. 2009;467(3):760–8.
20. Ganz R, et al. Surgical dislocation of the adult hip a technique with full access to the femoral head and acetabulum without the risk of avascular necrosis. J Bone Joint Surg Br. 2001;83(8):1119–24.
21. Scher DL, Belmont Jr PJ, Owens BD. Case report: osteonecrosis of the femoral head after hip arthroscopy. Clin Orthop Relat Res. 2010;468(11): 3121–5.
22. Sener N, et al. Avascular necrosis of the femoral head after hip arthroscopy. Hip Int. 2011;21(5): 623–6.
23. Naito M, et al. Acute effect of traction, compression, and hip joint tamponade on blood flow of the femoral head: an experimental model. J Orthop Res. 1992; 10(6):800–6.
24. Ong C, Hall M, Youm T. Surgical technique: arthroscopic treatment of heterotopic ossification of the hip after prior hip arthroscopy. Clin Orthop Relat Res. 2013;471(4):1277–82.
25. Bedi A, et al. The incidence of heterotopic ossification after hip arthroscopy. Am J Sports Med. 2012; 40(4):854–63.
26. Larson CM, Giveans MR. Arthroscopic management of femoroacetabular impingement: early outcomes measures. Arthroscopy. 2008;24(5):540–6.
27. Brooker AF, et al. Ectopic ossification following total hip replacement. Incidence and a method of classification. J Bone Joint Surg Am. 1973;55(8): 1629–32.
28. Randelli F, et al. Heterotopic ossifications after arthroscopic management of femoroacetabular impingement: the role of NSAID prophylaxis. J Orthop Traumatol. 2010;11(4):245–50.
29. Beckmann JT, et al. The effect of NSAID prophylaxis and operative variables on heterotopic ossification after hip arthroscopy. Am J Sports Med. 2014;42(6):1359–64.
30. Steppacher SD, et al. Surgical hip dislocation for treatment of femoroacetabular impingement: factors predicting 5-year survivorship. Clin Orthop Relat Res. 2014;472(1):337–48.
31. de Sa D, et al. Femoroacetabular impingement in skeletally immature patients: a systematic review examining indications, outcomes, and complications of open and arthroscopic treatment. Arthroscopy. 2014; 31:373–84.
32. Nwachukwu BU, et al. Complications of hip arthroscopy in children and adolescents. J Pediatr Orthop. 2011;31(3):227–31.
33. Dietrich F, et al. Complications in hip arthroscopy: necessity of supervision during the learning curve. Knee Surg Sports Traumatol Arthrosc. 2014; 22(4):953–8.
34. Park MS, et al. Hip arthroscopy for femoroacetabular impingement: the changing nature and severity of associated complications over time. Arthroscopy. 2014;30:957–63.
35. Gedouin JE, et al. Assessment of arthroscopic management of femoroacetabular impingement. A prospective multicenter study. Orthop Traumatol Surg Res. 2010;96(8 Suppl):S59–67.
36. Byrd JW, Jones KS. Arthroscopic management of femoroacetabular impingement in athletes. Am J Sports Med. 2011;39(Suppl):7S–13.
37. Pailhe R, et al. Pudendal nerve neuralgia after hip arthroscopy: retrospective study and literature review. Orthop Traumatol Surg Res. 2013; 99(7):785–90.
38. Telleria JJ, et al. Risk of sciatic nerve traction injury during hip arthroscopy-is it the amount or duration? An intraoperative nerve monitoring study. J Bone Joint Surg Am. 2012;94(22):2025–32.
39. Byrd JW. Hip arthroscopy utilizing the supine position. Arthroscopy. 1994;10(3):275–80.
40. Kruger DM, et al. Traction force profiles associated with the use of a fracture table: a preliminary report. J Orthop Trauma. 1990;4(3):283–6.
41. Mei-Dan O, McConkey MO, Young DA. Hip arthroscopy distraction without the use of a perineal post: prospective study. Orthopedics. 2013;36(1):e1–5.
42. Rupp R, Duggan B. Peripheral versus central compartment starting point in hip arthroscopy for femoroacetabular impingement. Orthopedics. 2012; 35(2):e148–53.
43. Griffin DR, Villar RN. Complications of arthroscopy of the hip. J Bone Joint Surg Br. 1999;81(4):604–6.
44. Sadri H. Complex therapeutic hip arthroscopy with the use of a femoral distractor. In: Sekiya JK et al., editors. Techniques in hip arthroscopy and joint preservation surgery. Philadelphia: Saunders; 2011. p. 113–20.
45. Byrd JW, Pappas JN, Pedley MJ. Hip arthroscopy: an anatomic study of portal placement and relationship to the extra-articular structures. Arthroscopy. 1995;11(4):418–23.
46. Elsaidi GA, et al. Complications associated with traction on the hip during arthroscopy. J Bone Joint Surg Br. 2004;86(6):793–6.
47. Oak N, et al. Complications in hip arthroscopy. Sports Med Arthrosc. 2013;21(2):97–105.
48. Badylak JS, Keene JS. Do iatrogenic punctures of the labrum affect the clinical results of hip arthroscopy? Arthroscopy. 2011;27(6):761–7.
49. Domb B, Hanypsiak B, Botser I. Labral penetration rate in a consecutive series of 300 hip arthroscopies. Am J Sports Med. 2012;40(4):864–9.
50. Byrd JW. Avoiding the labrum in hip arthroscopy. Arthroscopy. 2000;16(7):770–3.

51. Hernandez JD, McGrath BE. Safe angle for suture anchor insertion during acetabular labral repair. Arthroscopy. 2008;24(12):1390–4.
52. Lertwanich P, et al. Defining a safety margin for labral suture anchor insertion using the acetabular rim angle. Am J Sports Med. 2011;39(Suppl):111S–6.
53. Kocher MS, et al. Intra-abdominal fluid extravasation during hip arthroscopy: a survey of the MAHORN group. Arthroscopy. 2012;28(11):1654–60.e2.
54. Verma M, Sekiya JK. Intrathoracic fluid extravasation after hip arthroscopy. Arthroscopy. 2010;26(9 Suppl): S90–4.
55. Ribas M, et al. Hip osteoplasty by an anterior minimally invasive approach for active patients with femoroacetabular impingement. Hip Int. 2007;17(2): 91–8.
56. Lincoln M, et al. Combined arthroscopic and modified open approach for cam femoroacetabular impingement: a preliminary experience. Arthrocopy. 2009;25(4):392–9.
57. Cohen SB, et al. Treatment of femoroacetabular impingement in athletes using a mini-direct anterior approach. Am J Sports Med. 2012;40(7):1620–7.
58. Srinivasan SC, Hosny HA, Williams MR. Combined hip arthroscopy and limited open osteochondroplasty for anterior femoroacetabular impingement: early patient reported outcomes. Hip Int. 2013;23(2):218–24.
59. Peters CL, et al. Open treatment of femoroacetabular impingement is associated with clinical improvement and low complication rate at short-term followup. Clin Orthop Relat Res. 2010;468(2):504–10.
60. Botser IB, et al. Open surgical dislocation versus arthroscopy for femoroacetabular impingement: a comparison of clinical outcomes. Arthroscopy. 2011;27(2):270–8.
61. Kempthorne JT, et al. Surgical dislocation of the hip and the management of femoroacetabular impingement: results of the Christchurch experience. ANZ J Surg. 2011;81(6):446–50.
62. Bastian JD, et al. Stepped osteotomy of the trochanter for stable, anatomic refixation. Clin Orthop Relat Res. 2009;467(3):732–8.
63. Beaule PE, Le Duff MJ, Zaragoza E. Quality of life following femoral head-neck osteochondroplasty for femoroacetabular impingement. J Bone Joint Surg Am. 2007;89(4):773–9.

Revision FAI Surgery

18

James T. Beckmann and Marc R. Safran

Contents

J.T. Beckmann
Department of Orthopaedic Surgery, St. Luke's Health System, Boise, ID, USA
e-mail: jtbeckmann@gmail.com

M.R. Safran (✉)
Department of Orthopaedic Surgery, Stanford University, Redwood City, CA, USA
e-mail: msafran@stanford.edu

18.1 Introduction

Femoroacetabular impingement (FAI) is a cause of non-arthritic hip pain and progressive joint damage that has become increasingly recognized since Ganz et al.'s landmark paper in 2003 [1]. While most FAI patients improve substantially from surgical resection of the impinging bone together with the treatment of the resultant intra-articular damage, a subset of patients will not realize satisfactory results. Revision hip preservation surgeries have increased contemporaneously with primary FAI procedures to address these surgical failures. Failures can be defined by lack of symptom improvement, inability to return to a desired activity level, or poor postoperative patient satisfaction [2].

A systematic approach should be used to evaluate patients with failed hip FAI surgery. Basic principles are as follows: (1) diagnose the cause of failure, (2) formulate a treatment plan, and (3) recognize limitations to subsequent hip preservation procedures. The diagnosis should consider all intra-articular hip pathology and extra-articular pathology that may have been initially overlooked or developed postoperatively. Either open or arthroscopic surgical techniques can be used to address residual disease. Following these principles, improvements in patient-reported outcomes can be achieved, but typically the results are inferior to those from primary procedures [3, 4]. Some patients will not benefit from revision

O.R. Ayeni et al. (eds.), *Diagnosis and Management of Femoroacetabular Impingement*,
DOI 10.1007/978-3-319-32000-7_18

preservation techniques, especially when significant cartilage damage or radiographic osteoarthritis is present; total hip arthroplasty may be the only viable solution in these cases.

18.2 Historical Perspective

A historical awareness of arthroscopic hip techniques can be helpful in constructing an investigative framework into a failed primary FAI procedure. With improved understanding of hip pathomechanics, treatment approaches have evolved rapidly over the last decade. Hip-specific instrumentation, improved technical proficiency, and evidence-based outcome data have also contributed to temporal variations in FAI treatment strategies. Knowledge of these historical differences can clue in the revising surgeon to potential sources of continued symptomatology.

Early hip arthroscopy was primarily used for procedures such as loose body removal and isolated labral debridement, but now it is recognized that the impinging bony areas must be resected in addition to addressing the corresponding intra-articular pathology to achieve maximal improvement. Failure to adequately resect bony prominences can result in persistent impingement and continued symptoms requiring corrective FAI surgery [5]. Under-resection of the CAM lesion is the most commonly reported reason for revision (51–90 %) in most series [6]. Additionally, extra-articular impingement occurs in up to 4 % of cases, but is sometimes overlooked because it frequently coexists with intra-articular impingement [7].

More recently, awareness has been focused on soft tissue causes of failure, including labral deficiency and preservation as well as capsular insufficiency. Labral debridement with selective tissue resection was common before repair techniques were developed; however, labral preservation when possible helps to maintain joint fluid mechanics and hip stability through its suction-seal effect and increase in acetabular depth [8]. Symptomatic labral deficiency can be addressed with revision labral repair or reconstruction. Capsular insufficiency (primary or iatrogenic) can result in hip "microinstability" causing persistent pain or gross instability with joint subluxation or dislocation [9, 10]. Intraoperative capsular management consists of capsular repair or plication in patients that have signs of capsular laxity. Routine capsulotomy repair has been recommended in susceptible patient populations, particularly female patients with preoperative signs of instability, radiographic findings of dysplasia, or easily distractible hips upon traction application [11].

18.3 Patient Evaluation

18.3.1 General Considerations

A summary of potential sources of postoperative failures is summarized in Table 18.1. At least 6 months of nonsurgical therapy and three consecutive months lacking improvement should be undertaken before revision surgery is considered. Muscular weakness is a common cause of postoperative pain and must be corrected with directed

Table 18.1 Causes of postoperative failure following FAI surgery

Causes of FAI surgical failures
Bony under-resection
Acetabulum Femoral head-neck junction
Bony over-resection
Acetabulum Femoral head neck junction
Extra-articular impingement
Subspinous
Ischiofemoral Greater trochanter
Capsular insufficiency
Generalized ligamentous laxity
Failure to repair capsule
Labral insufficiency
Prior resection
Failed labral repair
Bony regrowth
Heterotopic ossification
Osseus regrowth of CAM
Postoperative adhesions
Extra-articular pathology
Misdiagnosed preoperatively
Developed postoperatively

physical therapy until full and symmetric strength is achieved. The patient evaluation for failed FAI surgery includes all aspects of a primary hip evaluation (see Chap. 5); components of the diagnostic evaluation that are specific to the revision setting will be discussed in this chapter.

18.3.2 History

The history should delineate between symptoms before and after the index FAI procedure. Ask the patient if their main complaint is pain, weakness, or stiffness/loss of motion and how these symptoms compare to their preoperative state. A distinct change in the quality, location, provocative positions, or timing of pain could indicate a new diagnosis or concomitant pathology. The temporal pattern of postoperative improvement – or lack thereof – can help to determine the cause of failure. A patient that has had no improvement should trigger an investigation into the original diagnosis and broaden the differential to extra-articular sources of pain. Conversely, a positive response to an intra-articular injection prior to the index procedure is usually reassuring that an intra-articular derangement such as FAI existed before the index surgery. Improvement following surgery, even if unsustained, should be investigated to determine the maximal amount of pain relief following surgery and the postoperative timing of maximal improvement. Activities that aggravated the hip symptoms during the recovery process can provide insight into the current diagnosis.

18.3.3 Physical Examination

A complete examination of the operative hip should be conducted and compared with the contralateral side. Standard aspects of the examination include gait analysis, hip range of motion, palpation of the muscular and bony prominences around the hip, and special tests for sources of referred pain including the spine and SI joints. Muscular weakness, which is common following hip arthroscopy, should be normalized to equal the opposite extremity when possible. Iliopsoas weakness from fractional iliopsoas lengthening can cause symptoms of early fatigue, abductor weakness may lead to peritrochanteric pain, and globalized weakness can exacerbate the symptoms associated with capsular instability. Residual impingement and labral stress signs are typically mild to moderately positive during the early recovery period, but, in the senior author's experience, should be decreased compared with preoperative levels at 6 months postoperatively. Markedly positive impingement signs that reproduce the patient's pain can indicate an incomplete bony resection, other types of impingement, or failed labral repair. Capsular instability may be suspected when generalized ligamentous laxity is present (>4/9 positive Beighton criteria) or specific examination maneuvers that stress the capsule elicit pain or subjective instability. The anterior capsule is stressed with external rotation and either abduction or neutral adduction-abduction with either neutral flexion-extension or hyperextension, whereas the posterior capsule is stressed with a posteriorly directed force in 90° of flexion and slight adduction.

18.3.4 Imaging

Radiographs should include an AP pelvis and lateral hip view. A Dunn lateral in 45° of flexion places the 1:30 position on the femoral head-neck junction on profile to evaluate for residual CAM deformity, which most commonly is seen at the 1:15 position in revision cases [6]. The false profile view can be helpful to determine anterior coverage and the morphology of the AIIS. Relief from an intra-articular injection of local anesthetic is useful to confirm an intra-articular source of pain, which can be performed under ultrasound guidance or fluoroscopy. Contrast injection during a fluoroscopically guided injection confirms an intra-articular location, but can result in a decreased negative predictive value due to contrast reaction. In the revision setting, 3D imaging with a CT scan or MRI provides extremely valuable information, and one should use a low threshold to order one or both of these tests. 3D imaging, in combination with collision software, helps to target incomplete resections, bony regrowth, and extra-articular sources of impingement (Fig. 18.1a–c).

18.3.5 Operative Report

Obtaining copies of the operative report and arthroscopic images is essential. Cartilage evaluation with MRA lacks sensitivity for identifying lesions and is best evaluated from arthroscopic pictures. Iatrogenic injuries to the cartilage or acetabular labrum can be visualized in some cases. Some degree of iatrogenic cartilage injury has been reported anecdotally in up to 64 % of cases; labral puncture during initial portal placement is also relatively common (up to 20 %), but has been shown to have no effect on patient outcome at 2 years following repair [12]. McCarthy et al. reported that the sensitivity of MRA for chondral lesions was only 65 % in their series [13]. A patient with severe cartilage damage at the time of index procedure is less likely to benefit from a revision hip preservation procedure. The condition of the labrum

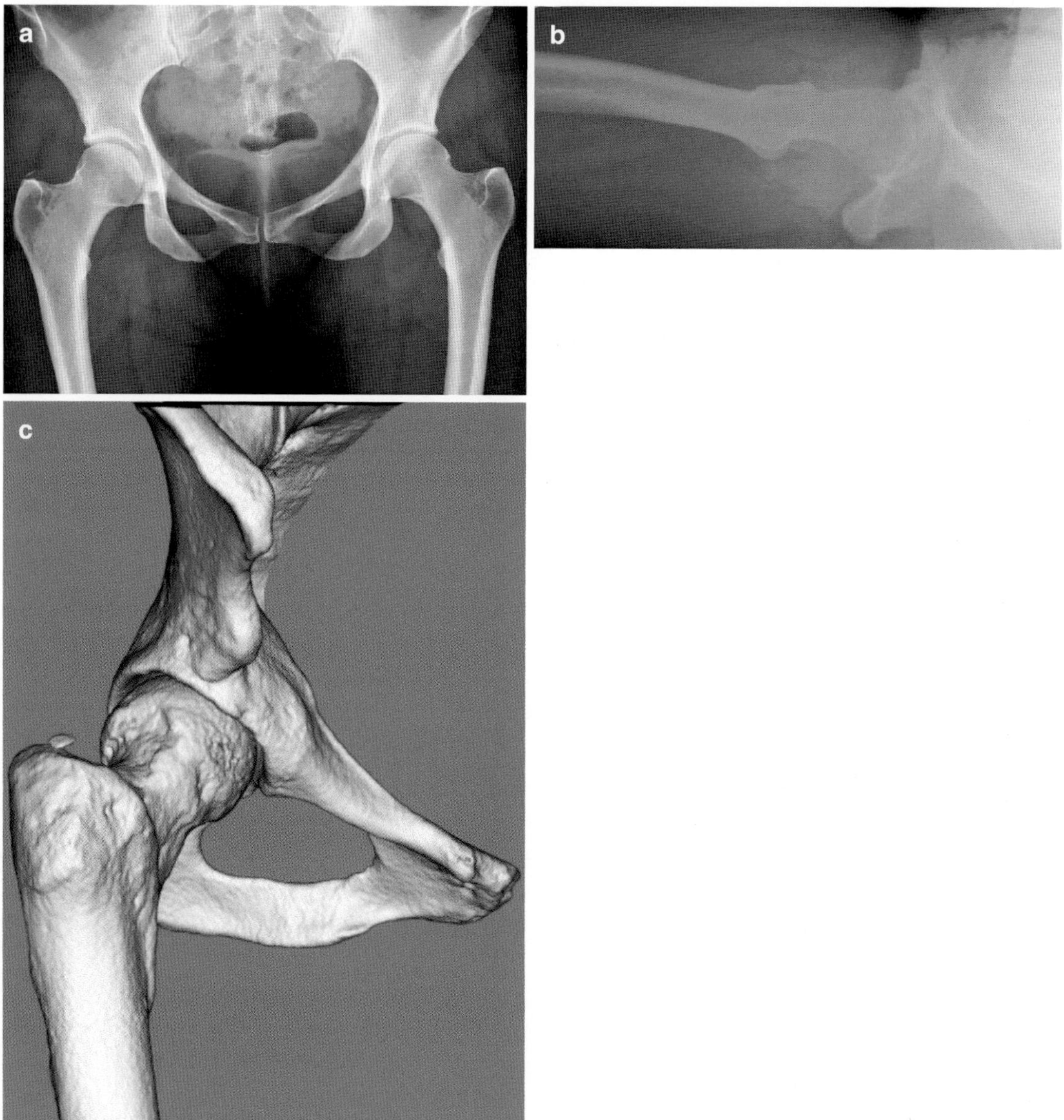

Fig. 18.1 AP (**a**), cross-table lateral (**b**), and 3D CT image (**c**) of a 32-year-old woman who had persistent symptoms of FAI 1 year following incomplete resection; an easily identifiable transition between the resected and residual CAM deformity occurs at the 1:30 position extending anteriorly to 3:00

can also be determined using the operative report, arthroscopic images, and postoperative imaging. Labral reconstruction may be indicated if operative reports or images indicate labral resection was performed without evidence of regrowth on current MRA or congenitally hypoplastic or attenuated labrum. Finally, the operative report will typically indicate if capsular repair was performed during the index procedure. Suspicion for microinstability is increased if no repair or plication was documented, though microinstability may exist even if the capsule was repaired.

18.4 Common Causes of Revision Surgery

18.4.1 Bony Under-resection

The most commonly reported reason for failure of FAI surgery is under-resection of the impinging bone (53–90 %) [5, 6]. Successful correction of FAI requires removal of the entire impinging area. Residual prominences following surgery can cause persistent symptoms even when much of the impinging location of the femoral head-neck junction has been resected. The most commonly reported location of residual FAI is the posterosuperior or lateral location along the femoral head-neck junction when an interportal capsulotomy is used [3]. It has been proposed that the substantial learning curve to perform hip arthroscopy could be culpable for this technical failure and need for revision surgery. Additionally, lack of recognition or ability to address acetabular over-coverage has been reported as another cause of undertreatment of FAI.

Philippon et al. found that 36 of 37 patients had persistent radiographic evidence of FAI in a series of revision hip arthroscopy cases between 2005 and 2006 [14]. Following correction, the modified Harris Hip Scores (mHHS) improved from 56 preoperatively to 77 postoperatively. Kelly et al. found that 79 % of early revision hip arthroscopies between 2003 and 2007 were due to under-addressed or untreated FAI [15]. Likewise, Clohisy et al. reported that 68 % of 60 revisions following primary hip arthroscopy were for residual or untreated FAI [16]. This series differs from the previously mentioned studies because all revision procedures – both open and arthroscopic – were included. In combination, these series report that residual FAI was the most common reason for early revision procedures; however, it is unknown if this trend has continued in recent years as more attention is placed on the underlying bony morphology responsible for labral tears and chondral injuries [17]. For example, in the series by Clohisy et al., osseous deformity was only addressed in 17 of 60 hips at the time of initial FAI surgery, which differs significantly from current practice. Further, as more surgeons are aware of FAI and more surgeons are more comfortable performing FAI surgery, it may be that lack of resection or under-resection of FAI bony anatomy is becoming a less prevalent cause of failed FAI surgery.

Open or arthroscopic methods can be used to address the underlying asphericity of residual bony impingement, but diligent preoperative planning is necessary to identify the location of the lesion. Three-dimensional CT- or MRI-based software can be extremely helpful to understand bony anatomy following previous FAI surgery. Static 2D radiographs show only shadows of the femoral head-neck anatomy corresponding to an orthogonal position from the direction of the X-ray beam. For example, an AP radiograph shows the 12:00 position, 45° Dunn shows the 1:30 position, and lateral views show the 3:00 position; however, the area of maximal deformity could occur anywhere between these positions. 3D reconstructions help map the bony topography and allow visualization of areas that can be missed on standard radiographic views. Figure 18.1 shows the AP, cross-table lateral, and 3D CT image of a patient who had persistent symptoms of FAI following incomplete resection; an easily identifiable transition between the resected and residual C deformity occurs at the 1:30 position extending anteriorly to 3:00. Milone et al. found that alpha angles were underestimated on plain radiographs by an average of 8.2° compared to 3D CT scan [18]. Software advances have recently enabled independent visualization of the femoral and acetabular sides, along with dynamic modeling of joint motion to locate

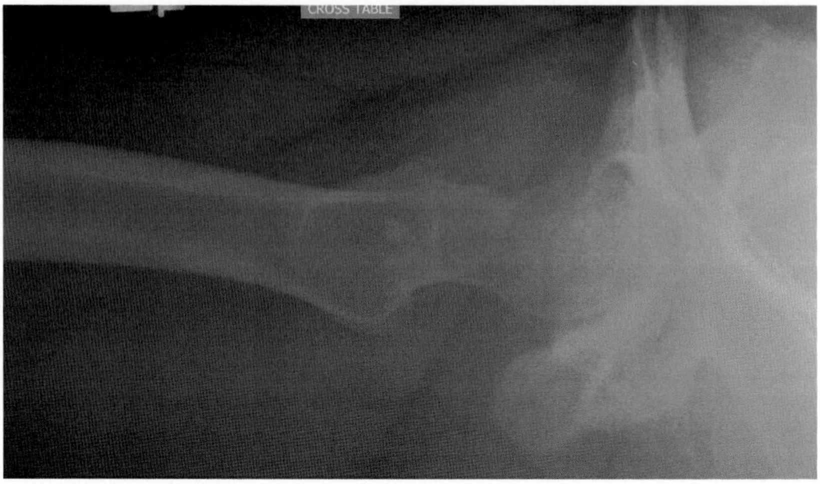

Fig. 18.2 Cross-table radiograph of a patient that previously underwent FAI surgery with large resection of the bone at the femoral head-neck junction. This resulted in loss of hip suction-seal effect in early flexion

potential sources of impingement. 3D CT evaluations should be considered part of the standard workup for failed FAI surgery to identify concerning areas for residual impingement. Reconstructed MRI images can be used in lieu of CT scans for younger patients where the lifetime risk of cancer from radiation exposure is higher.

18.4.2 Bony Over-resection

Although under-resection has been commonly reported as a source of failure, overaggressive bony resection can have its own set of detrimental consequences. Excessive deepening of the head-neck junction risks disruption of the labral suction seal that can reduce stability of the joint (Fig. 18.2). Biomechanical studies show an increased risk of femoral neck fracture if greater than one-third of the femoral neck is resected. Acetabuloplasty can change the contact pressures in the acetabulum resulting in edge loading and early wear mimicking developmental dysplasia of the hip. In extreme cases, instability and dislocation events are possible [19]. Correction of excessive acetabuloplasty may necessitate an open approach to the hip with osteochondral allograft or periacetabular osteotomy to restore normal contact pressures and joint stability. With time, joint damage can be unsalvageable necessitating total hip arthroplasty (Fig. 18.3).

18.4.3 Extra-articular Impingement

Extra-articular impingement refers to locations besides the proximal femur with the acetabular rim where hip motion may be symptomatically impeded. The most common location occurs when the femur impinges on the anterior inferior iliac spine (AIIS), but can also occur between the femur and the ischial tuberosity as well as with the greater trochanter colliding with the acetabulum. Extra-articular impingement is rare, occurring in only 4 % of patients with hip pain, but frequently coexists with CAM morphology and traditional FAI [7]. Patients with documented findings of extra-articular impingement are more likely to be young, female, and those who have undergone previous surgery. These patient demographics overlap substantially with the typical patient who has capsular laxity and may result in markedly increased hip motion allowing extra-articular impingement. It has been hypothesized that extra-articular impingement could create a potential fulcrum that exacerbates capsular stretching and pain via mechanoreceptors within the hip capsule [20].

Patients who should be suspected of having subspinous impingement are those who have a low-lying AIIS and pain with hip hyperflexion in neutral rotation. Pathologic AIIS morphology, particularly when the AIIS extends below the level of the acetabular rim, are often caused by a malunited rectus femoris avulsion injury, though

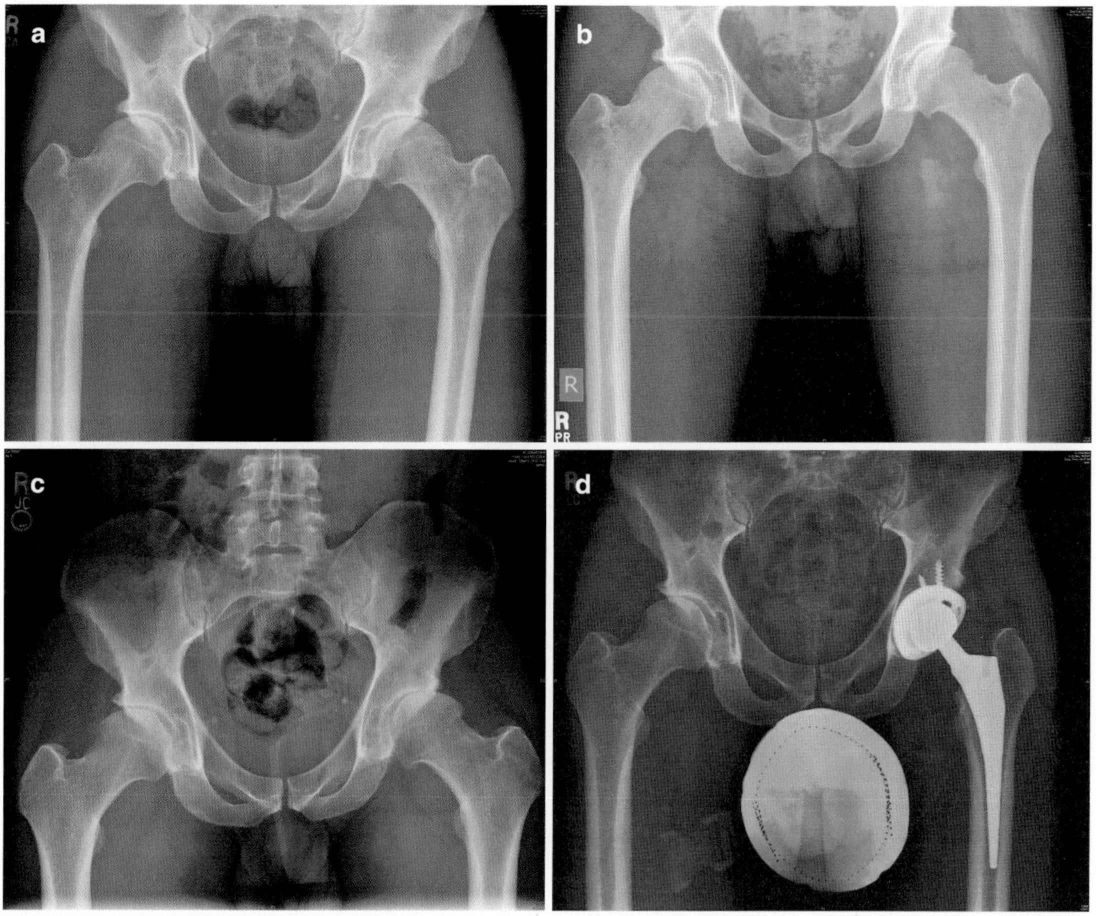

Fig. 18.3 Preoperative (**a**) and postoperative radiographs following acetabuloplasty at 3 months (**b**) and 1 year (**c**). Over-resection of the acetabular rim can result in altered loading properties. If recognized early, coverage can be restored through periacetabular osteotomy or bulk allograft. In this case, edge loading lead to accelerated cartilage damage necessitating total hip arthroplasty (**d**)

elongation of the AIIS may also be seen, and thought to be the result of sprinting and kicking activities as a child, resulting in overgrowth. A history of remote trauma from a previous hip strain can occasionally be elicited. In patients with suspected subspinous impingement, a false profile view or 3D CT scans should be obtained to evaluate AIIS morphology. Intraoperatively, the AIIS can be identified by tracing the direct head of the rectus back to its bony origin from either an extracapsular or intracapsular approach. An iliac oblique intraoperative fluorospot places the AIIS on profile and can be used to ensure adequate resection of the impinging area. Decompression of the AIIS was found to predict improvements in patient-reported outcomes in revision hip arthroscopy cases by Larson et al. [3].

Ischiofemoral impingement occurs when the quadratus femoris musculature is compressed between the lesser tuberosity and the ischium producing chronic groin or buttock pain. Pain is reproduced on physical examination by extension, external rotation, and adduction. Radiographs may reveal decreased femoral offset or evidence of altered bony anatomy such as previous ischial avulsion injury. MRI often shows increased signal within and around the quadratus on fluid-sensitive imaging indicative of compression injury. A diagnostic injection with local anesthetic using ultrasound or CT guidance is confirmatory for the diagnosis. Resection of the impinging bone can be performed endoscopically or through an open posterior approach.

18.4.4 Capsular Instability

The capsule is an important stabilizer of the hip joint that works in concert with static bony restraints, dynamic muscular forces, and the suction seal of the labrum to maintain the congruency of the joint throughout physiologic range of motion [21]. Hip instability results from an inability to maintain a concentric joint without undue stress [22]. Symptoms from instability range from pain only to hip joint unsteadiness or rarely joint dislocation [9]. The concept of hip instability is still early and somewhat controversial. Recent research confirms this evolving concept is a clinical entity. The term microinstability is used to denote pain without frank subluxation or dislocation.

Primary and iatrogenic capsular instability can be a source of persistent pain following surgical intervention. Capsulotomy is often performed to access the hip joint, but the importance of capsular closure has been highlighted in recent studies [11]. A standard capsulotomy between the anterolateral and mid-anterior portal places the iliofemoral ligament – the stoutest ligament in the human body – at risk for complete transection [21]. Failure to repair, or only partially repair the capsule, may lead to postoperative instability and decreased outcome scores compared to full repair [11]. In one study comparing partial versus complete closure of "T" capsulotomies, the complete closure group demonstrated significantly superior outcomes in the HOS-SS at 6 months that were sustained at 2.5 years (83.6 vs. 87.3; $p<.0001$) after surgery. All patients ($n=4$) requiring revision surgery were in the partial repair group.

Specific patient populations may be predisposed to capsular instability including those with baseline hyperlaxity or release of the psoas muscle due to its role as a secondary stabilizer of the hip [23]. Women have been consistently reported to have a higher incidence of capsular instability, which could explain the nearly three times increased revision rate reported by Domb et al. [4].

Capsular instability can be divided into three categories: primary capsular laxity related to innate ligamentous laxity, iatrogenic capsular laxity that can be repaired primarily, and iatrogenic capsular laxity with an irreparable capsular defect requiring grafting. When sufficient tissue is present, capsular shift or plication can be performed to tighten the capsule [24]. This can be performed at the location of the capsulotomy if present or through the lateral capsule or so-called rotator interval of the hip. For this closure, an oval section of capsule is excised using a suction shaver. The size of the oval is 8–10 mm by 12–15 mm. This rotator interval closure has been closed anterior to posterior (with length of the oval being proximal-distal) as well as proximal to distal (with the oval longer anterior to posterior), with no clinical difference identified. If the anterior capsule is intact, lateral plication offers the advantage of not having to transect the iliofemoral ligament [21]. Larson et al. showed that capsular plication during revision hip arthroscopy conferred a statistically significant improvement in postoperative mHHS scores compared to no plication in a cohort restricted to radiographically definable FAI [3]. While there is a lack of scientific study of hip instability and capsular plication, it should be noted that there is much work to be done to study the optimal technique for plication as well as amount. While it has been shown that capsular plication may limit hip range of motion [25], there are also concerns of overconstraining the hip joint, limiting the normal translational motion of the femoral head within the acetabulum [22]. Large capsular defects may be incapable of primary repair (Fig. 18.4a, b). In this case, arthroscopic or open reconstruction with allograft can restore continuity of the capsule to improve stability, though anecdotally discussed, no published clinical reports exist at this time.

18.4.5 Labral Insufficiency

Labral insufficiency is a potential cause of hip pain and microinstability following FAI surgery. It occurs most commonly following labral debridement or failed labral repair. Historically,

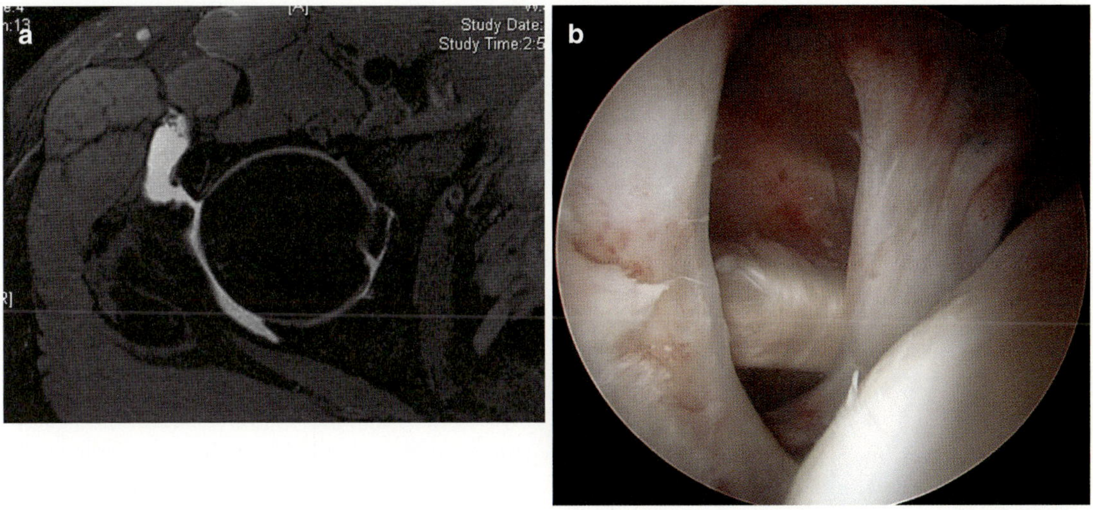

Fig. 18.4 MRI (**a**) of an extensive capsulotomy resulting in symptomatic microinstability. Primary capsular closure may be performed, as in this case. Alternatively, capsular plication may be performed through the interval between the iliofemoral and ischiofemoral ligament to restore the dynamic stabilizing effect of the capsule. Large symptomatic capsular defects (**b**) may require allograft reconstruction

labral debridement was used to treat labral tears before repair techniques were developed. Debridement may still be necessary for treatment of irreparable and degenerative labral tears as well as symptomatic labral ossification necessitating partial labrectomy. Labral retear was a common reason (33–85 %) for revision hip arthroscopy in two series [4, 15]. Symptomatic labral insufficiency can present similar to microinstability with loss of the normal suction seal [14]. The importance of the labrum as a stabilizing structure is magnified in the dysplastic or borderline dysplastic hip. A CEA angle of twenty-five degrees or less or a Tönnis angle (sourcil) of more than 14° should raise awareness of this possibility.

Reconstruction of the acetabular labrum may help restore the suction seal and normalize hip reactive forces. It is important to consider the potential for labral regrowth following partial labrectomy before planning surgical intervention. Abrams et al. showed that spontaneous labral regrowth with functional, normal-appearing tissue occurred in 21 of 24 patients investigated; however, Miozzari et al. found no labral regeneration in a similar study [26, 27]. If no functional tissue is present, labral reconstruction with either iliotibial band or semitendinosus reduced hip contact pressures in one in vitro study [28]. Reconstruction techniques have been developed using iliotibial band autograft or various tendon allografts (semitendinosus, gracilis, anterior tibialis); all of these options have similar tensile properties in a biomechanical analysis [29]. In lieu of reconstruction with allograft or distant tissue, labralization has been described with techniques that use local capsular autograft or a free chondral margin developed adjacent to the defect, but neither anatomic nor outcome follow-ups have been reported.

Arthroscopic reconstruction techniques are similar to labral repair techniques. The remnant labral tissue is debrided back to healthy bone, and the length of the reconstructed segment is estimated accounting for the curvature of the acetabular rim to allow for minimal overlap of the graft with the remnant labral tissue. A suture anchor is placed at the desired anchor point for the tissue graft. One end of an appropriately sized graft is then shuttled into the joint and tied into place. Some prefer to secure the opposite end of the graft using a SwiveLock anchor (Arthrex, Naples FL); the remainder of the graft is tacked down to the rim of the acetabulum using standard repair techniques (Fig. 18.5).

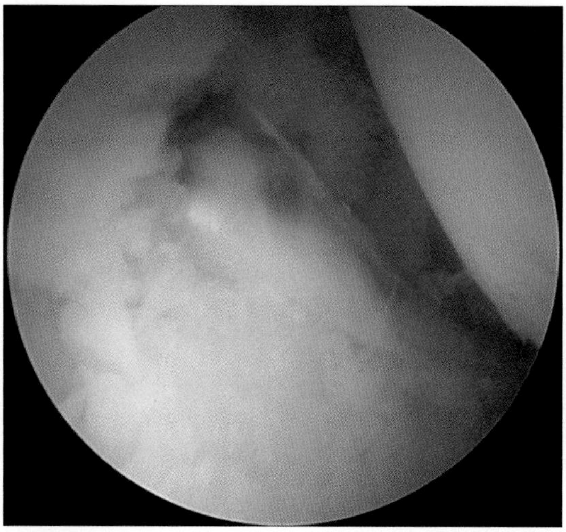

Fig. 18.5 Labral insufficiency treated with labral reconstruction. Allograft semitendinosus was used to recreate the deficient area and restore the suction-seal effect of the labrum

Clinical results following labral reconstruction are limited, but show promising short-term results. In a study by Boykin et al., 17 of 21 elite athletes were able to return to their previous level of competition after labral reconstruction, with improvements in both mHHS and HOS sports scores; however, two athletes required conversion to total hip arthroplasty [30]. Open technique for labral reconstruction achieved improvements in mean OHS and HOS scores (6.3 and 19.8 at 1-year follow-up) [31]. Another prospective study found that labral reconstruction was superior to debridement for segmental labral defects as determined by the Non-arthritic Hip Score at 2-year follow-up. Together, these studies show encouraging results for labral reconstruction in patients with symptomatic labral deficiency [30, 31].

18.4.6 Heterotopic Ossification

Heterotopic ossification (HO) is defined as the formation of histologically normal-appearing bone in an abnormal soft tissue location. HO is common after hip arthroscopy without prophylaxis, occurring in up to 44 % of individuals. NSAIDs have been shown to reduce the rate of HO to less than 10 % by blocking inductive signaling that is required for HO formation. HO is more likely to develop in male patients, after large osteochondroplasties and if acetabuloplasty is performed [32]. The location of HO is usually anterior to the joint, but has also been reported along portal tracts. It is currently unclear if small foci of HO (Brooker grades ≤2) are typically symptomatic. Only one study has compared outcomes between patients that developed HO postoperatively to those that did not and found no difference in PROs [33]. Other series report the need for resection in approximately 25 % of patient who develop HO because it was felt to be symptomatic [32, 34]. A careful investigation for other common sources of postoperative hip pain should be conducted prior to attributing symptoms to ectopic bone formation.

Resection of HO can be performed through open or arthroscopic approaches. It is advisable to wait at least 6 months, but preferably 1 year, until full bony maturation occurs to avoid recurrence. If in doubt in terms of the location of the ectopic bone, a CT scan can help guide surgical planning. Arthroscopic resection is performed by identifying the bony deposit from either an intra-articular or extra-articular approach. The nidus is dissected from engulfing tissue with an electrocautery device and removed in its entirety or segmentally once freed from the capsular tissue. One report of three patients that underwent HO resection showed postoperative improvements in outcome scores.

18.4.7 Cartilage Degeneration

Cartilage status is an important initial consideration in determining treatment options. Patients with extensive cartilage damage documented at the time of their index surgery may realize less benefit from further attempts at hip preservation procedures and may be candidates for joint replacement. In a systematic review, Saadat et al. found that indicators of cartilage loss at the time of surgery were predictive of need for total hip arthroplasty. Patients with < 2 mm of joint space remaining have a high likelihood of progressing to hip arthroplasty, and patients who underwent hip arthroscopy with Tönnis grade 2 changes had equal or worsened outcomes scores postoperatively [2]. Furthermore, patients who had microfracture during their index procedure were more likely to progress to THA in one study by Domb et al. [4]. Overall, 9.2 % of patients in that series went on to total hip replacement. Risk factors consistently identified on presentation include older age, history of microfracture, higher Tönnis grade, and history of acetabuloplasty. Intraoperative images can be helpful to document the degree of chondral damage, which is otherwise difficult on MRI or in early OA on plain radiography.

Conclusions

Revision hip preservation for failed FAI surgery will play a growing role as the numbers of primary procedures increase. Effective treatment requires diagnosing the cause of failure and formulating an appropriate treatment plan that considers all potential sources of intra-articular and extra-articular pathology. Most revisions can be performed through either an arthroscopic or open approach. Outcomes typically improve with revision surgery, but are inferior to the results seen with primary procedures. Extensive chondral injury or advanced arthritis (Tönnis grade > 1 or joint space < 2 mm) does not predictably improve with further preservation attempts and may be candidates for hip arthroplasty.

Take-Home Points

1. Residual FAI from incomplete bony resection is the most commonly reported reason for surgical failure in early series; changing patterns are anticipated with consistent bony resection and improved technical ability.
2. Muscular weakness is a common cause of persistent pain following hip arthroscopy that should be corrected if possible prior to consideration of a revision preservation procedure.
3. 3D imaging can be helpful to evaluate many sources of failure including residual impingement areas and extra-articular impingement.
4. Capsular insufficiency should be suspected in patients with borderline dysplasia, general ligamentous laxity, and pain with hip external rotation and extension on examination and when primary closure was not performed during the index procedure.
5. Patients with Tönnis grade > 1 or joint space < 2 mm do poorly with attempted revision preservation procedures.

Key Evidence Related Sources

1. Philippon MJ, Schenker ML, Briggs KK, Kuppersmith DA, Maxwell RB, Stubbs AJ. Revision hip arthroscopy. Am J Sports Med. 2007;35(11):1918–21. Level of Evidence: IV.
2. Bogunovic L, Gottlieb M, Pashos G, Baca G, Clohisy JC. Why do hip arthroscopy procedures fail? Clinical orthopaedicsrelatedresearch.2013;471(8):2523–9. Level of Evidence: IV.
3. Saadat E, Martin SD, Thornhill TS, Brownlee SA, Losina E, Katz JN. Factors associated with the failure of surgical treatment for femoroacetabular impingement: review of the literature. Am J Sports Med. 2013;42(6):1487–95. Level of Evidence: III.
4. Larson CM, Giveans MR, Samuelson KM, Stone RM, Bedi A. Arthroscopic hip revision surgery for residual femoroacetabular impingement (FAI): surgical outcomes compared with a matched cohort after primary arthroscopic FAI correction. Am J Sports Med. 2014;42(8):1785–90. Level of Evidence: III.
5. Cvetanovich GL, Harris JD, Erickson BJ, Bach BR, Jr., Bush-Joseph CA, Nho SJ. Revision hip arthroscopy: a systematic review of diagnoses, operative findings, and outcomes. Arthroscopy. 2015. In Press. Level of Evidence: IV.

References

1. Ganz R, Parvizi J, Beck M, Leunig M, Notzli H, Siebenrock KA. Femoroacetabular impingement: a cause for osteoarthritis of the hip. Clin Orthop Relat Res. 2003;417:112–20.
2. Saadat E, Martin SD, Thornhill TS, Brownlee SA, Losina E, Katz JN. Factors associated with the failure of surgical treatment for femoroacetabular impingement: review of the literature. Am J Sports Med. 2013;42(6):1487–95.
3. Larson CM, Giveans MR, Samuelson KM, Stone RM, Bedi A. Arthroscopic Hip Revision Surgery for Residual Femoroacetabular Impingement (FAI): Surgical Outcomes Compared With a Matched Cohort After Primary Arthroscopic FAI Correction. Am J Sports Med. 2014;42(8):1785–90.
4. Domb BG, Stake CE, Lindner D, El-Bitar Y, Jackson TJ. Revision hip preservation surgery with hip arthroscopy: clinical outcomes. Arthrosc : J Arthrosc Relat Surg : Off Pub Arthrosc Assoc N Am Int Arthrosc Assoc. 2014;30(5):581–7.
5. Cvetanovich GL, Harris JD, Erickson BJ, Bach Jr BR, Bush-Joseph CA, Nho SJ. Revision Hip arthroscopy: a systematic review of diagnoses, operative findings, and outcomes. Arthrosc : J Arthrosc Relat Surg : Off Pub Arthrosc Assoc N Am Int Arthrosc Assoc. 2015;31(7):1382–90.
6. Ross JR, Larson CM, Adeoye O, Kelly BT, Bedi A. Residual deformity is the most common reason for revision hip arthroscopy: a three-dimensional CT study. Clin Orthop Relat Res. 2015;473(4):1388–95.
7. Ricciardi BF, Fabricant PD, Fields KG, Poultsides L, Zaltz I, Sink EL. What are the demographic and radiographic characteristics of patients with symptomatic extraarticular femoroacetabular impingement? Clin Orthop Relat Res. 2015;473(4):1299–308.
8. Dwyer MK, Jones HL, Hogan MG, Field RE, McCarthy JC, Noble PC. The acetabular labrum regulates fluid circulation of the hip joint during functional activities. Am J Sports Med. 2014;42(4):812–9.
9. Shu B, Safran MR. Hip instability: anatomic and clinical considerations of traumatic and atraumatic instability. Clin Sports Med. 2011;30(2):349–67.
10. Magerkurth O, Jacobson JA, Morag Y, Caoili E, Fessell D, Sekiya JK. Capsular laxity of the hip: findings at magnetic resonance arthrography. Arthrosc : J Arthrosc Relat Surg : Off Pub Arthrosc Assoc N Am Int Arthrosc Assoc. 2013;29(10):1615–22.
11. Harris JD, Slikker 3rd W, Gupta AK, McCormick FM, Nho SJ. Routine complete capsular closure during hip arthroscopy. Arthrosc Tech. 2013;2(2):e89–94.
12. Badylak JS, Keene JS. Do iatrogenic punctures of the labrum affect the clinical results of hip arthroscopy? Arthrosc : J Arthrosc Relat Surg : Off Pub Arthrosc Assoc N Am Int Arthrosc Assoc. 2011;27(6):761–7.
13. McCarthy JC, Glassner PJ. Correlation of magnetic resonance arthrography with revision hip arthroscopy. Clin Orthop Relat Res. 2013;471(12):4006–11.
14. Philippon MJ, Schenker ML, Briggs KK, Kuppersmith DA, Maxwell RB, Stubbs AJ. Revision hip arthroscopy. Am J Sports Med. 2007;35(11):1918–21.
15. Heyworth BE, Shindle MK, Voos JE, Rudzki JR, Kelly BT. Radiologic and intraoperative findings in revision hip arthroscopy. Arthrosc : J Arthrosc Relat Surg : Off Pub Arthrosc Assoc N Am Int Arthrosc Assoc. 2007;23(12):1295–302.
16. Bogunovic L, Gottlieb M, Pashos G, Baca G, Clohisy JC. Why do hip arthroscopy procedures fail? Clin Orthop Relat Res. 2013;471(8):2523–9.
17. Wenger DE, Kendell KR, Miner MR, Trousdale RT. Acetabular labral tears rarely occur in the absence of bony abnormalities. Clin Orthop Relat Res. 2004;426:145–50.
18. Milone MT, Bedi A, Poultsides L, Magennis E, Byrd JW, Larson CM, et al. Novel CT-based three-dimensional software improves the characterization of cam morphology. Clin Orthop Relat Res. 2013;471(8):2484–91.
19. Mei-Dan O, McConkey MO, Brick M. Catastrophic failure of hip arthroscopy due to iatrogenic instability: can partial division of the ligamentum teres and iliofemoral ligament cause subluxation? Arthrosc : J Arthrosc Relat Surg : Off Pub Arthrosc Assoc N Am Int Arthrosc Assoc. 2012;28(3):440–5.
20. Gerhardt M, Johnson K, Atkinson R, Snow B, Shaw C, Brown A, et al. Characterisation and classification of the neural anatomy in the human hip joint. Hip Int: J Clin Exp Res Hip Pathol Ther. 2012;22(1):75–81.
21. Telleria JJ, Lindsey DP, Giori NJ, Safran MR. An anatomic arthroscopic description of the hip capsular ligaments for the hip arthroscopist. Arthrosc: J Arthrosc Relat Surg : Off Pub Arthrosc Assoc N Am Int Arthrosc Assoc. 2011;27(5):628–36.
22. Safran MR, Lopomo N, Zaffagnini S, Signorelli C, Vaughn ZD, Lindsey DP, et al. In vitro analysis of peri-articular soft tissues passive constraining effect on hip kinematics and joint stability. Knee Surg Sports Traumatol Arthrosc: Off J ESSKA. 2013;21(7):1655–63.
23. Duthon VB, Charbonnier C, Kolo FC, Magnenat-Thalmann N, Becker CD, Bouvet C, et al. Correlation of clinical and magnetic resonance imaging findings in hips of elite female ballet dancers. Arthrosc : J Arthrosc Relat Surg : Off Pub Arthrosc Assoc N Am Int Arthrosc Assoc. 2013;29(3):411–9.
24. Domb BG, Philippon MJ, Giordano BD. Arthroscopic capsulotomy, capsular repair, and capsular plication of the hip: relation to atraumatic instability. Arthrosc : J Arthrosc Relat Surg : Off Pub Arthrosc Assoc N Am Int Arthrosc Assoc. 2013;29(1):162–73.
25. Domb BG, Stake CE, Lindner D, El-Bitar Y, Jackson TJ. Arthroscopic capsular plication and labral preservation in borderline hip dysplasia: two-year clinical outcomes of a surgical approach to a challenging problem. Am J Sports Med. 2013;41(11):2591–8.
26. Abrams GD, Safran MR, Sadri H. Spontaneous hip labrum regrowth after initial surgical debridement. Clin Orthop Relat Res. 2013;471(8):2504–8.

27. Miozzari HH, Celia M, Clark JM, Werlen S, Naal FD, Notzli HP. No regeneration of the human acetabular labrum after excision to bone. Clin Orthop Relat Res. 2015;473(4):1349–57.
28. Lee S, Wuerz TH, Shewman E, McCormick FM, Salata MJ, Philippon MJ, et al. Labral reconstruction with iliotibial band autografts and semitendinosus allografts improves hip joint contact area and contact pressure: an in vitro analysis. Am J Sports Med. 2015;43(1):98–104.
29. Ferro FP, Philippon MJ, Rasmussen MT, Smith SD, LaPrade RF, Wijdicks CA. Tensile properties of the human acetabular labrum and Hip labral reconstruction grafts. Am J Sports Med. 2015;43(5):1222–7.
30. Boykin RE, Patterson D, Briggs KK, Dee A, Philippon MJ. Results of arthroscopic labral reconstruction of the hip in elite athletes. Am J Sports Med. 2013;41(10):2296–301.
31. Costa Rocha P, Klingenstein G, Ganz R, Kelly BT, Leunig M. Circumferential reconstruction of severe acetabular labral damage using hamstring allograft: surgical technique and case series. Hip Int : J Clin Exp Res Hip Pathol Ther. 2013;23 Suppl 9:S42–53.
32. Beckmann JT, Wylie JD, Kapron AL, Hanson JA, Maak TG, Aoki SK. The effect of NSAID prophylaxis and operative variables on heterotopic ossification after hip arthroscopy. Am J Sports Med. 2014;42(6):1359–64.
33. Rath E, Sherman H, Sampson TG, Ben Tov T, Maman E, Amar E. The incidence of heterotopic ossification in hip arthroscopy. Arthrosc : J Arthrosc Relat Surg: Off Pub Arthrosc Assoc N Am Int Arthrosc Assoc. 2013;29(3):427–33.
34. Bedi A, Zbeda RM, Bueno VF, Downie B, Dolan M, Kelly BT. The incidence of heterotopic ossification after hip arthroscopy. Am J Sports Med. 2012;40(4):854–63.

Future Directions of FAI Surgery: Diagnosis and Treatment

19

Michael J. Salata and W. Kelton Vasileff

Contents

The field of hip preservation surgery has undergone dramatic growth and development recently, particularly over the last decade. Through the efforts of many researchers, we have a much improved understanding how patients may present in the clinical setting, as well as a more nuanced appreciation of the varied pathology that patients may demonstrate. This increased knowledge base has vastly improved the care that we are able to provide our patients. As much growth as has been observed in the diagnosis and treatment of femoroacetabular impingement (FAI), there is a great deal of ongoing research and development into how best to diagnose and treat this disease process.

M.J. Salata, MD
Department of Orthopedic Surgery, University Hospitals Case Medical Center, Cleveland, Ohio, USA
e-mail: michaeljsalata@gmail.com

W.K. Vasileff, MD
The Ohio State University Wexner Medical Center, Ohio, USA

19.1 Epidemiology

As in all orthopedic disciplines, appropriate diagnosis is critical in providing optimal care for patients. Many authors have emphasized the importance of the physical exam in the diagnostic process, along with obtaining a full and complete history from the patient. Part of this is in understanding the general patient population that is seen in clinics with hip impingement complaints. Clohisy et al. have published a large study describing the cohort of patients from their large collaborative group [1]. They prospectively reviewed over 1000 patients undergoing surgery for FAI to examine the patient demographics, physical exam results, radiographic data, recorded diagnosis, surgical data, and patient reported outcomes (PROs). This large group of patients was 55 % female, with an average age of 28.4 years, and 87.8 % Caucasian. A family history of hip disease was reported in 19 % of the patients. Specific diagnosis assigned included CAM impingement in 48 %, mixed

O.R. Ayeni et al. (eds.), *Diagnosis and Management of Femoroacetabular Impingement*,
DOI 10.1007/978-3-319-32000-7_19

CAM/pincer in 45 %, and isolated pincer in only 8 %. History and radiographs showed 11 % with clear evidence of childhood hip disease. Intraoperatively, 93 % showed labral disease, and 83 % showed articular cartilage damage. Hip arthroscopy was performed in 50.4 % of patients, and surgical dislocation in 34.4 %. The remainder of the patients were treated with reverse periacetabular osteotomy or limited open osteochondroplasty in isolation or in conjunction with arthroscopy. Multiple outcome measures demonstrated significant limitation preoperatively. This study provides an excellent picture of patients undergoing surgery within this group, and further studies will certainly shed more light on patient populations most at risk for symptomatic FAI. Nepple et al. demonstrated via systematic review and meta-analysis that there is an increased risk of CAM morphology in male athletes compared to controls and that the risk increased with age and level of competition [2]. High-level impact sports such as hockey, basketball, and possibly soccer were also shown to increase the risk of development of CAM deformity. As studies provide a comprehensive view on this patient population, further efforts can be made to focus clinical programs such as effective screening.

19.2 Clinical Exam

Physical exam techniques continue to evolve and have improved the ability to diagnose symptomatic FAI as well as extra-articular impingement. Reiman et al. investigated various physical exam maneuvers with a systematic review and meta-analysis. They concluded that evidence for clinical tests was lacking to support clinical decision-making, suggesting these tests were only good enough for screening tests and that more high-quality studies needed to be performed [3]. Other researchers have investigated how a three-dimensional reachable workspace created with a Microsoft Kinect device can be utilized to examine range of motion and demonstrated moderate agreement with clinical examination [4]. More studies may open new avenues for accurate and reproducible automated digital range of motion examinations.

19.3 Imaging Assessment

Radiographic examination is vitally important in the clinical evaluation in patients with hip pain. Most physicians have a standard series of radiographs that they obtain in their initial evaluation. Almost all of these series include an anteroposterior projection of the pelvis, a lateral view of the proximal femur, and an oblique/lateral image of the acetabulum. While these images are helpful, they can be variable based on subtle differences in patient positioning [5], and certain parameters such as the "crossover sign" may be outright misleading [6]. Currently, efforts are being made to improve the imaging of the hip in a number of different ways. Some investigators have demonstrated how a relatively conventional MRI may be utilized to assess both femoral and acetabular morphology [7]. Using post-processing techniques, reconstructed images are created, which enabled both novice and experienced individuals to accurately identify multiple parameters.

Computed tomography (CT) imaging has proven to be a very useful tool to understand the morphology of the proximal femur and acetabulum. The images and data obtained from these scans can be reformatted in several ways to the advantage of the treating physician. Specific reconstructed planes allow the accurate measurement of several radiographic indices of FAI as well as version on the femoral and pelvic side. Three-dimensional images that can be manipulated by the viewer about several axes can also aid in the diagnosis and treatment of both standard and atypical pathological patterns. More recent developments for CT protocols have allowed for reduction of the radiation dosage exposed to patients. The amount of radiation received by patients during these contemporary exams is now very similar to plain radiography [8]. Other researchers have developed a stereoradiography system for preoperative planning that can produce three-dimensional images via biplanar x-rays with very low radiation exposure [9]. One advantage of this imaging may be that it can be performed with the patient in an upright weight-bearing position which may prove to be useful in the clinical setting.

As has been discussed by many authors, one of the limitations of standard imaging techniques is that static pictures are created in an attempt to understand a dynamic problem. Several different tactics are being utilized to help with this inherent problem with static imaging. A potential utilization of MRI technology is to create "dynamic" range of motion images. Protocol parameters have been developed by some to create sequential images in a specific plane and sequence through a set range of motion. This creates several images at multiple points within the full arc of motion, which can aid with diagnosing both more typical FAI impingement and extra-articular impingement patterns [10]. Another technology that continues to expand is dynamic computer-based three-dimensional modeling software systems. These systems allow the creation of a three-dimensional virtual model from CT scans, which can then be manipulated in space. This allows for the measurement and appreciation of femoral anatomic changes better than two-dimensional radiographs, as well as acetabular orientation, where potential bony conflict may arise between them during dynamic range of motion [11]. The software also allows the operator to perform "virtual surgery" for the resection of CAM or pincer lesions and evaluate the potential improved range of motion and the alleviation of prior points of bony impingement [12]. The utility of this preoperative planning tool may lie in the ability to compare preoperative resection plan to intraoperative results.

Ultrasound imaging, as a dynamic technique, may be able to address some of the inherent imaging limitations with other static techniques such as radiography and MRI. Ultrasound can be used to evaluate a number of pathologies around the hip as well as determine the range of motion of the hip [13, 14]. Bony morphology of the acetabulum and femur including multiple standard radiographic indices of FAI can be evaluated using 3D ultrasound techniques and in the future may be used to evaluate pre- and post-operative changes [15] [16]. Tendinosis of the multiple tendons crossing the hip joint as well as snapping hip syndromes can be reliably imaged with ultrasound, which has the advantage of being able to capture the pathology in question as it occurs in real time [13,17]. Abductor and gluteal muscle injuries as well as their tendon insertions can be imaged in much the same way as rotator cuff muscles and tendon insertions [18, 19]. Recent technological advantages have allowed for the creation of ultrasound/MRI fusion imaging. This type of imaging has been shown to be useful for guided biopsies and also to add to the diagnostic yield in the ultrasound suite [20, 21]. In addition to the diagnostic utility, ultrasound can be utilized to guide injections into the hip joint proper as well as other areas around the hip with local anesthetic agents, anti-inflammatories, or other materials such as platelet-rich plasma [22].

One of the most persistent issues with the currently available imaging modalities is the relative inability to accurately assess the state of the articular cartilage surface and its health. Several different three-dimensional isotropic MRI sequences are currently under development with higher resolution. Most of these sequences are either gradient return echo or fast spin echo based and will make it easier to differentiate between native and repair cartilage, subchondral bone, and intra-articular fluid [23]. In an effort to assess the biochemical makeup of articular cartilage and repair tissue, attempts are being made to evaluate the proteoglycans, collagen, and water distribution. Imaging studies specific to proteoglycans include delayed gadolinium-enhanced magnetic resonance imaging for cartilage (dGEMRIC), T1ρ mapping, and sodium (23Na) MRI. T2 mapping, magnetization transfer contrast imaging, and diffusion weighted imaging may be used to evaluate collage and water distribution as well as free water movement [23]. MRI utilizing dGEMRIC techniques is one of the more fully developed and has been shown to be effective in differentiating healing autologous chondrocyte transplantation tissue from adjacent healthy cartilage [24]. Another MRI technique that may prove useful in evaluating cartilage changes in the hip is T1ρ sequencing. T1ρ pulse sequences are able to quantify biochemical changes in articular cartilage, which can help to visualize arthritic changes at an early stage, as well as evaluate focal chondral lesions and the status of repair tissue. Most of the research has been performed in the knee joint, but can be translated to hip imaging in the future [25]. Glycosaminoglycan content of the cartilage can be quantitatively evaluated using 23Na MRI sequencing. These types of images have been shown to be able to evaluate cartilage lesions, as well as microfracture and matrix-associated autologous chondrocyte transplantation repair tissue. Investigators have shown the utility of this sequencing using 3-Tesla as well as 7-Tesla scanners in knee and ankle cartilage [26, 27]. MR imaging with T2* mapping has been shown to be able to detect changes in articular cartilage, and creation of a flattened acetabular map projection can allow for appreciation of areas of unhealthy cartilage. One study in FAI-type pathology demonstrated excellent correlation with the T2* mapping technique and changes directly observed at the time of arthroscopy [28]. Higher-strength MR imaging scanning techniques have been investigated as well to evaluate the status of articular cartilage after injury and during the healing process. A mouse model has been utilized to study 9.4 T MR imaging and shown that it is able to detect changes in the articular cartilage after an induced injury and also may be used to track the healing process as it is able to differentiate healing tissue from native cartilage [29]. MR arthrography (MRA) can be utilized to evaluate the cartilage as well as the acetabular labrum. Investigators have compared MRA with CT arthrography (CTA) for the evaluation of hip conditions. CTA was shown to be superior to MRA for evaluating labral pathology but slightly inferior for evaluation of cartilage injury on the femoral and acetabular sides of the joint [30].

Rapid prototyping, a technology that allows for the creation of realistic models via three-dimensional printing, is beginning to make further inroads in. Its use has been explored in orthopedic surgery as well as other medical specialties [31]. Newer printers are able to be used in an office setting, and some are even small enough to be utilized on a tabletop. Surgeons have used CT images to create full-size models of different body parts, including the pelvis and proximal femur. This has allowed for improved treatment in difficult reconstructive cases, including the creation of custom implants and enhanced preoperative planning and simulated surgery. In another application of the technology, other investigators have used the printers to create 3D models of the pelvis following complex fractures involving the pelvis and acetabulum [32]. The models they created were utilized for preoperative planning, as well as intraoperative fracture reduction assessment, as they were sterilizable. In addition, a mirror image model of the uninjured hemipelvis was created to allow for precontouring of reconstruction plates and planning of screw placement and trajectory. These technologies may be applied to FAI surgery and allow the creation of models of the hip joint which would allow surgeons to appreciate the true 3D nature of the pathology involved and simulate surgical procedures. This may help to alleviate some of the more common complications of FAI surgery, specifically under- and over-resection of CAM and pincer lesions.

19.4 Treatment

The diagnosis of FAI has been changing rapidly and so have the methods utilized for treatment of the condition. Nonoperative treatment is commonly used in the initial stages of the management of patients with FAI. One of these types of treatment involves different substances being injected into the hip joint proper, frequently with ultrasound or fluoroscopic guidance. Corticosteroid and local anesthetic injections are used regularly for therapeutic as well as diagnostic purposes, but their reliability for either use has been questioned recently [33, 34]. Viscosupplementation injections, which have been used for a number of years in the knee, as well as other large joints, have been explored for use in the hip. Multiple studies have been conducted to evaluate the efficacy of these types of injections and have had somewhat mixed results [35]. These types of injections do appear to provide short-term relief in patients with mild to moderate arthritic symptoms, although there is no consensus on the ideal formulation of material for injection or the number of injections that should be provided. As further evidence emerges, viscosupplementation may prove to be a useful adjunctive treatment for patients with intra-articular hip pain. Another type of injection involves the production of autologous-derived material, typically in the form of platelet-rich plasma (PRP), a platelet gel, or a condition serum. Similar to the literature in other large joints with these types of injections, results have been equivocal, at least in part due to a lack of standardized product for injection. Certain studies have shown definite pain relief with platelet gel and PRP injections, but showed that the cartilage surfaces do not significantly heal or change in patients with chondral damage and degradation [36]. Larger-scale reviews showed that PRP is efficacious at reducing pain within the 6–12-month window in the hip and knee, but were unable to make recommendations regarding the use of PRP due to a lack of quality clinical evidence definitively showing benefits in patients with arthritis-type pain [37]. Autologous conditioned serum has also been investigated for use in the hip and shown to significantly decrease pain scores in patients with cartilage degenerative type pain in their hip and that the benefits lasted at least 14 months [38]. Other authors have utilized PRP injections in patients undergoing hip arthroscopy and labral repair, but showed no improvement over local anesthetic injection postoperatively [39]. A large amount research is currently under way to determine what specific biochemical components of these injections are leading to symptomatic relief of pain and which may help the healing process postoperatively. As these studies yield results and identify the most efficacious products, injections may be more feasible as nonoperative treatment measures and also as adjuncts to operative intervention.

The idea of using computer-assisted navigation intraoperatively has been applied to several areas of orthopedics including hip and knee arthroplasty and spine surgery. Utilizing some of the same systems that were discussed previously for the creation of dynamized 3D models from 2D CT or MRI scans, precise preoperative plans can be created, leading to improved surgery [40]. Several different systems have been developed with the goal of creating intraoperative navigation systems. The overarching goal of these systems is to improve the outcomes from the procedure without increasing the risks of surgery. Navigation systems may improve surgical outcomes by ensuring appropriate bony resection, reducing surgical times, and reducing iatrogenic joint damage. One CT-based system was developed and was shown in a small cohort to not significantly change the rate of sufficient CAM resection from non-navigated procedures but that this also did not alter the patient reported outcomes [41]. Another system has been developed again utilizing CT or MRI to create 3D models. Following this, an encoder linkage was created, affixing an encoder base pin to the pelvis and other encoders attached to the appropriate arthroscopic instruments. The main outcomes reported in the model they created were a 38 % reduction in time to task completion and 71.8 % decrease in tool path length when utilizing this navigation system [42]. Although there is promise in these technologies, they are limited in that there has yet to be a proven improvement in the clinical outcomes. Furthermore, these systems can be costly, with an associated steep learning curve, and also are unable to factor in soft tissue impingement [43].

Robotic-assisted arthroplasty has been well studied and shown by some to improve surgical technical results, while improved patient outcomes are less well demonstrated. The Mako tactical guidance system has been used in hip and knee arthroplasty and has shown good results in terms of component position, accuracy, and reproducibility using a CT scan-based mapping system [44]. This type of system may be able to be translated into FAI surgical procedures in the future, as the main advantage of the system as it exists currently is a controlled, accurate bony resection in the knee and hip arthroplasty setting. Research will need to be done to determine the feasibility of using this system with arthroscopic instrumentation and whether this improves technical results or subsequent patient outcomes.

19.5 Labrum

One of the most frequently performed procedures as a part of FAI surgery involves treating the acetabular labrum. The labrum has been shown to be an important structure for the hip for a number of reasons. The fluid seal function of the labrum has been well described and is disrupted by labral tears caused by impingement and instability. Multiple studies have shown improved clinical results with labral repair when compared to debridement and segmental resection of torn labral tissue [45]. This coincides with anatomic cadaver studies that have shown that debridement of labral tears disrupts the fluid seal of the hip and leads to increased distractibility of the hip. At the same time, labral repair partially restores the native seal and distractive stability functions, while labral reconstruction was also able to improve the fluid seal and stability of the hip as much or more when compared to the repaired labrum [46, 47]. Other cadaveric studies have been done to evaluate the effects of labral resection and reconstruction on contact pressures and contact areas within the hip joint. These authors demonstrated that segmental labrum resection significantly alters the contact pressures and areas in the hip and that labrum reconstruction with allograft was able to restore some of the biomechanical properties of the intact labrum, but not all [48]. Multiple studies have been performed evaluating the outcomes of labral reconstruction compared to labral debridement and repair. These studies are limited due to short-term follow-up of 2–3 years and variability in types of graft tissue used. One study demonstrated improved outcomes with reconstruction when compared to segmental resection at a minimum 2-year follow-up using patient reported outcomes [49]. In a slightly larger study with at least 3 years of follow-up, significantly improved function and satisfaction were reported in the 76 % of patients with IT band autograft reconstruction patients who did not progress to hip arthroplasty [50]. Another study with over 2 years of follow-up in patients with gracilis autograft reconstruction compared to labral refixation showed equivalent and superior outcomes despite the reconstruction patients starting with more severe labral injury and inferior non-arthritic hip score [51]. In a group of elite athletes undergoing labral reconstruction, the patients reported high satisfaction rates and outcome measures as well as an 85 % rate of return to play [52]. Open surgical hip dislocation has also been utilized as an approach for labral reconstruction, and authors have reported good results utilizing ligamentum teres and fascia lata autograft as donor graft tissue [53]. Other researchers have advocated for quadriceps tendon autograft based on low donor-site morbidity, size of graft tissue available, and tensile strength [54]. Current indications for reconstruction include deficient labrum due to previous resection or debridement or irreparable tears in relatively young patients without evidence of significant arthritis [55]. Future studies will assist in determining ideal patients and indications for this procedure, along with improved surgical techniques and graft choices. In addition, other biologic adjuvant treatments may be introduced to aid labral healing, as well as the use of tissue scaffolds for the purposes of labral reconstruction.

19.6 Ligamentum Teres

Injuries to the ligamentum teres have been discussed with increasing frequency in the literature, as have techniques designed for repair and reconstruction of the structure. One study compared the results of standard MR arthrogram with anatomy and pathology visualized at the time of arthroscopy. These authors determined that MRA was an accurate and useful modality for imaging the ligamentum teres and determining whether or not a tear was present [56]. One of the earlier descriptions of this procedure includes four patients treated with an IT band autograft reconstruction. The presumption made is that when femoroacetabular impingement occurs, a levering force is produced, creating instability and introducing the ligamentum teres as a secondary stabilizing force that may be damaged over time. Early reported results in the study were positive, in conjunction with the other pathologies treated in these patients, including other FAI-type procedures [57]. In another earlier study, a single patient was treated with a double-stranded semitendinosus autograft affixed on the acetabular side with bone anchors and through a bone tunnel on the femoral side. The patient improved clinically, although at repeat arthroscopy 15 months after surgery, the graft was found to have resorbed and the sutures were functioning as a checkrein ligament [58]. The use of semitendinosus allograft and autograft with bone tunnels has been advocated by a group of authors. In this technique, the femoral tunnel is drilled through the trochanter and fovea and the acetabular tunnel is drilled transfemoral using anatomic safe zones described in the arthroplasty literature for screw placement. Cortical suspensory fixation is utilized to secure the acetabular portion of this graft construct [59]. Another newer technique describes the use of posterior tibialis and semitendinosus allograft for ligamentum teres reconstruction. These authors utilize all-suture anchors for the acetabular fixation, which has the advantage of being used with bone tunnels and the creation of a wider footprint, as well as the fact that if the anchor dislodges, it would be less damaging to the articular cartilage surfaces [60]. Other authors have reviewed the literature and suggested that the current indications for debridement include patients who have failed conservative treatment and have partial-thickness tears of the ligamentum teres. Reconstruction of the ligamentum teres is suggested in patients who have a combination of a full-thickness tear, have failed prior debridement or have symptomatic instability, and do not have advanced arthritis [61]. Although small studies have shown that ligamentum teres debridement and reconstruction can be effective at reducing pain and improving short-term outcomes, further research will better define the role of ligamentum teres pathology in the patient with hip pain and instability as well as refine appropriate patient selection and surgical technique.

19.7 Capsule

The management of hip joint capsular tissue continues to evolve along with many other portions of FAI surgery. The capsule is a complex anatomic structure and its contribution to normal hip kinematics and stability is beginning to be more completely understood. The capsule itself has different components and varied thickness at different points between the acetabulum and femoral insertion. In addition, the iliocapsularis, reflected head of the rectus femoris, and gluteus minimus all appeared to have consistent capsular contributions in a recent anatomic study [62]. The capsule appears to play a significant role in the stability of the hip, as a transverse capsulotomy performed as it would during an arthroscopic FAI surgery introduced changes in both the translational and rotational kinematics of the hip at different points throughout a range of motion in a cadaveric study [63]. Several studies have described patients who underwent hip arthroscopy and developed iatrogenic instability postoperatively related to capsule management, leading to poor outcomes and need for further surgery [64]. Several different methods have been described for capsule repair at the conclusion of surgical treatment as well as capsular plication for patients with borderline dysplastic hips. Some of these methods have utilized suture anchors and sutures to repair the capsule as a part of the labral repair [65]. Other studies have described multiple techniques for all-suture repairs routinely performed during all cases, with focus on the medial portion of the capsule containing the majority of the iliofemoral ligament [66, 67]. In patients with evidence of borderline dysplasia, instability becomes even more of a concern than in most patients, and some authors have advocated for capsular plication during these cases and demonstrated success at 2-year follow-up [68]. Most recently, the usage of retractor devices intraoperatively has been described, obviating the need for capsulotomy at all during arthroscopic FAI surgery, including osseous procedures in the peripheral compartment [69]. A clinical study was performed which did show improved clinical outcomes in patients undergoing complete repair of T-capsulotomy when compared to those who only had a partial repair performed [70]. As more basic science literature emerges and a more full understanding of both the anatomy and kinematic properties of the hip capsule is gained, along with further clinical outcomes data and innovative surgical techniques, clinicians will be better able to determine the best course of action in regard to capsule management during hip arthroscopy for FAI treatment.

19.8 Cartilage

One of the more difficult aspects of FAI surgery is the management of cartilage defects and focal cartilage loss. Lesions can be found on the femoral head and are also commonly seen along the acetabular rim as a part of the spectrum of chondrolabral destabilization regularly observed alongside labral tears. Although research is growing, currently little evidence exists to direct the management of these lesions. Subsequently, most of the techniques have been adapted from those utilized in other joints, particularly the knee. One of the first-line treatments for chondral defects is microfracture. Results of microfracture in the knee are well established, but the literature is less robust concerning the hip. Several studies have demonstrated reasonable success in patients who underwent microfracture in terms of cartilage fill and patient reported outcomes [71–73]. Autologous chondrocyte implantation is another form of cartilage restoration that is increasingly being applied to the hip. The literature is sparse, and more of the recent research has focused on techniques utilizing scaffolds and matrices for the chondrocytes as opposed to the traditional periosteal patch. These matrix-assisted autologous chondrocyte implantation (MACI) techniques are standard two-stage procedures, which have shown good results when compared to debridement alone [74]. A more recent technique maintains both stages, but utilizes three-dimensional spheroids in an all-arthroscopic fashion, with good short-term results [75]. Mosaicplasty is a technique that has certain advantages over ACI and MACI procedures. One advantage is the single-stage nature of surgery, as well as the utilization of native articular cartilage as opposed to reliance on type II fibrocartilage (repair cartilage), although the risks related to donor-site morbidity are introduced. The technique has been used successfully on femoral lesions and requires open surgical exposure as opposed to arthroscopic interventions [76]. For larger full-thickness lesions, fresh osteochondral allograft transplantation is another technique that has shown reasonable success in limited studies. While this technique does eliminate the issue of donor-site morbidity, it does introduce issues with potential disease transmission and the difficulty in obtaining graft tissue and challenging logistics of patient care [77]. Several different cartilage products have also been developed and utilized in the knee and ankle. Particulated juvenile cartilage has been used successfully in the knee for full-thickness cartilage lesions and shown good clinical, radiographic, and histological results at 2-year follow-up [78]. Another recently developed product utilizes micronized allograft cartilage matrix in an arthroscopic fashion for full-thickness lesions. Studies have included knee and talar lesions, but few results of the technique have been published [79]. Further refinement of these techniques will continue and provide for improved patient care. Additionally, further studies will be conducted on these various cartilage restoration and repair techniques, in particular for the hip joint. Further, new cartilage restoration products will be developed and applied to the hip joint, further enhancing the spectrum of care provided within the realm of hip preservation surgery (Fig. 19.1) (Table 19.1).

19.9 Biomarkers of FAI

Circulating biomarkers have been investigated as a noninvasive tool to examine the health of articular cartilage. Several studies have been performed and shown that there are several different compounds that may be used as markers of cartilage and bone health, as well as show evidence of breakdown [80, 81]. As the basic science literature becomes more refined, we will be able to identify the most useful of these markers as it pertains to the hip joint. With this

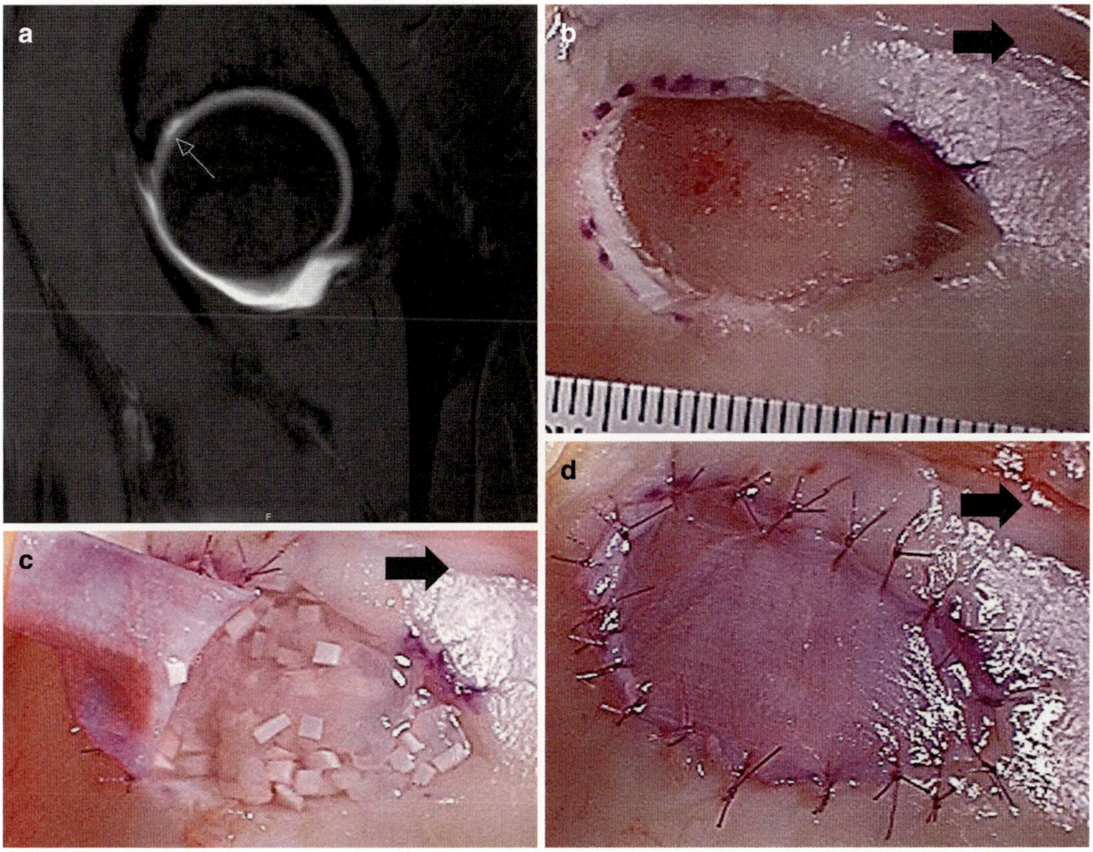

Fig. 19.1 (**a**) Sagittal T1 fat-saturated MRI image of acetabular cartilage lesion. (**b**–**d**) Cartilage lesion after debridement and subsequent particulated juvenile cartilage repair technique. Acetabular labrum indicated with *black arrows*

Table 19.1 Current and developing diagnostic and treatment techniques for the treatment of femoroacetabular impingement pathology

Diagnostic imaging	Injections	Labrum tears	Cartilage injuries
3D CT	Corticosteroid	Debridement	Debridement
Dynamic computer models	Viscosupplementation	Labral repair	Microfracture
Dynamic ultrasound	Platelet-rich plasma	Labral reconstruction	ACI/MACI
Dynamic MRI	Autologous conditioned plasma		Osteochondral autograft
MRI with cartilage sequences			Osteochondral allograft
Computer navigation			Particulated juvenile cartilage
Robotic-assisted surgery			Micronized allograft cartilage matrix

knowledge, these chemical tests could be used to screen and evaluate patients and stratify their risk for developing arthritic hip disease, allowing the targeting of patients who would benefit most from surgical interventions. One of the more innovative uses of new technology is the development of bioprinters. This technology aims to utilize thermoplastic fibers and cell-laden hydrogels to create tissue constructs. These techniques have been developing rapidly, and it is possible to create tissue with specific mechanical properties in order to mimic native structures containing different cell types and bioactive factors [82]. Newer developments have allowed the creation of multiple-layer skin-like soft tissue models including human fibroblasts and keratinocytes in a standardized and reproducible fashion [83]. In the future, this type of technology may allow for the creation of grafts for the repair of articular cartilage lesions and soft tissue injuries such as labral tears that are custom-made for individual patients, enhancing the ability to treat FAI injuries of the hip:

Take-Home Points

1. Diagnostic imaging techniques, particularly MRI, are becoming more effective for FAI diagnosis and the evaluation of cartilage lesions.
2. Three-dimensional imaging techniques will continue to grow and enhance the ability to accurately diagnose and treat FAI pathology, including the development of navigation systems.
3. The treatment of the hip capsule is rapidly evolving, and evidence is beginning to emerge for the biomechanical and clinical benefits of capsular repair and plication.
4. Labral tears are treated commonly during FAI surgery, and as the treatment methods have evolved from simple debridement to include base refixation and reconstruction, clear indications will emerge and new techniques will develop.
5. Cartilage repair and reconstruction techniques are growing in use in the hip, to include autograft, allograft, and newer cartilage matrix products to augment traditional microfracture procedures.

Key Evidence Related Sources

1. Reiman MP, Goode AP, Cook CE, Hölmich P, Thorborg K. Diagnostic accuracy of clinical tests for the diagnosis of hip femoroacetabular impingement/labral tear: a systematic review with meta-analysis. Br J Sports Med. 2015;49(12):811.
2. Harris-Hayes M, Commean PK, Patterson JD, Clohisy JC, Hillen TJ. Bony abnormalities of the hip joint: a new comprehensive, reliable and radiation-free measurement method using magnetic resonance imaging. J Hip Preserv Surg. 2014;1(2):62–70.
3. Milone MT, Bedi A, Poultsides L, Magennis E, Byrd JW, Larson CM, Kelly BT. Novel CT-based three-dimensional software improves the characterization of cam morphology. Clin Orthop Relat Res. 2013;471(8):2484–91.
4. Lazik A, Körsmeier K, Claßen T, Jäger M, Kamminga M, Kraff O, Lauenstein TC, Theysohn JM, Landgraeber S. 3 Tesla high-resolution and delayed gadolinium enhanced MR imaging of cartilage (dGEMRIC) after autologous chondrocyte transplantation in the hip. J Magn Reson Imaging. 2015;42(3):624–33.
5. Tannenbaum EP, Ross JR, Bedi A. Pros, cons, and future possibilities for use of computer navigation in hip arthroscopy. Sports Med Arthrosc. 2014;22(4):e33–41.
6. Domb BG, Stake CE, Lindner D, El-Bitar Y, Jackson TJ. Arthroscopic capsular plication and labral preservation in borderline hip dysplasia: two-year clinical outcomes of a surgical approach to a challenging problem. Am J Sports Med. 2013;41(11):2591–8.
7. Bedi A, Lynch EB, Sibilsky Enselman ER, Davis ME, Dewolf PD, Makki TA, Kelly BT, Larson CM, Henning PT, Mendias CL. Elevation in circulating biomarkers of cartilage damage and inflammation in athletes with femoroacetabular impingement. Am J Sports Med. 2013;41(11):2585–90.

References

1. Clohisy JC, Baca G, Beaulé PE, et al. Descriptive epidemiology of femoroacetabular impingement: a North American cohort of patients undergoing surgery. Am J Sports Med. 2013;41(6):1348–56.
2. Nepple JJ, Vigdorchik JM, Clohisy JC. What is the association between sports participation and the development of proximal femoral cam deformity? A systematic review and meta-analysis. Am J Sports Med. 2015;43(11):2833–40.
3. Reiman MP, Goode AP, Cook CE, Hölmich P, Thorborg K. Diagnostic accuracy of clinical tests for the diagnosis of hip femoroacetabular impingement/labral tear: a systematic review with meta-analysis. Br J Sports Med. 2015;49(12):811.
4. Lahner M, Mußhoff D, von Schulze Pellengahr C, et al. Is the kinect system suitable for evaluation of the hip joint range of motion and as a screening tool for femoroacetabular impingement (FAI)? Technol Health Care. 2015;23(1):75–81.
5. Ross JR, Tannenbaum EP, Nepple JJ, Kelly BT, Larson CM, Bedi A. Functional acetabular orientation varies between supine and standing radiographs: implications for treatment of femoroacetabular impingement. Clin Orthop Relat Res. 2015;473(4):1267–73.
6. Zaltz I, Kelly BT, Hetsroni I, Bedi A. The crossover sign overestimates acetabular retroversion. Clin Orthop Relat Res. 2013;471(8):2463–70.
7. Harris-Hayes M, Commean PK, Patterson JD, Clohisy JC, Hillen TJ. Bony abnormalities of the hip joint: a new comprehensive, reliable and radiation-free measurement method using magnetic resonance imaging. J Hip Preserv Surg. 2014;1(2):62–70.
8. Saltybaeva N, Jafari ME, Hupfer M, Kalender WA. Estimates of effective dose for CT scans of the lower extremities. Radiology. 2014;273(1):153–9.
9. Rousseau MA, Brusson A, Lazennec JY. Assessment of the axial rotation of the pelvis with the EOS® imaging system: intra- and inter-observer reproducibility and accuracy study. Eur J Orthop Surg Traumatol. 2014;24(6):891–5.
10. Singer A, Clifford P, Tresley J, Jose J, Subhawong T. Ischiofemoral impingement and the utility of full-range-of-motion magnetic resonance imaging in its detection. Am J Orthop. 2014;43(12):548–51.
11. Milone MT, Bedi A, Poultsides L, Magennis E, Byrd JW, Larson CM, Kelly BT. Novel CT-based three-dimensional software improves the characterization of cam morphology. Clin Orthop Relat Res. 2013;471(8):2484–91.
12. Masjedi M, Mandalia R, Aqil A, Cobb J. Validation of the 'FeMorph' software in planning cam osteochondroplasty by incorporating labral morphology. Comput Methods Biomech Biomed Engin. 2016;19(1):67–73 doi: 10.1080/10255842.2014.986654.
13. Dawes AR, Seidenberg PH. Sonography of sports injuries of the hip. Sports Health. 2014;6(6):531–8.
14. Larkin B, van Holsbeeck M, Koueiter D, Zaltz I. What is the impingement-free range of motion of the asymptomatic hip in young adult males? Clin Orthop Relat Res. 2015;473(4):1284–8.
15. Mabee M, Dulai S, Thompson RB, Jaremko JL. Reproducibility of acetabular landmarks and a standardized coordinate system obtained from 3D hip ultrasound. Ultrason Imaging. 2015;37(4):267–76.
16. Buck FM, Hodler J, Zanetti M, Dora C, Pfirrmann CW. Ultrasound for the evaluation of femoroacetabular impingement of the cam type. Diagnostic performance of qualitative criteria and alpha angle measurements. Eur Radiol. 2011;21(1):167–75.
17. Azizi HF, Lee SW, Oh-Park M. Ultrasonography of snapping hip syndrome. Am J Phys Med Rehabil. 2015;94(1):e10–1.
18. Whittaker JL, Emery CA. Sonographic measures of the gluteus medius, gluteus minimus, and vastus medialis muscles. J Orthop Sports Phys Ther. 2014;44(8):627–32.
19. Kong A, Van der Vliet A, Zadow S. MRI and US of gluteal tendinopathy in greater trochanteric pain syndrome. Eur Radiol. 2007;17(7):1772–83.
20. Khalil JG, Mott MP, Parsons 3rd TW, Banka TR, van Holsbeeck M. 2011 Mid-America Orthopaedic Association Dallas B. Phemister Physician in Training Award: can musculoskeletal tumors be diagnosed with ultrasound fusion-guided biopsy? Clin Orthop Relat Res. 2012;470(8):2280–7.
21. Vollman A, Hulen R, Dulchavsky S, Pinchcofsky H, Amponsah D, Jacobsen G, Dulchavsky A, van Holsbeeck M. Educational benefits of fusing magnetic resonance imaging with sonograms. J Clin Ultrasound. 2014;42(5):257–63.
22. Mautner K, Colberg RE, Malanga G, Borg-Stein JP, Harmon KG, Dharamsi AS, Chu S, Homer P. Outcomes after ultrasound-guided platelet-rich plasma injections for chronic tendinopathy: a multicenter, retrospective review. PM R. 2013;5(3):169–75.
23. Ronga M, Angeretti G, Ferraro S, DE Falco G, Genovese EA, Cherubino P. Imaging of articular cartilage: current concepts. Joints. 2014;2(3):137–40.
24. Lazik A, Körsmeier K, Claßen T, Jäger M, Kamminga M, Kraff O, Lauenstein TC, Theysohn JM, Landgraeber S. 3 Tesla high-resolution and delayed gadolinium enhanced MR imaging of cartilage (dGEMRIC) after autologous chondrocyte transplantation in the hip. J Magn Reson Imaging. 2015;42(3):624–33.
25. Wang L, Regatte RR. T1ρ MRI of human musculoskeletal system. J Magn Reson Imaging. 2015;41(3): 586–600.
26. Zbýň S, Brix MO, Juras V, Domayer SE, Walzer SM, Mlynarik V, Apprich S, Buckenmaier K, Windhager R, Trattnig S. Sodium magnetic resonance imaging of ankle joint in cadaver specimens, volunteers, and patients after different cartilage repair techniques at 7 T: initial results. Invest Radiol. 2015;50(4):246–54.
27. Widhalm HK, Apprich S, Welsch GH, Zbyn S, Sadoghi P, Vekszler G, Hamböck M, Weber M, Hajdu S, Trattnig S. Optimized cartilage visualization using 7-T sodium ((23)Na) imaging after patella disloca-

tion. Knee Surg Sports Traumatol Arthrosc. 2016; 24(5):1601–9 doi: 10.1007/s00167-014-3455-x. Epub 2014 Nov 28.
28. Morgan P, Spiridonov S, Goebel R, Nissi M, Frei R, Ellermann J. MR imaging with T2*- mapping for improved acetabular cartilage assessment in FAI-a case report with arthroscopic correlation. Orthop Traumatol Surg Res. 2014;100(8):971–3.
29. Mak J, Leonard C, Foniok T, Rushforth D, Dunn JF, Krawetz R. Evaluating endogenous repair of focal cartilage defects in C57BL/6 and MRL/MpJ mice using 9.4T magnetic resonance imaging: a pilot study. Magn Reson Imaging. 2015;33(5):690–4.
30. Sahin M, Calisir C, Omeroglu H, Inan U, Mutlu F, Kaya T. Evaluation of labral pathology and Hip articular cartilage in patients with femoroacetabular impingement (FAI): comparison of multidetector CT arthrography and MR arthrography. Pol J Radiol. 2014;79:374–80.
31. Schwartz A, Money K, Spangehl M, Hattrup S, Claridge RJ, Beauchamp C. Office-based rapid prototyping in orthopedic surgery: a novel planning technique and review of the literature. Am J Orthop (Belle Mead NJ). 2015;44(1):19–25.
32. Niikura T, Sugimoto M, Lee SY, Sakai Y, Nishida K, Kuroda R, Kurosaka M. Tactile surgical navigation system for complex acetabular fracture surgery. Orthopedics. 2014;37(4):237–42.
33. Krych AJ, Griffith TB, Hudgens JL, Kuzma SA, Sierra RJ, Levy BA. Limited therapeutic benefits of intra-articular cortisone injection for patients with femoro-acetabular impingement and labral tear. Knee Surg Sports Traumatol Arthrosc. 2014;22(4):750–5.
34. Ayeni OR, Farrokhyar F, Crouch S, Chan K, Sprague S, Bhandari M. Pre-operative intra-articular hip injection as a predictor of short-term outcome following arthroscopic management of femoroacetabular impingement. Knee Surg Sports Traumatol Arthrosc. 2014;22(4):801–5.
35. Rivera F. Can viscosupplementation be used in the hip? An Italian perspective. Orthopedics. 2014;37(1):48–55.
36. Rizzo C, Vetro R, Vetro A, Mantia R, Iovane A, Di Gesù M, Vasto S, Di Noto L, Mazzola G, Caruso C. The role of platelet gel in osteoarticular injuries of young and old patients. Immun Ageing. 2014;11(1):21.
37. Tietze DC, Geissler K, Borchers J. The effects of platelet-rich plasma in the treatment of large-joint osteoarthritis: a systematic review. Phys Sportsmed. 2014;42(2):27–37.
38. Baltzer AW, Ostapczuk MS, Stosch D, Seidel F, Granrath M. A new treatment for hip osteoarthritis: clinical evidence for the efficacy of autologous conditioned serum. Orthop Rev (Pavia). 2013;5(2):59–64.
39. Redmond JM, Gupta A, Stake CE, Hammarstedt JE, Finch NA, Domb BG. Clinical results of hip arthroscopy for labral tears: a comparison between intraoperative platelet-rich plasma and bupivacaine injection. Arthroscopy. 2015;31(3):445–53.
40. Tannast M, Kubiak-Langer M, Langlotz F, Puls M, Murphy SB, Siebenrock KA. Noninvasive three-dimensional assessment of femoroacetabular impingement. J Orthop Res. 2007;2(1):122–31.
41. Brunner A, Horisberger M, Herzog RF. Evaluation of a computed tomography-based navigation system prototype for hip arthroscopy in the treatment of femoroacetabular cam impingement. Arthroscopy. 2009;25(4):382–91.
42. Monahan E, Shimada K. Verifying the effectiveness of a computer-aided navigation system for arthroscopic hip surgery. Stud Health Technol Inform. 2008;132:302–7.
43. Tannenbaum EP, Ross JR, Bedi A. Pros, cons, and future possibilities for use of computer navigation in hip arthroscopy. Sports Med Arthrosc. 2014;22(4):e33–41.
44. Werner SD, Stonestreet M, Jacofsky DJ. Makoplasty and the accuracy and efficacy of robotic-assisted arthroplasty. Surg Technol Int. 2014;24:302–6.
45. Larson CM, Giveans MR, Stone RM. Arthroscopic debridement versus refixation of the acetabular labrum associated with femoroacetabular impingement: mean 3.5-year follow-up. Am J Sports Med. 2012;40(5):1015–21.
46. Philippon MJ, Nepple JJ, Campbell KJ, Dornan GJ, Jansson KS, LaPrade RF, Wijdicks CA. The hip fluid seal – part I: the effect of an acetabular labral tear, repair, resection, and reconstruction on hip fluid pressurization. Knee Surg Sports Traumatol Arthrosc. 2014;22(4):722–9.
47. Nepple JJ, Philippon MJ, Campbell KJ, Dornan GJ, Jansson KS, LaPrade RF, Wijdicks CA. The hip fluid seal – part II: the effect of an acetabular labral tear, repair, resection, and reconstruction on hip stability to distraction. Knee Surg Sports Traumatol Arthrosc. 2014;22(4):730–6.
48. Lee S, Wuerz TH, Shewman E, McCormick FM, Salata MJ, Philippon MJ, Nho SJ. Labral reconstruction with iliotibial band autografts and semitendinosus allografts improves hip joint contact area and contact pressure: an in vitro analysis. Am J Sports Med. 2015;43(1):98–104.
49. Domb BG, El Bitar YF, Stake CE, Trenga AP, Jackson TJ, Lindner D. Arthroscopic labral reconstruction is superior to segmental resection for irreparable labral tears in the hip: a matched-pair controlled study with minimum 2-year follow-up. Am J Sports Med. 2014;42(1):122–30.
50. Geyer MR, Philippon MJ, Fagrelius TS, Briggs KK. Acetabular labral reconstruction with an iliotibial band autograft: outcome and survivorship analysis at minimum 3-year follow-up. Am J Sports Med. 2013;41(8):1750–6.
51. Matsuda DK, Burchette RJ. Arthroscopic hip labral reconstruction with a gracilis autograft versus labral refixation: 2-year minimum outcomes. Am J Sports Med. 2013;41(5):980–7.
52. Boykin RE, Patterson D, Briggs KK, Dee A, Philippon MJ. Results of arthroscopic labral reconstruction of the hip in elite athletes. Am J Sports Med. 2013;41(10):2296–301.
53. Walker JA, Pagnotto M, Trousdale RT, Sierra RJ. Preliminary pain and function after labral recon-

struction during femoroacetabular impingement surgery. Clin Orthop Relat Res. 2012;470(12):3414–20.
54. Park SE, Ko Y. Use of the quadriceps tendon in arthroscopic acetabular labral reconstruction: potential and benefits as an autograft option. Arthrosc Tech. 2013;2(3):e217–9.
55. Ayeni OR, Alradwan H, de Sa D, Philippon MJ. The hip labrum reconstruction: indications and outcomes – a systematic review. Knee Surg Sports Traumatol Arthrosc. 2014;22(4):737–43.
56. Chang CY, Gill CM, Huang AJ, Simeone FJ, Torriani M, McCarthy JC, Bredella MA. Use of MR arthrography in detecting tears of the ligamentum teres with arthroscopic correlation. Skeletal Radiol. 2015;44(3): 361–7.
57. Philippon MJ, Pennock A, Gaskill TR. Arthroscopic reconstruction of the ligamentum teres: technique and early outcomes. J Bone Joint Surg Br. 2012;94(11): 1494–8.
58. Amenabar T, O'Donnell J. Arthroscopic ligamentum teres reconstruction using semitendinosus tendon: surgical technique and an unusual outcome. Arthrosc Tech. 2012;1(2):e169–74.
59. Lindner D, Sharp KG, Trenga AP, Stone J, Stake CE, Domb BG. Arthroscopic ligamentum teres reconstruction. Arthrosc Tech. 2012;2(1):e21–5.
60. Mei-Dan O, McConkey MO. A novel technique for ligamentum teres reconstruction with "all-suture" anchors in the medial acetabular wall. Arthrosc Tech. 2014;3(2):e217–21.
61. de SA D, Phillips M, Philippon MJ, Letkemann S, Simunovic N, Ayeni OR. Ligamentum teres injuries of the hip: a systematic review examining surgical indications, treatment options, and outcomes. Arthroscopy. 2014;30(12):1634–41.
62. Walters BL, Cooper JH, Rodriguez JA. New findings in hip capsular anatomy: dimensions of capsular thickness and pericapsular contributions. Arthroscopy. 2014;30(10):1235–45.
63. Bayne CO, Stanley R, Simon P, Espinoza-Orias A, Salata MJ, Bush-Joseph CA, Inoue N, Nho SJ. Effect of capsulotomy on hip stability-a consideration during hip arthroscopy. Am J Orthop (Belle Mead NJ). 2014;43(4):160–5.
64. Mei-Dan O, McConkey MO, Brick M. Catastrophic failure of hip arthroscopy due to iatrogenic instability: can partial division of the ligamentum teres and iliofemoral ligament cause subluxation? Arthroscopy. 2012;28(3):440–5.
65. Slikker 3rd W, Van Thiel GS, Chahal J, Nho SJ. The use of double-loaded suture anchors for labral repair and capsular repair during hip arthroscopy. Arthrosc Tech. 2012;1(2):e213–7.
66. Harris JD, Slikker 3rd W, Gupta AK, McCormick FM, Nho SJ. Routine complete capsular closure during hip arthroscopy. Arthrosc Tech. 2013;2(2):e89–94.
67. Chow RM, Engasser WM, Krych AJ, Levy BA. Arthroscopic capsular repair in the treatment of femoroacetabular impingement. Arthrosc Tech. 2013;3(1):e27–30.
68. Domb BG, Stake CE, Lindner D, El-Bitar Y, Jackson TJ. Arthroscopic capsular plication and labral preservation in borderline hip dysplasia: two-year clinical outcomes of a surgical approach to a challenging problem. Am J Sports Med. 2013;41(11):2591–8.
69. Fiz N, Sánchez M, Pérez JC, Guadilla J, Delgado D, Azofra J, Aizpurua B. A less-invasive technique for capsular management during hip arthroscopy for femoroacetabular impingement. Arthrosc Tech. 2014;3(4):e439–43.
70. Frank RM, Lee S, Bush-Joseph CA, Kelly BT, Salata MJ, Nho SJ. Improved outcomes after hip arthroscopic surgery in patients undergoing T-capsulotomy with complete repair versus partial repair for femoroacetabular impingement: a comparative matched-pair analysis. Am J Sports Med. 2014; 42(11):2634–42.
71. Karthikeyan S, Roberts S, Griffin D. Microfracture for acetabular chondral defects in patients with femoroacetabular impingement: results at second-look arthroscopic surgery. Am J Sports Med. 2012;40(12):2725–30.
72. McDonald JE, Herzog MM, Philippon MJ. Performance outcomes in professional hockey players following arthroscopic treatment of FAI and microfracture of the hip. Knee Surg Sports Traumatol Arthrosc. 2014;22(4):915–9.
73. Domb BG, Redmond JM, Dunne KF, Stake CE, Gupta A. A matched-pair controlled study of microfracture of the hip with average 2-year follow-up: do full-thickness chondral defects portend an inferior prognosis in hip arthroscopy? Arthroscopy. 2015;31(4):628–34.
74. Fontana A. A novel technique for treating cartilage defects in the hip: a fully arthroscopic approach to using autologous matrix-induced chondrogenesis. Arthrosc Tech. 2012;1(1):e63–8.
75. Körsmeier K, Claßen T, Kamminga M, Rekowski J, Jäger M, Landgraeber S. Arthroscopic three-dimensional autologous chondrocyte transplantation using spheroids for the treatment of full-thickness cartilage defects of the hip joint. Knee Surg Sports Traumatol Arthrosc. 2014.
76. Girard J, Roumazeille T, Sakr M, Migaud H. Osteochondral mosaicplasty of the femoral head. Hip Int. 2011;21(5):542–8.
77. Khanna V, Tushinski DM, Drexler M, Backstein DB, Gross AE, Safir OA, Kuzyk PR. Cartilage restoration of the hip using fresh osteochondral allograft: resurfacing the potholes. Bone Joint J. 2014;96-B(11 Supple A):11–6.
78. Farr J, Tabet SK, Margerrison E, Cole BJ. Clinical, radiographic, and histological outcomes after cartilage repair with particulated juvenile articular cartilage: a 2-year prospective study. Am J Sports Med. 2014;42(6):1417–25.
79. Desai S. Surgical treatment of a tibial osteochondral defect with debridement, marrow stimulation, and micronized allograft cartilage matrix-an All-arthroscopic technique: a case report. J Foot Ankle Surg. 2016;55(2):279–82.
80. Bedi A, Lynch EB, Sibilsky Enselman ER, Davis ME, Dewolf PD, Makki TA, Kelly BT, Larson CM,

Henning PT, Mendias CL. Elevation in circulating biomarkers of cartilage damage and inflammation in athletes with femoroacetabular impingement. Am J Sports Med. 2013;41(11):2585–90.
81. Yamaguchi R, Yamamoto T, Motomura G, Ikemura S, Iwasaki K, Zhao G, Doi T, Iwamoto Y. Bone and cartilage metabolism markers in synovial fluid of the hip joint with secondary osteoarthritis. Rheumatology (Oxford). 2014;53(12):2191–5.
82. Schuurman W, Khristov V, Pot MW, van Weeren PR, Dhert WJ, Malda J. Bioprinting of hybrid tissue constructs with tailorable mechanical properties. Biofabrication. 2011;3(2):021001.
83. Rimann M, Bono E, Annaheim H, Bleisch M, Graf-Hausner U. Standardized 3D Bioprinting of Soft Tissue Models with Human Primary Cells. J Lab Autom. 2015. pii: 2211068214567146. [Epub ahead of print].

Future Directions in Training FAI Surgeons

20

Justin W. Arner, Raymond Pahk, Vonda Wright, Craig Mauro, and Volker Musahl

Contents

J.W. Arner, MD • R. Pahk, MD • C. Mauro, MD
Department of Orthopaedic Surgery, University of Pittsburgh, Pittsburgh, PA, USA
e-mail: maurocs@upmc.edu; pahkrb@upmc.edu; rnerjw@upmc.edu

V. Wright, MD
Department of Orthopaedic Surgery, University of Pittsburgh, 3471 Fifth Avenue, Pittsburgh, PA 15213, USA

V. Musahl, MD (✉)
Orthopaedic Surgery and Bioengineering, UPMC Center for Sports Medicine, University of Pittsburgh, Pittsburgh, PA, USA
e-mail: musahlv@upmc.edu

20.1 Current FAI Education

Hip arthroscopy presents unique technical obstacles, even for surgeons who are familiar with arthroscopy of the knee and shoulder [1–10]. Among these are the use of the 70° arthroscope, traction, orientation about the hip joint, establishing and maintaining portals, mastering different portals and compartments, as well as triangulation in an anatomically deep and constrained location. Additionally, hip arthroscopists must optimize efficiency in order to limit hip distraction time and reduce risks such as pudendal nerve neuropraxia. These factors contribute to the challenge of training future open and arthroscopic FAI surgeons.

Education in hip arthroscopy and FAI is handled differently both in residency and fellowship. Depending on the program, hip arthroscopy and FAI management are taught, without standardization, often on various subspecialty services/rotations (sports medicine, pediatrics, trauma, and/or joint reconstruction). Recently, the Accreditation Council for Graduate Medical Education (ACGME), with the support of the American Board of Orthopaedic Surgery (ABOS) and the Residency Review Committee for Orthopaedic Surgery (RRCOS), created the Orthopaedic Surgery Milestone Project which outlines requirements for orthopedic surgeon competency [11]. Although created by American organizations, these principals can be applied throughout the world. However, most of these recommendations

O.R. Ayeni et al. (eds.), *Diagnosis and Management of Femoroacetabular Impingement*,
DOI 10.1007/978-3-319-32000-7_20

are anecdotal [11]. According to ACGME recommendations, residents should be able to classify FAI at level 2, defined as a pre-midlevel resident's knowledge. Hip arthroscopy and FAI treatment are not addressed in the ACGME residency milestones, and no hip arthroscopy training is required prior to graduation [12, 13]. Likewise, orthopedic training in Canada is taught under the auspices of the Royal College of Physicians and Surgeons of Canada (RCPSC) and the Specialty Committee for Orthopaedic Surgery (SCOS), who have developed the CanMED competencies [14]. The competencies make no specific mention of FAI or hip arthroscopy [15]. Australian orthopedic education is directed by the Surgical Education and Training (SET) syllabus established by the Australian Orthopaedic Association/New Zealand Orthopaedic Association (AOA/NZOA) [16], which requires a trainee in the fourth to fifth year of specialist training to demonstrate knowledge of "specific and broad concepts" of the anatomy and "aetiologies of femoro-acetabular impingement (FAI)" and the "arthroscopic classification of hip labral pathology" [16] but does not otherwise outline requirements for hip arthroscopy training. FAI education may be somewhat more standardized in the United Kingdom. Orthopedic training in the United Kingdom is overseen by the General Medical Council (GMC), who have produced a curriculum that calls on trainees to demonstrate "a knowledge of the indications for, and principles of, complex femoral osteotomies, hip arthroscopy, reconstruction of the hip in young adults (JCA and hip dysplasia, etc), [and] complex hip revision surgery" [17]. An advanced hip and groin course including training in hip arthroscopy is offered by the Royal College of Surgeons of England [18]. FAI is mentioned as a cause of possible hip pain with its own section in Orthopaedic Knowledge Update 10 where types, symptomatology, clinical evaluation, radiographic evaluation, and treatment options are outlined [19]. This resource is commonly used by residents, particularly in the United States as it provides a succinct update of relevant orthopedic topics. It is unknown how many hip arthroscopies for FAI treatment an average resident assists or performs. An informal poll of residents in a United States and a Canadian program found, on average, residents assisted or performed 18.4 hip arthroscopies, almost all for the treatment of FAI [20].

According to the Orthopaedic Sports Medicine Milestone Project, fellows should be competent to perform hip arthroscopy at level 3, which is defined as the fellow being able to perform the majority of milestones targeted by fellowships. The graduation target for ACGME accredited sports fellowships, level 4, is where the fellow is able to surgically treat hip labral pathology as well as FAI. However, no number of hip arthroscopy procedures or FAI surgeries is required for graduation [21]. As of 2014, according to the Arthroscopic Association of North America (AANA)/American Orthopaedic Society for Sports Medicine (AOSSM) match, there are 90 accredited sports fellowships and three unaccredited fellowships in the United States [22]. The International Society for Hip Arthroscopy website recognizes nine fellowship programs worldwide for hip arthroscopy [23]. It is unknown how many of these include treatment of FAI management as no training standard exists. Only two formal hip preservation fellowships exist in the United States that are 1 year in duration and likely there is the same number internationally [24]. These are defined as multidisciplinary centers incorporating multiple specialties and resources with the goal of early diagnosis and treatment to prevent hip degeneration.

Pediatric, arthroplasty, and other structured "mini-fellowships" exist which teach hip arthroscopy for FAI, but no data is available regarding the number or the standards of these experiences. These are usually limited to, at most, 1 or 2 months of treatment of hip preservation in general [24]. Continuing education courses also exist through AANA and AOSSM. These hip arthroscopy courses are mostly intensive 2-day master's courses run by experienced hip arthroscopists with the goal of updating and improving hip arthroscopy techniques. The topics include preoperative evaluation, indications, patient positioning, portal placement, anatomy, and the breadth of treatment options with arthroscopy. FAI treatment is only a small part of the course [25]. Courses sponsored by industry also exist [26].

20.2 Becoming a Competent FAI Surgeon

Currently, there is no agreed-upon curriculum or length of study, and it is unknown if a surgeon would be capable of unrestricted practice in this field with a given exposure to FAI treatment and arthroscopy. Historically, surgeons with successful hip preservation practices were self-driven learners who distilled their training from visitation to mentors, cadaveric study, and collaboration. However, few formal avenues to accomplish this exist. [24] Few studies exist regarding the number of hip arthroscopies that are required before one becomes proficient. It is assumed that proficiency requires significantly more experience when compared with knee or shoulder arthroscopy based on higher complication rates and operative times. It is thought that, with experience, these complications decrease significantly [1]. However, few studies thoroughly examine clinical outcome related to learning experiences.

Arthroscopic FAI treatment is also considered more difficult due to the joint access and difficulty visualizing intra-articular structures. Most studies evaluating the learning curve of hip arthroscopy do not involve the more difficult treatment of FAI (versus loose body removal, labral debridement) and therefore may even be an underestimate of the skill required to be competent [3]. One study evaluated the learning curve of arthroscopic treatment of FAI by comparing the complications from the first 61 patients treated by a young hip arthroscopist under supervision of a senior hip arthroscopist and the first 61 patients treated by this senior surgeon. The authors found a lower complication rate with the senior surgeon overseeing the junior hip arthroscopist (4.9 %) when comparing the senior surgeon's first cases (7.0 %). The authors concluded that because the junior surgeon spent 6 months performing arthroscopic FAI surgery under senior supervision and had a decreased number of complications, he benefited from senior oversight. They advise that those new to arthroscopic FAI surgery participate in specialized courses and learn the skill in a specialty center where many surgeries are performed but do not offer recommendations beyond that [3]. Another study evaluated a single surgeon and his improvement over time with hip arthroscopy without bony or synovial work. They found a decrease in complications, surgical time, and patient satisfaction and therefore concluded that performing approximately 30 cases makes one proficient in central compartment hip arthroscopy. They also found a decreased surgical time of 40 % and believe this indicated rapid learning. The author found a separate learning curve with similar improvements regarding bony work after 60 patients [4]. A group from Mexico has similar outcomes with decreased operative time and complications after 30 cases [5]. Another group found that 20 cases were required before satisfactory clinical outcomes were expected and 30 cases for failure rates to be minimal. Most of these studies include only simple arthroscopic debridement without any labral repair or osteoplasty and are performed by a single surgeon [2]. One study, however, found that the number of complications persisted with treatment of 194 patients over 9 years, only the severity of complications and surgical time decreased. They believe this was due to the increasing complexity of cases, including FAI, that were treated as the surgeon became more comfortable with hip arthroscopy with time [27]. Nevertheless, these few limited studies show the learning curve required is significantly higher than that reported of other arthroscopic procedures [6, 28]. Although the few existing studies cite 30 as the point where the learning curve plateaus, this should be interpreted with caution as no validation exists, and only entry level arthroscopy was reported. This number likely should be at least doubled for reconstructive surgical cases (N=60–80) (Table 20.1) [2–4, 7–10, 27, 29].

20.3 Accessory FAI Training

Because of the difficult learning curve associated with hip arthroscopy and limited exposure to cases during residency training, alternative training options such as cadaveric skills labs and arthroscopic simulator training should be explored (Fig. 20.1). These methods offer an

Table 20.1 Summary of current literature evaluating the learning curve for hip arthroscopy/FAI

Author	Date	Learning curve	Way of measuring learning curve	# of cases	Types of cases	Surgeon's experience
Boden et al.	2014	First 20 vs. 21–120	Non-arthritic hip score	120	Hip arthroscopy	Unknown
Dietrich et al.	2014	First 61 patients of surgeon with and without oversight	Complications of surgeon with and without oversight	61	FAI	With oversight vs. none
Lee et al.	2013	First 20 vs. 21–40	Failure rate, modified Harris hip score	40	Hip arthroscopy	Hip fellowship
Comba et al.	2012	First 30 vs. 31–202	Complications, operative time, traction time	232	Hip arthroscopy	Observation of 25 hip arthroscopies, instructional courses
Konan et al.	2011	First 30 vs. 31–100, groups of 10	Complications, operative time, patient satisfaction	100	Hip arthroscopy	Instructional courses
Sobau et al.	2011	First 100 vs. 101–400	Complications	400	FAI	Unknown
Souza et al.	2010	Consecutive groups of 30	Complications	194	Hip arthroscopy	Unknown
Vilchez et al.	2010	First 30 vs. 31–97	Complications, operative time, traction time	97	Hip arthroscopy	Observation of 15 hip arthroscopies, instructional courses

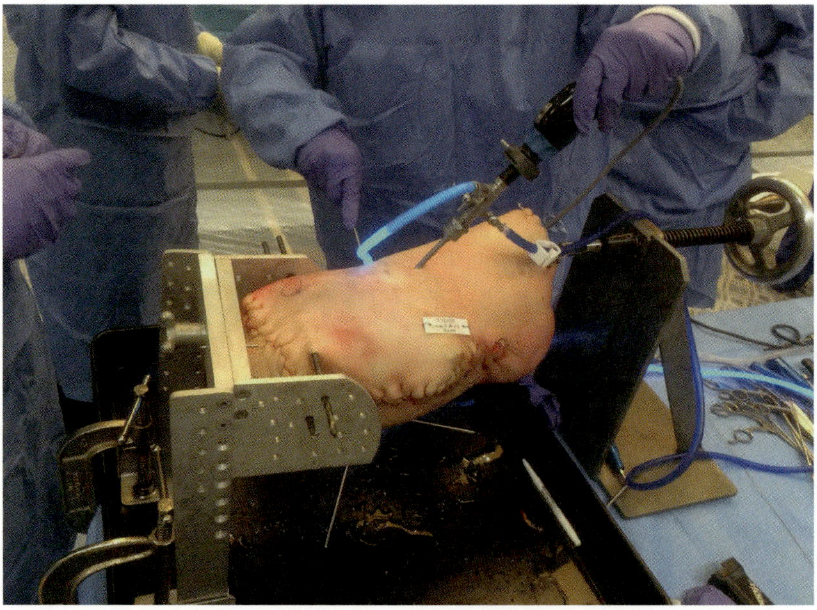

Fig. 20.1 Hip arthroscopy cadaveric skills lab

environment in which the nascent hip arthroscopist has the opportunity to learn and practice valuable skills without exposing a patient to potential harm or consuming valuable time in the operating room. A systematic review of arthroscopic simulator training studies concluded that training on knee simulator improves performance on simulators, but could not definitively establish that such training improves skill in the operating room [29]. However, a number of studies in the general surgery literature have demonstrated the transfer validity of simulator training to surgical procedures [15–17]. Although the orthopedic literature is more limited, there is evidence that arthroscopy simulation training likewise translates to improved technical ability in the operating room. Cannon et al. demonstrated the transfer validity of arthroscopic simulation in a randomized study of orthopedic residents trained on a virtual knee simulator [18]. Postgraduate year 3 orthopedic residents at seven institutions were randomized into simulator-trained and control groups. Simulator-trained residents were trained in knee diagnostic arthroscopy using the ArthroStim™ (Touch of Life Technologies, Aurora, Colorado) virtual-reality arthroscopic knee simulator an average of 11 h. Both groups then performed a diagnostic knee arthroscopy procedure on a live patient and were evaluated by expert arthroscopists who were blinded to the residents' identities. Simulator-trained residents were found to perform significantly better in the operating room than their peers when rated according to an internal procedural checklist. Howell et al. also found significant improvement in psychomotor skills in a randomized study of junior orthopedic residents who were trained on a benchtop knee arthroscopy simulator. This again translated to superior performance in the operating room on an actual patient.

Arthroscopic hip simulators are relatively new and have not been as well studied as those for the knee and shoulder in orthopedic education. One such device is the Sawbones® (Malmo, Sweden) hip arthroscopy simulator (Fig. 20.2). [30, 32] used this simulator to train residents in hip arthroscopy, studying differences in learning curve patterns for residents trained in supine versus lateral positions. Subjects were assessed using 3D motion analysis, using the parameters of time taken to perform the procedure, number of hand movements, and total path length of hand movements. Residents were noted to have a learning curve similar to those established in studies of laparoscopic procedures and arthroscopy of the knee and shoulder. Subjects in both groups demonstrated significant objective improvement in all parameters, which appeared to plateau after nine training sessions. Those trained in the lateral position initially encountered more difficulty, which the authors surmised was due to disorientation, but rapidly achieved parity with the supine group. Junior trainees were also found to perform at a similar level to more senior trainees by the end of the study period. While the evidence is limited, these studies suggest that simulator training improves technical skill that is transferrable to the operating room and may present a supplemental avenue for training hip arthroscopists.

20.4 FAI Teaching Recommendations

Although the literature is limited on how hip arthroscopy and FAI surgery is or should be taught, teaching to the appropriate level is important. This too depends on whether a resident partakes in any hip arthroscopy at all or participates and becomes competent. Further, difficulties exist in standardizing education, as differences exist internationally with regard to exposure [24]. Resident education may benefit from teaching technical steps in a stepwise progression, beginning with patient positioning and use of traction and progressing to joint access, capsulotomy, rim preparation, labral and chondral work, femoral work, and capsule work [30, 31]. Such a progression might allow trainees to absorb and emulate the technical aspects of FAI treatment in a reproducible fashion. Some opt for a standardized technique such as the 23-point hip arthroscopy procedure which may allow easier teaching and standardization for those learning the technique [31]. This is difficult, however, because no standardized techniques exist as there is great

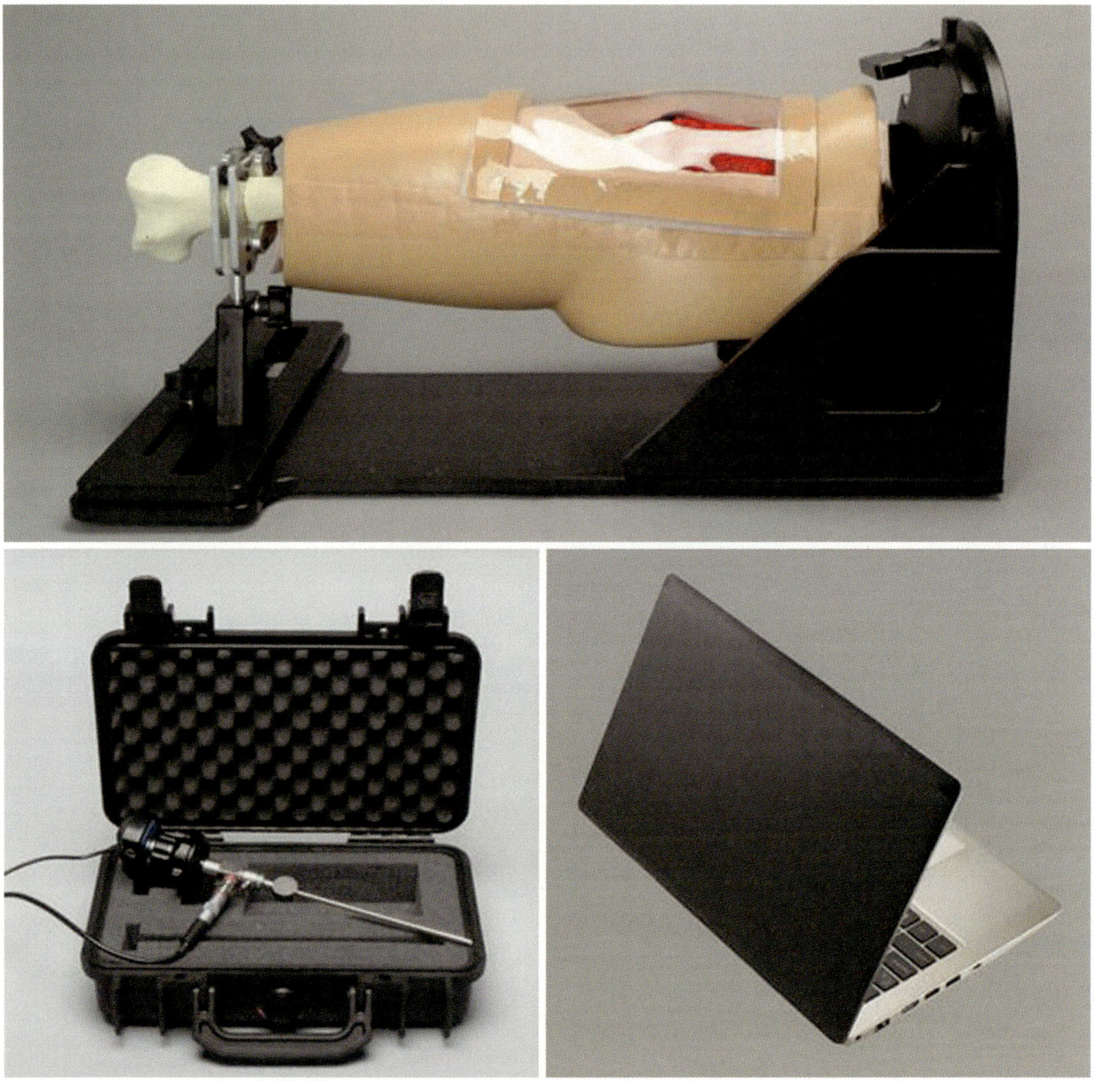

Fig. 20.2 Sawbones hip arthroscopy simulator (Sawbones AB, Malmo, Sweden)

variability, for example, in hip arthroscopy access and number of portals used, if capsulotomy is done and if the capsule is closed.

Without a standardized model, programs have a varying focus on open, mini-open, and arthroscopic treatment of hip pathology and FAI [24]. It is recommended that a curriculum be developed where a junior resident is able to recognize the condition, be proficient in physical examination, and know indications for operative intervention and where a senior resident focuses on basic surgical techniques. This would provide a good foundation for both the surgeon pursuing further fellowship training or for the general orthopedist interested in diagnosis and nonoperative treatments. Fellowship training could be focused on improving surgical skills to treat a wide variety of hip conditions requiring arthroscopic or open treatment, including FAI. This would allow mentorship to continue after fellowship, which has been key to the success of many current hip surgeons. Ideally, this could be driven and standardized by an international hip surgery group (such as ISHA), which would provide guidelines, accreditation, and future collaboration [24].

We recommend a multifaceted hip model where midlevel residents are introduced to FAI and hip arthroscopy with dedicated time in both an office and operating room setting. This is critical, as we believe the clinic experience is essential in understanding the management of FAI particularly in understanding the indications. Emphasis should be placed on evidence-based practice. Familiarity with current literature, research methodologies, and outcome scores should be encouraged, which is important for both education and informing future research efforts. Further, understanding the indications for hip arthroscopy and FAI surgery is imperative. Education in diagnosis, imaging, and nonoperative management, simulator training, and wet lab experiences are important components of introductory exposure to hip surgery. Senior-level rotations or electives should start with diagnostic hip arthroscopy and progress to more advanced procedural exposure to hip arthroscopy, graduating to more technically challenging procedures such as FAI surgery. Exposure to multiple hip practices in residency and fellowship is essential. Fellows should have the opportunity to rotate with open pediatric or young adult hip surgeons. Flexibility should exist for those with more interest in FAI treatment to spend more dedicated time with faculty who have high volume hip practices. Also, support for travel to courses and for dedicated post-fellowship hip preservation mini-fellowships is important. Trainees should be encouraged to engage with faculty in hip and FAI research, which will shape the future of FAI surgery.

Take-Home Points

1. Hip arthroscopy and FAI treatment present challenges to mastery as well as to education.
2. Studies suggest competency in hip arthroscopy after 30 procedures. This should be interpreted with caution, however, as few studies exist and most involve one surgeon with simple arthroscopic cases only. Likely, 60–90 reconstructive procedures are required for competence due to the technical complexity of chondral and labral surgery and osteoplasty. This means likely it takes double the amount of hip scopes as knee scopes to be competent.
3. Skills labs and simulation may offer avenues for supplemental training in hip arthroscopy.
4. More studies should be conducted to establish scientific-based recommendations for education of FAI treatment.
5. Standardization of teaching FAI treatment and hip arthroscopy is lacking and should be established and required based on level of training, continued education, and collaboration. Knowledge of current literature, research methodologies, and outcome scores is important for both education and informing future research efforts.

Key Evidence Related Sources

1. Hoppe DJ, de Sa D, Simunovic N, et al. The learning curve for hip arthroscopy: a systematic review. Arthroscopy J Arthrosc Relat Surg Off Publ Arthroscopy Assoc North Am Int Arthroscopy Assoc. 2014;30(3):389–97.
2. Samora JBBP, Jones A, Milbrandt T, Mazzocca AD, Quinn RH. Orthopaedic graduate medical education: a changing paradigm. JBJS Rev. 2014;e1(11).
3. Wadey VMR, Dev P, Buckley R, Walker D, Hedden D. Competencies for a Canadian orthopaedic surgery core curriculum. J Bone Joint Surg (Br). 2009; 91(12):1618–22.
4. Peters CL, Beaule PE, Beck M, Tannast M, Jiranek W, Sierra RJ. Report of breakout session: strategies to improve hip preservation training. Clin Orthop Relat Res. 2012;470(12):3467–9.
5. Pollard TC, Khan T, Price AJ, Gill HS, Glyn-Jones S, Rees JL. Simulated hip arthroscopy skills: learning curves with the lateral and supine patient positions: a randomized trial. J Bone Joint Surg Am. 2012;94(10):e68.

References

1. Sampson TG. Complications of hip arthroscopy. Clin Sports Med. 2001;20(4):831–5.
2. Lee YK, Ha YC, Hwang DS, Koo KH. Learning curve of basic hip arthroscopy technique: CUSUM analysis. Knee Surg Sports Traumatol Arthrosc Off J ESSKA. 2013;21(8):1940–4.

3. Dietrich F, Ries C, Eiermann C, Miehlke W, Sobau C. Complications in hip arthroscopy: necessity of supervision during the learning curve. Knee Surg Sports Traumatol Arthrosc Off J ESSKA. 2014;22(4):953–8.
4. Konan S, Rhee SJ, Haddad FS. Hip arthroscopy: analysis of a single surgeon's learning experience. J Bone Joint Surg Am. 2011;93 Suppl 2:52–6.
5. Vilchez F, Erquicia J, Tey M. Learning curve of arthroscopic hip surgery. Acta Ortop Mex. 2010;24(3):177–81.
6. Hodgins JL, Veillette C, Biau D, Sonnadara R. The knee arthroscopy learning curve: quantitative assessment of surgical skills. Arthroscopy J Arthrosc Relat Surg Off Publ Arthroscopy Assoc North Am Int Arthroscopy Assoc. 2014;30(5):613–21.
7. Hoppe DJ, de Sa D, Simunovic N, et al. The learning curve for hip arthroscopy: a systematic review. Arthroscopy J Arthrosc Relat Surg Off Publ Arthroscopy Assoc North Am Int Arthroscopy Assoc. 2014;30(3):389–97.
8. Boden RA, Wall AP, Fehily MJ. Results of the learning curve for interventional hip arthroscopy: a prospective study. Acta Orthop Belg. 2014;80(1):39–44.
9. Comba F, Quinteros M, Martorell G, Buttaro M, Piccaluga F. Prospective analysis of complications after hip arthroscopy: the influence of the learning curve. Paper presented at: The international society of hip arthroscopy meeting, Boston; 2012.
10. Sobau C, Miehlke W. Complications in hip arthroscopy treating femoroacetabular impingement. Paper presented at: 8th biennial ISAKOS congress, Rio de Janeiro; 2011.
11. Samora JBBP, Jones A, Milbrandt T, Mazzocca AD, Quinn RH. Orthopaedic graduate medical education: a changing paradigm. JBJS Rev. 2014;e1(11).
12. P S. The Orthopaedic Surgery Milestone Project. A Joint Initiative of The Accreditation Council for Graduate Medical Education and The American Board of Orthopaedic Surgery. 2013. http://www.acgme.org/portals/0/pdfs/milestones/orthopaedicsurgerymilestones.pdf.
13. Case Log Guidelines. Accreditation Council for Graduate Medical Education. 2014. https://www.acgme.org/acgmeweb/Portals/0/PFAssets/ProgramResources/260_Case_Log_Guidelines.pdf.
14. Wadey VMR, Dev P, Buckley R, Walker D, Hedden D. Competencies for a Canadian orthopaedic surgery core curriculum. J Bone Joint Surg (Br). 2009;91(12):1618–22.
15. Objectives of training in the specialty of orthopedic surgery. Copyright © 2010 The Royal College of Physicians and Surgeons of Canada. Referenced and produced with permission.
16. Australian Orthopaedic Association. https://www.aoa.org.au/docs/default-source/ecm-files/training_aoa-nzoasyllabus_mar2011.pdf?sfvrsn=2. Date last accessed 19 Jan 2015.
17. Pitts D, Rowley DI, Marx C, Sher L, Banks T, Murray A. A competency based curriculum for specialist training in trauma and orthopaedics. Copyright © 2006 The British Orthopaedic Association.
18. The Royal College of Surgeons of England. https://www.rcseng.ac.uk/courses/course-search/advanced-hip-and-groin. Date last accessed 19 Jan 2015.
19. Sierra R, Della Valle C. Hip and pelvic reconstruction and arthroplasty. Orthopaedic Knowledge Update. 2011;10:414–7.
20. Musahl VAF. Evaluation of resident hip arthroscopy experience in two North American academic institution. informal resident poll performed by University of Pittsburgh and McMaster University 2014.
21. Kenter K. The Orthopaedic Sports Medicine Milestone Project. A Joint Initiative of The Accreditation Council for Graduate Medical Education and The American Board of Orthopaedic Surgery. 2013. https://www.acgme.org/Portals/0/PDFs/Milestones/OrthopaedicSportsMedicineMilestones.pdf.
22. RA A. Fellowship Listing. 2014. http://www.sportsmed.org/apps/fellowships/fellowship_listing.aspx.
23. J OD. Fellowships, Training/Education. 2014. http://www.isha.net. Accessed 10/30, 2014.
24. Peters CL, Beaule PE, Beck M, Tannast M, Jiranek W, Sierra RJ. Report of breakout session: strategies to improve hip preservation training. Clin Orthop Relat Res. 2012;470(12):3467–9.
25. 2015 AANA Masters Experience Courses. 2014. https://www.aana.org/CMECoursesMeetings/MastersExperience/2015CourseAgendas/tabid/946/Default.aspx.
26. Arthrex Training & Courses. 2014. http://www.arthrex.com/medical-education/training-and-courses. Accessed 10/30, 2014.
27. Souza BG, Dani WS, Honda EK, et al. Do complications in hip arthroscopy change with experience? Arthroscopy J Arthrosc Relat Surg Off Publ Arthroscopy Assoc North Am Int Arthroscopy Assoc. 2010;26(8):1053–7.
28. Guttmann D, Graham RD, MacLennan MJ, Lubowitz JH. Arthroscopic rotator cuff repair: the learning curve. Arthroscopy J Arthrosc Relat Surg Off Publ Arthroscopy Assoc North Am Int Arthroscopy Assoc. 2005;21(4):394–400.
29. Park MS, Yoon SJ, Kim YJ, Chung WC. Hip arthroscopy for femoroacetabular impingement: the changing nature and severity of associated complications over time. Arthroscopy J Arthrosc Relat Surg Off Publ Arthroscopy Assoc North Am Int Arthroscopy Assoc. 2014;30(8):957–63.
30. Bedi A, Galano G, Walsh C, Kelly BT. Capsular management during hip arthroscopy: from femoroacetabular impingement to instability. Arthroscopy J Arthrosc Relat Surg Off Publ Arthroscopy Assoc North Am Int Arthroscopy Assoc. 2011;27(12):1720–31.
31. Bond JL, Knutson ZA, Ebert A, Guanche CA. The 23-point arthroscopic examination of the hip: basic setup, portal placement, and surgical technique. Arthroscopy J Arthrosc Relat Surg Off Publ Arthroscopy Assoc North Am Int Arthroscopy Assoc. 2009;25(4):416–29.
32. Pollard TC, Khan T, Price AJ, Gill HS, Glyn-Jones S, Rees JL. Simulated hip arthroscopy skills: learning curves with the lateral and supine patient positions: a randomized trial. J Bone Joint Surg Am. 2012;94(10):e68.

